A Uro-Oncology Nurse Specialist's Reflection on her Practice Journe

T0093747

Beverley Anderson

A Uro-Oncology Nurse Specialist's Reflection on her Practice Journey

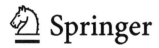 Springer

Beverley Anderson
Uro-Oncology Department
Epsom and St. Helier University Hospitals NHS Trust
Carshalton, Surrey, UK

ISBN 978-3-030-94198-7   ISBN 978-3-030-94199-4   (eBook)
https://doi.org/10.1007/978-3-030-94199-4

This Springer imprint is published by the registered company Springer Nature Switzerland AG
The registered company address is: Gewerbestrasse 11, 6330 Cham, Switzerland

Preface

Although I may not have been consciously aware at the time, I suppose I had first thought of becoming a nurse in Jamaica, when I was 6 years old, on the weekly visit to the local market town, sitting outside the health centre and watching the nurses come and go. I was fascinated by their white uniforms and white shoes and hats, looking smart and efficient, and young as I was, being mesmerised by what the grown-up notion of a nurse would entail. Five years later, I had travelled to the UK to be with my family. At 11 years old, I had to complete my schooling years, during which my desire to become a nurse had remained steadfast. At 18 years old, the notion of becoming a nurse had been realised as I embarked on my nursing journey—a journey that was far from smooth. There were moments when I had questioned whether this was truly the path for me.

Reflection is a powerful tool, one that over the years has enabled me to contemplate on the observations and examinations of ongoing lived experiences. It helped me to identify problems and concerns and accordingly devise strategies to bring about change and/or make improvements as appropriate. Thus, during my nursing career, these strategies included the writing and subsequent publication of articles and sharing the outcomes with my immediate colleagues and within the wider circle of the nursing profession. To date, I have written 20 publications in various nursing journals, and this book has evolved as a result of one of those publications, namely *'An insight into the patient's response to a urological cancer diagnosis', British Journal of Nursing (BJN), May 2017*. This publication caught the interest of a representative at the British Association of Urological Nursing (BAUN) and resulted in an invitation to present this paper at their yearly conference in 2018. Consequently, I was contacted by the Head of the Nursing Program at Springer Nature Publishers with the proposed offer of writing a book on urology-oncology nursing. After a period of consideration, writing a book about my nursing journey presented as a challenging, yet exciting, opportunity.

Reflection underlines my journey from the beginning (1973) through to my retirement (2019), including post-retirement updates up to April 2021. The storytelling encompasses the progression of my role from a novice to a specialist nurse, highlighting salient issues and experiences and changes to nursing and the nurse's role over the past 50 years, including how science, technology, research and academia have contributed to such.

The objective of this book is to provide a wide range of healthcare readers, nursing students, qualified nurses, those considering a change of nursing speciality or allied healthcare professionals with an honest and timely recounting of my experiences throughout my practice journey.

The book will also act as a useful reference point to access information that has the potential to support their learning. As such, I believe that the reflective narratives of the book could also lead to the readers' self-awareness and deepen their insight into themselves and their patients, which would contribute to the improvement of their competency as a practitioner.

Carshalton, UK   Beverley Anderson

Acknowledgements

Looking back on my career over the past 46 years, while I am very proud of what I have achieved, I am also aware that my achievements were not obtained in isolation. I have been fortunate to have received, and be still receiving, the support of some key individuals, some of whom have moved on to pastures new. These include the following:

- **Librarians**: Potenza Atiogbe and Marisa Martinez Ortiz, whose ongoing support in the undertaking of relevant searches and obtaining articles as and when required, as well as helping with referencing, has been invaluable.
- **Nursing colleagues**: Janet Pinfield (JP), urology clinical nurse specialist (UCNS), whose role as my mentor from 1998 to 2002 had contributed significantly to my academic journey, specifically in regard to my early studies, developing patient information and learning about urology nursing.

Dr. Wendy Naish (WN), urology nurse consultant (UNC), whose support and encouragement have been instrumental in my study undertakings—both as a mentor in my academic undertakings and as sub-author of four article publications.

Yvonne Mason (YM), UCNS, who as my ward manager had been the initiator of encouraging my steps on the academic ladder—first with undertaking the Accreditation of Prior Experiential Learning (AP(E)L) study and towards achieving my Diploma in Nursing Degree. Yvonne, together with Joanna Cooper (JC), UCNS, and Daphne Colpman (DC), UNC, has been the source of support and encouragement in the undertaking of academic tasks, namely, with proofreading of my various writing aspirations. Their support and feedback comments provided working-level credence to the written word.

A special thank you to my family, particularly my husband, Wil, for his patience and support over the years, specifically in proofreading various academic undertakings and writing aspirations and for never doubting my ability to succeed. To my son Owen, I thank him for giving me the opportunity and trusting me to write about his cancer experience. To my son Ciaran and my daughter Kheyla, who have never been less than a constant source of encouragement, since starting this book.

I would like to thank my nursing colleague, and a very good friend, Lorraine Denny (Lor), who has been with me from the beginning. Our nursing journey highlights many wonderful memories—memories that, then and today, incited much fun and laughter in a profession where stress, anxiety, sadness and disillusionment had often prevailed. Her belief in my capability and steadfast support is duly noted.

A very special thank you is extended to Dr. Sylvie Marshall-Lucette (SM-L) for her invaluable help and support throughout this journey. Dr. Lucette's support commenced with her role as my supervisor, initially in the undertaking of the BSc Hons. Nursing Degree and then the MSc Advanced Practice Degree. I also acknowledge her guidance and support with the research project as sub-author in the writing and publication of research findings, and accompanying me to Panama to present study findings at the International Conference on Cancer Nursing (ICCN) in September 2014, and as sub-author of the follow-up study—Prostate Cancer Among Jamaican Men, published in October 2016. Her support in proofreading various articles prior to their publication is also duly noted. Over the past 15 years, she has inspired confidence in my ability to rise to any given challenge and to always deliver my best effort.

I wish to acknowledge the part played by the Macmillan Cancer Support and Prostate Cancer UK (PCUK) in this academic journey.

Acknowledgements also include the funding of my research project and subsequently for the study results to be presented to the ICCN in Panama City. The provision of various study sessions for the CNS, as well as relevant patient information on urological cancers within the Trust and the wider circle, is also acknowledged.

Acknowledgement is further extended to the Hospital Trust for enabling appropriate study leave sessions and funding towards completion of nursing degrees: MSc Advanced Practice, BSc Hons. Nursing and Diploma Nursing.

Finally, I would like to extend my thanks to Springer Publishers for giving me this wonderful opportunity. The writing of this book provides completeness to a nursing journey spanning nearly 47 years and along the way enables to tap into some wonderfully poignant memories.

Beverley Anderson

About this Book

Reflection is a multidimensional learning tool that I have used to underline my nursing journey from 1973 until now, illustrating what I had learnt and how the experiences gained contributed to my personal and professional development and the nurse I eventually became.

My intention is to provide the reader with a rounded perspective of my journey as a mother, as a secretary, in running my own business and as a teacher, reinforcing how I integrated these experiences as a whole.

In terms of my academic journey, content includes the various studies undertaken and how these contributed to my professional development and improving patient and practice outcomes.

I have discussed my sabbatical from nursing alongside my achievements and how I grew during this time as well as my return to nursing and the subsequent progression of my career.

However, as the title suggests, cancer care is the theme that runs through this story, and while I have provided a true and honest depiction of my personal and professional experiences with various cancers, in this context, the main focus is placed on the urology multidisciplinary team and my role as the Macmillan Uro-Oncology Cancer Nurse Specialist (MUCNS) in managing patients diagnosed with urological cancers and highlighting the many elements of the role.

Integral to this management are my prior experiences of urology nursing and the principles of practice within the urology ward, honing in on the delivery of service and the various attributes that made this area of practice so rewarding.

In an attempt to highlight both the positive and negative aspects in this nursing journey, I have chosen to address the uncomfortable truth, that is, racism within the NHS, particularly the impact on myself as well as people from various ethnic backgrounds.

In taking light of current affairs, with the country (UK) facing so much change due to Brexit and the recent onslaught of the coronavirus pandemic, I feel it is imperative to discuss their impact, not just on the NHS but also on the country and the wider community.

In the delivery of nursing care, I have acknowledged the role of government targets and, in the performance of my role as MUCNS, the part played by the Macmillan Cancer Support and Prostate Cancer UK (PCUK).

It is my hope that in the recounting of the events of this journey, I have provided evidence of my ability to show compassion as a caregiver as well as my developing maturity and its contribution to my personal and professional growth as a practitioner.

Beverley Anderson

Contents

About the Author

Beverley Anderson My name is Beverley Anderson. When I retired in October 2019, I had been a nurse for 46 years and 7 months. During the course of this journey, my role evolved from that of a novice to an expert, advanced nurse practitioner.

My achievements comprise Registered General Nurse (RGN), MSc Advanced Practice, BSc Hons. Nursing and Diploma in Higher Education (Dip. H.E. Nursing).

On 1st August 2005, I was appointed to the role of Macmillan Uro-Oncology Clinical Nurse Specialist (MUCNS). I worked within secondary care at a multisite district general hospital as a member of the urology department. I held this role for over 14 years. This involved me working in a multidisciplinary context within the tertiary and primary care sectors and the community.

My professional background encompassed a range of abilities, including 21 years' in-depth experience of nursing patients with both urological dysfunction and urological cancers at varying stages of the disease. As an MUCNS, my role was pivotal in the diagnosis and management of those patients diagnosed with urological cancers and in providing them with optimal support. Integral to this was audit and research and my application of these in the completion of various academic undertakings and journal publications.

I am of African-Caribbean descent, originally from Jamaica, West Indies, and I arrived in the UK, aged 11 years old. I am married to Wil, my husband for 41 years. We have three adult children and four grandchildren.

You can contact me via my email address at b.v.anderson@btinternet.com.

List of Boxes

List of Figures

List of Tables

Introduction

1

Reflection is defined 'as a process of consciously examining what has occurred in terms of thoughts, feelings and actions against underlying beliefs, assumptions and knowledge as well as against the backdrop in which specific practice has occurred' (Kim 1999). In nursing, reflection is considered beneficial to enabling nurses to consciously think about an activity or incident, and accordingly, considering what was positive or challenging, and if appropriate, plan how it might be enhanced, improved or done differently in the future (Royal College of Nursing 2020). It is through a process of critical reflection on experience that nurses develop an awareness of the broader social and political issues which influence their practice and which are affected by it (Atkins and Murphy 1995). However, as pointed out by Moon (Moon 2007) reflection is not a clearly defined and enacted concept. Not only will the individual's perception of the reflected experience vary considerably, but it may also be quite subjective. In the recounting of the events in this book, distinction will be made between reflection during practice and reflection occurring in 'thinking back on practice' (Kim 1999), as it seems to be the most appropriate approach to highlighting the experiences and the learning gained and how these translated into practice throughout this journey (Royal College of Nursing 2020).

Reflective practice is the ability to reflect on one's actions so as to engage in a process of continuous learning (Oelofsen 2012). This activity is designed to gain insight into one's own practice with the intention of improving it, but it also has the potential to raise questions, answers to which must be supported by other evidences such as research (Parahoo 2006).

Throughout my academic journey, I have utilised a number of reflective models, of which the most frequently used has been Gibbs (Fig. 1.1) (Gibbs 1988). This is a cyclical process that enables continual retrospective reflection.

Emotional Aspects of Reflective Practice Throughout this book, the issue of pain, whether it be physical or emotional, is acknowledged and contextualised in terms of its relevancy to the topic area (i.e. the receipt of bad news or coping with the threat of/actuality of loss) being discussed.

© Springer Nature Switzerland AG 2022
B. Anderson, *A Uro-Oncology Nurse Specialist's Reflection on her Practice Journey*, https://doi.org/10.1007/978-3-030-94199-4_1

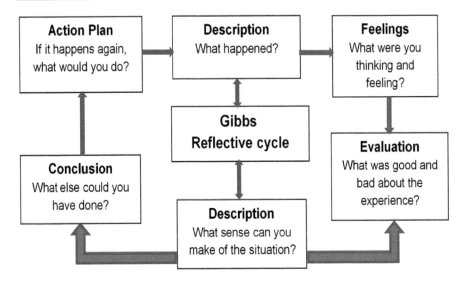

Fig. 1.1 The Gibbs' reflective cycle [adapted from Gibbs (Gibbs 1988)]

There is evidence to suggest that reflection is a difficult exercise, one that can evoke uncomfortable and painful feelings (Atkins and Murphy 1995; Cox et al. 1991), feelings that as human beings, if we are forced to confront, we will try to avoid, both instinctively and consciously (Farnham Street Learning Community 2020). It has been shown that 'our painful moments are important moments, in that when we confront something painful, we are left with a choice between viewing it as an ugly and painful truth or a beautiful delusion'. Unsurprisingly, many of us will opt for the latter, and run from the pain. However, only by reflecting on, and exploring the pain and discomfort, confronting the encountered thoughts and feelings, as well as being critically honest in understanding their meaning, can we truly start to evolve (Cox et al. 1991; Farnham Street Learning Community 2020). I believe that while these words of wisdom may be true, it is understandable that as human beings, we may seek the easier path—to avoid the pain, for a while, at least.

Thinking back on my nurse training, I can appreciate that in some ways, training helped me to better cope with some of the more uncomfortable issues in nursing. In terms of patient interaction, the initial advice from my nursing tutor, not to get too personally or emotionally invested in the individual's situation, still resonates. However, in my experience, as a human being and a nurse, it is virtually impossible to be totally unaffected by an individual's emotions, all of the time. There will be moments when a patient's diagnosis and the ensuing fallout from this will be particularly harrowing (Hemming 2017). I have also found that when dealing with emotional issues, patients want their health professional (nurse or doctor) to be just that—professionals who understand their dilemma and are caring and considerate, yet strong enough to withstand the ensuing emotions, and basically stop them from falling apart (Anderson 2014). In these moments, a breakthrough in my carefully established emotional barrier was not unusual, although, as I soon realised, these emotions were a show of strength, not a weakness. They are after all part and parcel of showing compassion, a trait that is very human, and an integral part of being a nurse.

Observations and Reflections on My Practice According to Helyer (Helyer 2015), done well and effectively, reflective practice can be an enormously powerful tool to examine and transform practice. In this context, reflective practice relates to observations and reflections on my practice, in that whenever I observed something unusual or thought-provoking in practice, it usually sparked a natural curiosity to gain insight into the arising issues, and accordingly share the outcomes through various publications, both in-house with my colleagues and with the wider circle. My ability for writing was first realised in May 2005, following the successful publication of my first article, 'Nutrition and Wound Healing: A Need for Assessment' (Anderson 2005), by the British Journal of Nursing (BJN). This was an extremely rewarding experience that inspired me to continue to journey down this path, and over the past 14 years has resulted in 20 article publications (*Appendix A*). Strangely enough, the Anderson (Anderson 2017) article had been the most challenging to write—in fact, at one point, I did consider abandoning the project. However, with encouragement from one particular reviewer, and the BJN's Editor, I persevered, which in hindsight was the correct decision. Reference will be made to all publications throughout the book.

My Intriguing Observation Over the years, I have found that in the undertaking of various academic studies and writing aspirations, the inspirations for their conception and how they subsequently developed were usually triggered by social activities/hobbies, such as reading a book, walking, watching television or just relaxing at home. However, some of the most constructive inspirations were often triggered during my sessions at the local gym, a space in which I receive clarity, empowerment as well as a release from day-to-day stressors. Usually while on the treadmill, cross-trainer, in the swimming pool or even in the spa. Even more interesting is that the arrival of such inspiration(s) was usually very relevant to enhancing the topic area being discussed. In fact, I would argue that inspirations had dictated the format in which the relevant document should develop. It is no surprise, then, that they have continued to drive the format in the writing of this book.

Work-based learning (WBL) is defined as any formal higher education learning that is based wholly or predominantly in a work setting (Helyer 2015). This activity enables workers to hone their reflective skills, and in so doing to critically appraise what has been experienced via practice, and accordingly use the information to improve practice (Helyer 2015). This form of reflection is in fact experiential learning (Billet 2011). As part of my ongoing professional development, and my attempts to improve both patient and practice outcomes, I have used WBL as a tool in my undertaking of a number of activities for the accreditation of prior learning (AP(E)L) project, and stand-alone projects for the completion of various degrees:

Nursing Diploma, BSc Hons Nursing and MSc Advanced Practice. These are presented as appropriate throughout the book. My intention is to explain how these assignments contributed to enhancing my learning and accordingly improving the care I delivered to my patients. To deepen the storytelling, I have used case study presentations and scenarios to emphasise the true essence of the experiences and their impact, from both the patient and the MUCNS perspectives.

Real Time Where appropriate, reflective accounts, discussions and supporting evidence for these activities are depicted in real time, that is, the actual year and date of their conception, with a subsequent conclusion that acknowledges lessons learnt and changes over this time.

1.1   Change, Audit and Research

Change is defined as making something different from the way it was originally, and may be planned or unplanned. Unplanned change brings about unpredictable outcomes, while planned change is a sequence of events implemented to achieve established goals (Oguejiofo 2018). My personal definition of change is of a relentless entity that is a naturally occurring part of the status quo. We cannot stop it, nor can we avoid its inevitability. According to Burns (Burns 1993), change is one of life's transitions, and one that is inherent in the healthcare setting (Haynes 1992), especially in nursing, where it is deemed an integral part of practice (Nemeth 2003). Based on my experience, clinical practice is not a 'static' exercise. The process is changeable; therefore, protocols need to be constantly updated by the regular monitoring of practice to ensure that improvements are accordingly instigated to maintain standards. Integral to this monitoring is audit, not only in highlighting change, but also in its subsequent implementation into practice, and at which point, emphasis is placed on effective leadership and management skills to achieve the desired outcomes (Burns 1993). It has been shown that change that is implemented too quickly will cause increased stress and ensuing resistance (Lancaster and Lancester 1982). To avoid resistance, it is important to remember that in the same way that we need time to plan and implement the change, the same is also true following its implementation. As recipients of the change, we will also need time to come to terms with, and to adjust to, its imposition (Lancaster and Lancaster 1982).

Audit and Research Evidence-based practice is broadly defined as 'the use of the best clinical evidence in making patient care decisions' (Polit and Beck 2006). Evidence-based practice was first recognised during the nineteenth century, when Florence Nightingale collected data on soldier morbidity and mortality during the Crimean War and, utilising an evidence-based approach to care, evaluated the treatment that was given to patients, and accordingly used the information to instigate changes to improve care in areas that were below standard (Burns and Grove 2001). Integral to this concept is change, research and audit. According to Tourish and Hargie (Tourish and Hargie 1996), change is a core management concern within the

NHS, in which, argues Cormack (Cormack 1991), research is acknowledged as having an important role in determining its direction. While the principle of examining nursing practice has been in existence for over 140 years and historically undertaken through research (Tourish and Hargie 1996), there is evidence to suggest that in conducting an examination of most nursing practices, research may not necessarily be the best approach (Hegyvary 1991). A more simplistic approach is through audit—'a multi-professional, patient-focused process that leads to cost-effective, high-quality care delivery in clinical teams' (Morrell and Harvey 1996). Thus, when considering a change in practice, audit is an important place to start, as not only could it indicate the need for change, but could also bring about change in an acceptable and workable manner (Irvine and Irvine 1997).

My audit and research activities will be illustrated as appropriate throughout the book.

Noteworthy Legislation   Over the past 50 years, measures to improve the quality and standard of the services provided to the general public have resulted in the introduction of legislation such as the Citizen's Charter (HMSO 1991) and the Patient's Charter (Department of Health 1991). The Patient's Charter puts the Citizen's Charter into practice in the NHS. First published in October 1991, the Patient's Charter had aimed to improve the quality of health service delivery to patients, in which it outlined patients' rights in the NHS and standards of service they could expect to receive in areas addressing, among others, waiting times, information about services and treatment, patient choice and privacy and dignity issues. A revised Charter, issued in 1995, had drawn together the rights and standards set out in the original Charter together with improvements made since 1991. These legislation included Clinical Governance … defined as 'a framework through which NHS organisations are accountable for continually improving the quality of their services, and safeguarding high standards of care by creating an environment in which excellence in clinical care will flourish'. This includes clinical effectiveness and risk management (Department of Health 2020). Basically, these legislation placed the onus on the NHS to meet this challenge (Burns and Grove 2001). I can still remember when these legislation were introduced into practice and the ensuing changes as a result. For some patients and their relatives, legislation gave them the confidence to question issues of concerns in regard to the care received. There was a distinct shift in the balance of power between the patient and the healthcare professional (i.e. the nurse), a shift that placed the onus on the patient's demand for higher standards and quality of care and accordingly on the healthcare professional to deliver.

1.2   Cancer (Oncology) Management

Macmillan nurses are specialist nurses who are employed throughout the UK and whose role is mainly focused on cancer and palliative care. A key feature of the role is influencing patient care by offering indirect and direct services to patients and their families (Trevatt and Leary 2010a). Macmillan is the largest group of specialist nurse roles (for various cancer types), in both hospital and community settings, and as an organisation has responded over the years to the ever-increasing demands of society in meeting the changing dynamics of cancer, and cancer care delivery, including information and financial support (Trevatt and Leary 2010a).

Cancer is a complex illness that over the years has provoked much fear and speculation for those afflicted by this disease. However, we cannot deny that compared to 50 years ago, there have been some outstanding achievements in its management (Zinser and Hsieh 2007) central to which are the Cancer Networks (Macmillan Cancer Support 2012). Macmillan has placed great faith in these networks effecting reform in the NHS, specifically in driving up standards and quality of care and improving overall outcomes for cancer patients (Macmillan Cancer Support 2012). As a result of increased screening programmes, improved technologies and improved awareness, prevalence in the diagnosis of new cancers has risen to record levels (Cancer Research UK 2020). Earlier detection, and significant improvements in treatment modalities, has also meant that more people are now surviving cancer and go on to live longer and healthier lives (Zinser and Hsieh 2007; Davis 2009), which in some cases extend to 20 years or more, over their life expectancy (McDaid and Oliver 2005). Unfortunately, with such successes, there have been penalties, namely the cost implications of delivering optimal care to patients (Department of Health 2005).

Guidelines have been set for the management of all cancers in the UK, denoting specifications for each cancer type (National Institute for Health and Care Excellence) (National Institute for Clinical Excellence [NICE] 2002). The overall objective of this management is to ensure that individuals are provided with appropriate support and representation during the cancer journey, from the point of diagnosis, throughout treatment, and survival beyond the disease (survivorship) (Macmillan Cancer Support 2014). Intrinsic to cancer management are the multidisciplinary teams (MDTs) (in which the cancer clinical nurse specialist (CNS) is pivotal) (Macmillan Cancer Support 2014), and the government's austerity measures (targets) (Department of Health 2011) (Table 1.1). In this context, the MDT facilitates individual disciplines working in partnership. Attempts to meet stated goals are interrelated and are reliant on a performance that is geared towards delivering optimal care to patients in line with meeting the specified target (Taylor et al. 2010).

The Role of the Cancer CNS It is well noted that the CNS's knowledge, experience, skills and expertise are vital to improving a patient's cancer experience and quality-of-life outcomes (Macmillan Cancer Support 2014); hence, patients who are allocated to a CNS respond far more positively to a cancer diagnosis than those who are not (Tarrant et al. 2008). There are many elements to the cancer CNS role, but the primary focus is helping patients understand their disease and treatment options following the receipt of a diagnosis (the breaking of bad news) (Hemming 2017),

Table 1.1 Government waiting time targets

2-week rule	Patient must receive an appointment to see a consultant or a nurse for an investigation within 2 weeks of referral
31-day rule	From the decision to treat, you have 31 days to commence treatment
62-day rule	Patient must receive full treatment within 62 days, including both the 2-week and 31-day rule

Source: NICE (Department of Health 2011) [Suspected Cancer Referral Guidelines published in 2015, updated in 2017]

and acting as the patient's key worker in line with national guidance (Macmillan Cancer Support 2014). A 'key worker' is defined as someone who, with the patient's consent and agreement, plays a principal role in coordinating patient care, promoting continuity and ensuring that the patient knows whom to contact for required support (Macmillan Cancer Support 2014).

Intrinsic to this support is effective communication and informational support (Ali 2017; McClain 2012), which is vital to counteracting the effect of the bad news following the receipt of a diagnosis (Hemming 2017). In the delivery of subsequent care, a holistic approach (which constitutes an assessment of the physical, psychological/emotional, psychosocial, spiritual and cultural components of the individual's health needs) is beneficial in identifying patients' concerns and considering how these might be addressed (Doyle and Henry 2014). Holistic care has become more and more popular, and is perceived to result in decreased in-patient times and better health outcomes (UKEssays 2018).

Interestingly, despite the CNS role being well noted in the management of cancer patients, there is still the concern that CNS provision is insufficient, inconsistent and inequitable (Trevatt and Leary 2010b), and is thus unable to meet the increasing demand for specialist cancer nursing care across the UK (Prostate Cancer UK et al. 2014). Based on my experience, this is a concern with which I fully concur, specifically that CNS provision is insufficient. As observed in local practice, while the CNS will always strive to support patients, time constraints, overbooked clinics, increased workloads and reductions in CNS availability have often impinged on their efforts to provide this support to all patients.

The general consensus is that in 'the breaking of bad news', the cancer CNS is better placed to provide patients with more constructive support following the receipt of bad news than is the consultant (Hemming 2017). This consensus is based on the belief that the consultant has less time to interact with the patient, while the CNS has more time and is thus able to interpret and understand the ensuing fallout to the news (Hemming 2017). However, in my experience, being the sole CNS responsible for providing this support in the outpatient department (often to several patients in the same session) required a good deal of juggling to ensure that all patients were equally supported. The following patient scenario provides an example of how I provided the said support in local practice.

Patient Scenario

Mr. Levy was a 71-year-old gentleman who was diagnosed with locally advanced prostate cancer, and for whom the agreed management was hormone or androgen deprivation therapy (ADT) to be commenced in clinic, and chemotherapy. Additional management included participation in the STAMPEDE trial (a trial comparing hormone therapy alone with a combination of hormone therapy and one or more other treatments for prostate cancer).

By sitting in with the consultant while he delivered the diagnosis to Mr. Levy, I was able to observe his response to the diagnosis; to note the ensuing impact of the news on him in terms of fear, anxiety and distress; and accordingly to provide him with the support that was targeted to meeting his specific needs.

Following the receipt of his diagnosis, I then proceeded to see Mr. Levy in another room where I spent significant time (over an hour) with him. Conversations revealed his evident shock and dismay at the news; it was clearly not what he expected. It was also clear that he had not fully understood all the information received from the consultant, nor had he absorbed all the explanations given. However, spending time with Mr. Levy; re-explaining the diagnosis and the plan of care; answering his questions and concerns; explaining the treatment options and the relevant risks and benefits of these, several times over; then signposting him to the pharmacy to fill prescription for the first part of his treatment—hormone therapy; arranging subsequent follow-up; and giving him my contact details did seem to allay some of his fears and anxiety. However, at his subsequent follow-up appointment, his lack of memory in regard to the diagnosis and the additional treatment with chemotherapy was surprising, a surprise that had led me to question whether his response to the diagnosis was genuine and just how much information he absorbed. These questions resulted in the publication of Anderson (Anderson 2017), in which Mr. Levy's case study was used to explore this interesting phenomenon and my role in supporting him.

Nurse-led Services The demand for nurse-led services has increased since it was acknowledged that not only was this service beneficial to increasing the patient's experience and clinical outcomes, but it was also beneficial in reducing the pressures on doctors (Anderson 2010). Central to this service is the cancer CNS, on whom specific focus is placed in the delivery of health education and promotion and its importance in raising and increasing the individual's awareness of issues likely to impact their overall health, and accordingly enabling them to make the appropriate lifestyle choices (Anderson 2009).

Targets were initially designed to increase competition among healthcare providers, and accordingly to ensure that those individuals who are affected by cancer received care that was of the highest quality, delivered in a timely manner, and tailored to meeting their individual needs (Sprinks 2010; Tan and Mays 2014). My earliest memory of targets and their impact on healthcare delivery pertains to the 4-h waiting time target (Department of Health 2001) and payment by results (PbR) (Department of Health 2005), for which emphasis was placed on the patient being in the forefront in the provision of high-quality, cost-effective care (Department of Health 2005). The reality, however, is that we live in a culture, where the provision of such care is governed not so much by quality, but by whether the provision is cost effective (Hewett and Ross 2012). Ultimately, in attempts to remain financially viable, we witnessed the imposition of remedial strategies to recoup and retain vital funds (Sprinks 2010; Tan and Mays 2014). These strategies included cuts in services and manpower (i.e. nurses, doctors), both of which led to increased stress and anxiety for the health professional, and reductions in their efforts to deliver optimal care to patients (Handley 2010; Leary et al. 2010). In regard to the cancer CNS role, my memory identifies with moments when I, as well as my colleagues, had been in the midst of change that was the direct result of targets. Unfortunately, because specialist nurses were perceived to attract a higher level of pay, there was a significant challenge to be faced in enlightening health service managers that we were a valuable resource, and consequently we were easy targets in cost-saving exercises (Handley 2010; Leary et al. 2010). Of specific note was the evident upset that resulted from attempts to reconfigure the CNS role in 2007. These attempts placed CNSs in the worrying position of having to reapply for their jobs—an action that raised doubts regarding not only our competency, but also whether the role was worthy of the proposed higher level of pay. Not only did the uncertainty of the situation heighten our fears in regard to financial security, as a result of potentially losing our jobs, but also the exercise left us feeling demoralised and undervalued. Today, the CNS post still attracts scrutiny, and government targets continue to dictate the organisation's management and delivery of its services (Handley 2010; Leary et al. 2010; Anderson 2016; Campbell 2016).

In this book, the focus will be placed on the role of the urology multidisciplinary team (UMDT) and the Macmillan uro-oncology CNS (MUCNS) in the management of patients diagnosed and treated for urological cancers.

The provision of support to patients following the breaking of bad news is an integral part of the MUCNS role; as such, this theme will be recurrent throughout the book.

1.3   Conclusion and Lessons Learnt

This chapter has shown that reflection continues to be an integral part of health professionals', specifically the nurse's, role. As an activity, the belief is that to truly appreciate the emanating emotions it should be painful. The process is key to enabling individuals to observe and reflect on their practice, to identify problems or concerns and accordingly to initiate change, usually through audit or research, with the objective being to secure improvement in patient and overall practice outcomes. Integral to this are my publications whose conceptions were strongly influenced by my social activities that almost always delivered the appropriate 'Aha!' (epiphanic) moment. The roles of the MDT and the cancer CNS remain pivotal in the delivery of effective and expedient holistic care to patients. Integral to this is the CNS provision of appropriate support (effective communication and information) following the receipt of bad news. Nurse-led services continue to prove beneficial in improving patient care and clinical practice outcomes. We currently live in a society in which funding is essentially the key driver of healthcare, an objective in which government targets continue to dictate its delivery, and seemingly will continue to do so for the foreseeable future.

Chapter 2 provides an in-depth recounting of my early years in the nursing journey and highlights how the experiences and learning gained have contributed to my personal and professional development throughout this journey.

References

Ali M (2017) Communication skills 1: benefits of effective communication for patients. Nurs Times 113(12):18–19

Anderson B (2005) Nutrition and wound healing: the necessity of assessment. Br J Nurs (Tissue Viability Suppl) 14(19):S30–S38

Anderson B (2009) Understanding the role of smoking in the aetiology of bladder cancer. Br J Community Nurs 14(9):385–392. [Internet]. https://doi.org/10.12968/bjcn.2009.14.9.43805

Anderson B (2010) The benefits to nurse-led telephone follow-up for prostate cancer. Br J Nurs 19(17):1085–1090. [Internet]. https://doi.org/10.12968/bjon.2010.19.17.78565

Anderson B (2014) Challenges for the clinical nurse specialist in uro-oncology care. Br J Nurs 23(Sup10):S18–S22. [Internet]. https://doi.org/10.12968/bjon.2014.23.Sup10.S18

Anderson B (2016) Cancer management: the difficulties of a target-driven healthcare system. Br J Nurs (Urol Suppl) 25(9):S36–S40

Anderson B (2017) An insight into the patient's response to a diagnosis of urological cancer. Br J Nurs 26(18):S4–12. [Internet] http://www.ncbi.nlm.nih.gov/pubmed/29034698

Atkins S, Murphy K (1995) Reflective practice. Nurs Stand 9(45):31–37

Billet S (2011) final report: curriculum and pedagogic bases for effectively integrating practice based experiences [Internet]. [cited 2020 Oct 20]. https://www.academia.edu/13432747/Curriculum_and_pedagogic_bases_for_effectively_integrating_practice_based_experiences

Burns N, Grove SK (2001) The practice of nursing research: conduct, critique & utilization, 4th edn. Saunders, Philadelphia, PA

Burns R (1993) Managing people in changing times : coping with change in the workplace : a practical guide. Allen & Unwin, St.Leonards, NSW

Campbell D (2016) Hospitals told to cut staff amid spiralling NHS cash crisis [internet]. The Guardian. [cited 2020 Oct 20]. https://www.theguardian.com/society/2016/jan/29/hospitals-told-cut-staff-nhs-cash-crisis#:~:text=Hospitals are being told to, at risk of the sack

Cancer Research UK. Bladder Cancer: risks and causes [Internet]. cancerresearchuk.org. 2019 [cited 2020 Oct 24]. https://www.cancerresearchuk.org/about-cancer/bladder-cancer/risks-causes

Cormack DF (1991) The research process in nursing, 2nd edn. Blackwell, Oxford

Cox H, Hickson P, Taylor P (1991) Exploring reflection: knowing and constructing practice. In: Pratt G, Gray R (eds) Towards a discipline of nursing. Churchill Livingstone

Davis C (2009) Increasing awareness of prostate cancer. Cancer Nurs Pract 8(5):12–15

Department of Health (1991) The patient's charter

Department of Health (2001) Reforming emergency care

Department of Health (2005) Payment by results consultation: preparing for 2005, London

Department of Health (2011) Review of cancer waiting times standards improving outcomes: a strategy for cancer [Internet]. Gov.uk. [cited 2020 Oct 24]. https://assets.publishing.service. gov.uk/government/uploads/system/uploads/attachment_data/file/213787/dh_123395.pdf

Department of Health. A First Class Service: quality in the new NHS [Internet]. 1998 [cited 2020 Oct 20]. https://webarchive.nationalarchives.gov.uk/+/http://www.dh.gov.uk/en/ Publicationsandstatistics/Publications/PublicationsPolicyAndGuidance/DH_4006902

Doyle N, Henry R (2014) Holistic needs assessment: rationale and practical implementation [internet]. Cancer Nurs Pract 13:16–21. [cited 2020 Oct 23] http://rcnpublishing.com/doi/ abs/10.7748/cnp.13.5.16.e1099

Farnham Street Learning Community (2020) Pain plus reflection equals progress [Internet]. fs.blog. [cited 2020 Oct 13]. https://fs.blog/2018/06/pain-reflection/

Gibbs G (1988) Learning by doing: a guide to teaching and learning methods [internet]. FEU, London. [cited 2020 Oct 13]. https://www.amazon.co.uk/Learning-doing-teaching-learning-methods/dp/1853380717/ref=sr_1_1?dchild=1&keywords=Learning+by+Doing%3A+a+Gui de+to+Teaching+and+Learning+Methods%2C&qid=1602590449&s=books&sr=1-1

Handley A (2010) Specialists face up to more cuts. Nurs Stand 24(20):20–21

Haynes S (1992) Let the change come from within: the process of change in nursing. Prof Nurse 7(10):635–638

Hegyvary ST (1991) Issues in outcomes research. J Nurs Qual Assur [Internet] 5(2):1–6. http:// www.ncbi.nlm.nih.gov/pubmed/1984024

Helyer R (2015) Learning through reflection: the critical role of reflection in work-based learning (WBL). J Work Manage 7(1):15–27. [Internet]. https://doi.org/10.1108/JWAM-10-2015-003/ full/html

Hemming L (2017) Breaking bad news: a case study on communication in health care. Gastrointest Nurs 15(1):43–50. [Internet]. https://doi.org/10.12968/gasn.2017.15.1.43

Hewett J, Ross E (2012) Views of specialist head and neck nurses about changes in their role [internet]. Cancer Nurs Pract 11:34–37. [cited 2020 Oct 23]. https://doi.org/10.7748/ cnp2012.03.11.2.34.c8989

HMSO (1991) The citizen's charter: raising the standard, Cm 1599. HMSO, London

Irvine D, Irvine S (eds) (1997) Making sense of audit [internet], 2nd edn. Radcliffe Medical Press, Abingdon, Oxon. [cited 2020 Oct 13]. https://www.amazon.co.uk/Making-Sense-Business-General-Practice/dp/1857751191/ref=sr_1_1?dchild=1&keywords=Making+Sense+of+Audit .&qid=1602589654&s=books&sr=1-1

Kim HS (1999) Critical reflective inquiry for knowledge development in nursing practice. J Adv Nurs 29(5):1205–1212. [Internet]. https://doi.org/10.1046/j.1365-2648.1999.01005.x

Lancaster J, Lancester W (eds) (1982) Concepts for advanced nursing practice: nurse as a change agent [Internet]. Mosby, St Louis, MO. [cited 2020 Oct 13]. https://www.amazon.co.uk/ Concepts-Advanced-Nursing-Practice-Change/dp/0801628326/ref=sr_1_1?dchild=1&keywor ds=The+Nurse+as+a+Change+Agent%3A+Concepts+for+Advanced+Nursing+Practice&qid =1602589840&s=books&sr=1-1

Leary A, Oliver S, Forum RC of NRN (2010) Clinical nurse specialists: adding value to care, an executive summary [Internet]. [cited 2020 Oct 24]. http://alisonleary.co.uk/docs/ RCNStudyAddingValuetoCaretheworkoftheCNS.pdf

Macmillan Cancer Support (2014) Cancer clinical nurse specialists [Internet]. macmillan.org. uk. https://www.macmillan.org.uk/documents/aboutus/research/impactbriefs/impactbriefs-clinicalnursespecialists2014.pdf

Macmillan Cancer Support (2012). The role of cancer networks in the new NHS [Internet]. [cited 2020 Oct 20]. https://www.macmillan.org.uk/documents/getinvolved/campaigns/theroleofcan-cernetworksinthenewnhs.pdf

McClain G (2012) Healthcare professionals: acknowledging emotional reactions in newly-diagnosed patients [Internet]. justgotdiagnosed.com. https://justgotdiagnosed.com/resources/ professionals-acknowledging-emotional-reactions-newly-diagnosed-patients/

McDaid D, Oliver A (2005) Inequalities in health international patterns and trends: international patterns and trends. In: Scriven A, Garman S (eds) Promoting health: global perspectives. Palgrave Macmillan, Basingstoke

Moon J (2007) Getting the measure of reflection: considering matters of definition and depth [internet]. J Radiother Pract 6:191–200. [cited 2020 Oct 1] https://www.cambridge.org/core/product/identifier/S1460396907006188/type/journal_article

Morrell C, Harvey G (1996) Clinical audit. Nurs Stand 10(17):38–42

National Institute for Clinical Excellence [NICE] (2002). Improving outcomes in urological Cancers; Cancer service guideline [CSG2] [Internet]. National Institute for Clinical Excellence [cited 2020 Oct 13]. http://guidance.nice.org.uk/CSGSP/Guidance/pdf

Nemeth LS (2003) Implementing change for effective outcomes. Outcomes Manag 7(3):134–139

Oelofsen N (2012) Using reflective practice in frontline nursing. Nurs Times 108(24):22–24

Oguejiofo N (2018) Change theories in nursing [Internet]. bizfluent.com. [cited 2020 Oct 13]. https://bizfluent.com/about-5544426-change-theories-nursing.html

Parahoo K (2006) Nursing research : principles, process and issues. Palgrave Macmillan, Basingstoke

Polit DF, Beck CTB (2006) Essentials of nursing research: methods, appraisal, and utilization [internet], 6th edn. Lippincott Williams and Wilkins, Philadelphia, PA, pp 458–465. [cited 2020 Oct 13] https://www.amazon.co.uk/Essentials-Nursing-Research-Appraisal-Utilization/dp/0781749727/ref=sr_1_1?dchild=1&keywords=Essentials+of+Nursing+Research.+Methods%2C+Appraisal%2C+and+Utilization.&qid=1602591204&s=books&sr=1-1

Prostate Cancer UK, British Association of Urological Nurses, Mouchel, Plymouth University, London South Bank University. The specialist nursing workforce caring for men with prostate cancer in the UK: research report 2014 [Internet]. 2014 [cited 2020 Oct 13]. https://prostate-canceruk.org/media/2491517/2631-urology-nurse-workforce-research-report__web.pdf

Royal College of Nursing. Revalidation requirements: reflection and reflective discussion [Internet]. rcn.org.uk. 2020 [cited 2020 Oct 20]. https://www.rcn.org.uk/professional-development/revalidation/reflection-and-reflective-discussion

Sprinks J (2010) Drive to abolish "politically motivated" NHS targets raises serious clinical issues. Nurs Stand [Internet] 24(49):14. http://www.ncbi.nlm.nih.gov/pubmed/20831106

Tan S, Mays N (2014) Impact of initiatives to improve access to, and choice of, primary and urgent care in England: a systematic review. Health Policy (New York) [Internet] 118(3):304–315. https://linkinghub.elsevier.com/retrieve/pii/S0168851014001766

Tarrant C, Sinfield P, Agarwal S, Baker R (2008) Is seeing a specialist nurse associated with positive experiences of care? The role and value of specialist nurses in prostate cancer care. BMC Health Serv Res 8(1):65. [Internet]. https://doi.org/10.1186/1472-6963-8-65

Taylor C, Munro AJ, Glynne-Jones R, Griffith C, Trevatt P, Richards M et al (2010) Multidisciplinary team working in cancer: what is the evidence? [internet]. BMJ 340:c951. (Clinical research ed.) http://www.ncbi.nlm.nih.gov/pubmed/20332315

Tourish D, Hargie O (1996) Communications audit and the management of change: a case study from an NHS unit of management. Health Serv Manage Res 9(2):125–135

Trevatt P, Leary A (2010a) A census of the advanced and specialist cancer nursing workforce in England, Northern Ireland and Wales. Eur J Oncol Nurs 14:68. [Internet]

Trevatt P, Leary A (2010b) Commissioning the specialist cancer nursing workforce. Cancer Nurs Pract 9(5):23–26. [Internet]. https://doi.org/10.7748/cnp2010.06.9.5.23.c7815

UKEssays (2018) Reflecting on one's practice nursing essay [Internet]. ukessays.com. [cited 2020 Oct 13]. https://www.ukessays.com/essays/nursing/reflecting-on-ones-practice-nursing-essay.php?vref=Feb;14(1):68–73

Zinser L, Hsieh P (2007). Moral Health Care vs. "Universal Health Care" Objective standard, [Internet]. theojectivestandard.com. [cited 2020 Oct 20]. https://theobjectivestandard.com/2007/11/moral-vs-universal-health-care/

The Early Years

2

Youth Experience has shown that while youth is a wonderful stage in one's development, it is an equally complex stage that encompasses certain vulnerabilities which for the young may be difficult to understand. It is a period of exploring and of finding out what makes us 'tick'. Arguably, the young can be quite naïve—often acting in haste and neglecting to consider the consequences of their actions. It is important not to generalise in all cases, but based on my experience, the young tend not to dwell too much on serious issues—seeking instead the fun and the thrill of the moment. As a young woman barely 18 years old I did not, or could not, fully comprehend the full implications of what being a nurse would entail, not until much later, and only after I matured and acquired some much-needed life experience. With this experience, I learned to be less selfish and accordingly developed a sense of caring for others. Arguably, this is a subjective view, but I truly believe that caring is an innate skill—which in nursing defines our ability to deliver compassionate care to our patients. These elements of youth—naivety, inexperience, having fun and not taking things too seriously, as well as demonstrating compassion—are illustrated in this chapter.

2.1   1973–1975: Enrolled Nurse Training and Related Factors

My reflection on the early years of my nursing journey highlights some poignant memories and explains how the various experiences and learning gained during this stage contributed to my professional development over the past 46 years. Practice commenced as a trainee pupil nurse to qualifying and working as an enrolled nurse (EN).

Group Demographics The 1973 pupil nurse intake comprised 23 pupils, all of whom were at varying ages and life experiences, from the less mature 18-year-old pupils to the more mature 30-year-old-plus pupils, who were married with children, and most of whom had resided in their own home. For today's nurses' intake, it

B. Anderson, *A Uro-Oncology Nurse Specialist's Reflection on her Practice Journey*, https://doi.org/10.1007/978-3-030-94199-4_2

could be argued that the demographics of these groups are more representative of an older, more mature individuals, who are likely to have had previous career pathways. As such, their life experiences and work ethics position them in good stead for a caring profession in today's climate.

The Nurses' Homes During this training, a majority of pupils resided in the nurses' home, where they were allocated rooms within the group of hospitals, where they had checked in on the previous day, second March 1973, prior to commencing induction training on third March 1973. There were six of us in my group. We were all allocated rooms in a wing connected to the care home for the elderly, which was attached to the main geriatric hospital. From the various venues, we travelled to the training venue that hosted the teaching sessions throughout the 2 years, in this case, a room situated on the third floor within the surgical hospital. Today, nurses do not have to live on-site. Most nursing homes are flatlets, where three or more persons (not just nurses, doctors as well) are likely to share accommodation, and the rules in terms of visitors are less regimented.

Training Programme Training lasted for 2 years (1973–1975), during which time 3-monthly rotational placements occurred between the four hospitals within the group. First rotation included a 6-week induction in school, followed by a 6-week placement on the ward. For my group, our first rotational placement took place in the geriatric hospital (later changed to Care of The Elderly (COTE)); second, in the surgical hospital; third, back in the geriatric hospital; fourth, back in the surgical hospital; and final rotation in the main training hospital, where we completed the 2 years of training, me, on a 32-bedded orthopaedic ward. The 2-year EN training programme was intense, but it enabled us to be more hands-on in our approach to care. It was also hugely beneficial in extending my knowledge and experience of various fields of nursing practice.

Initial Group Meeting and Interactions It was a sunny spring day on third March 1973, the first day of induction. The time was 09.00, and the venue, a room based on the third floor, was within the hospital. Twenty-three pupils were dressed in 'civvies', sitting in their seats, chairs in a row, one behind the other. Each of us, understandably, was nervous and apprehensive, but also excited at the prospect of embarking on an unfamiliar journey. Even though the windows were opened, the room was still quite warm. The tutor, a tall and buxom lady with red hair, and wearing black-framed spectacles, seemed friendly enough, but with a sternness of face that intimated a zero tolerance for any nonsense. During the 6 weeks of induction, she gave us some useful advice relating to our placements on the wards and of the potential issues we might face. This advice included subtle nuances such as 'Your face will not always fit'. 'It may not be your fault'. 'Try not to take remarks too personally', or 'not to get too personally invested in a patient's situation'. Beneficial advice, but at 18 years old, it was hard to appreciate the wisdom of its true meaning.

This occurred some years later, after I acquired some much-needed life experience. Thinking back on this period, I realise that even at that early stage, my tutor had instilled in me a sense of self-worth, pride and a determination to succeed.

Strict Code of Conduct—The Traditional Matron When I reflect on nursing in the 1970s, I clearly remember a strict code of conduct and an expectation to behave in a manner, which ultimately elevated the nurse's image and how we were perceived by patients and the general public. Specific to enforcing this objective was the traditional matron, who, for me, epitomised the true meaning of what nursing represented at that time. Matrons tended to be strict disciplinarians, who for the most part were fair in enforcing such discipline, and in doing so also demonstrated leadership qualities that commanded respect. Over the years, there had been a significant shift, both in the definition of the role of the matron and the expectation of the role, as well as questions being raised in regard to the quantity of matrons in employment, seemingly too many in comparison to nurses (Patterson 2012; UKEssays 2018). From a personal perspective, I believe that despite these senior professionals' previous role as ward-based nurses, who acquired a certain degree of knowledge and expertise (in terms of nursing and principles of practice), in obtaining the matron's role, they 'donned another hat', so to speak. Therefore, in the performance of the matron's role, their focus was more on the objectives of funding and targets, rather than on how these objectives would impact on the health professional, and more importantly on the patient and clinical outcomes. Nonetheless, this is a conclusion with which I can sympathise, since ultimately performance was driven by the expectation of meeting the target and avoiding any subsequent fine.

Uniform Policy The strict code of conduct also related to the uniform policy and ensuring that nurses adhered to the stated guidance. The pupil nurse uniform comprised a dress—light green and white stripes, white collar and white belt with silver buckle, paper hat, pocket watch, name badge, tights or stockings, comfortable flat heels, leather shoes (must be quiet, not squidgy), starched white apron, plus a black cape with red lining. I remember learning to make up the paper hat, which was held in place with two white hair grips. Nails were cut short with no trace of nail varnish in sight. There was a sense of pride and importance, and always the onus on ensuring that our actions reflected well on the profession. This professionalism was heeded during such times when we ventured out publicly, in our uniforms, for instance, at lunch time, going down to the local market, with uniform intact, including hat, but loosely covered with the black, red fabric-lined cape. Aaaah, loved that cape. In those days, there was an evident demonstration of the public's appreciation and respect for the nurse, which was usually clarified by a reduction in fees on subsequent purchases. On accomplishing the enrolled nurse (EN) role, the uniform policy still included all of the above-stated items, but the dress changed to a plain, mid-green colour, and a dark-green belt with a brass buckle. Looking smart and efficient, and proud as punch!

Changes to Nurse's Uniforms The evidence has shown that between the 1960s and 2019, there have been changes to the uniform policy. These included a change in the traditional dress and stockings; dresses became a little shorter and the white caps began to lose importance in some hospitals across the country. The 1980s saw an end of the nursing caps/hats altogether, and nurses began wearing disposable aprons rather than cloth aprons. Medical facilities were much less militant in regard to restrictions on jewellery and cosmetics. During the 1990s onwards, nursing dresses were replaced with more user-friendly scrub suits that are available in a wide variety of colours and styles. Some hospitals have specific scrub suit colours for different types of hospital staff, and others allow nurses and other staff to choose colours and styles that appeal to them. Today's nursing uniforms are designed more for function than form, but are also considered much more comfortable than those worn throughout history (UKEssays 2018). Thinking back on the nurse's uniform in the 1970s and 1980s, I suppose one of the reasons for these changes could be attributed to the risk of infection, a risk that has been exemplified by the wearing of uniforms (usually inadequately covered) on the road and when travelling on public transport. Admittedly, this was not a practice that I remember in the 1970s and 1980s.

When I commenced the MUCNS role in 2005, my uniform was befitting of my role. I had the choice of wearing my own clothes, 'civvies', for 4 days of the week, but on the day that I ran the nurse-led chemotherapy clinic, the expectation was that I would wear my uniform. In 2019, as I was about to embark on the next stage of my journey (my retirement), there was yet another change to the nurse's uniform. In attempts to 'out' the intrusion of the 'civvies attire', and to make the CNS appearance more professional, and more easily recognisable by patients and the general public, the CNS uniform was upgraded and implemented into practice. This time, the expectation was that these would be permanently worn by the CNS group for all aspects of care delivery. Alas, this was a change, for which my impending retirement had given me a pass.

Injecting a Sense of 'FUN' into the Equation The following recounting of the events illustrates that while certain elements of nursing were daunting and stressful, we managed to have fun along the way. I am not suggesting that nurses in the twenty-first century do not have fun; what I am saying is that as clarified in Anderson (Anderson 2010), they are more likely to experience a significant increase in stress levels, reduction in self-esteem and morale and consequently emotional burnout.

The Nurses' Home The following reflections relate to my placement in the main teaching hospital in the second year of training. This nurse's home consisted of four floors, spreading across several wings, that facilitated various access points. My memory of this period is of supporting, togetherness, cooking, sharing, laughing, exploring, learning and growing, both physically and emotionally, and for the younger pupil nurses, a feeling of being unencumbered and of not taking things too seriously. My memory of cooking is especially satisfying, since I managed to avoid doing my fair share. However, because all the nurses in my group could cook, we ate relatively well. As shown in the following account, there were fewer satisfying moments too.

Annoying Behaviour   Stealing food was an annoying behaviour that was imbedded in the nurse's home ethos. The nurse's home consisted of one main kitchen, situated on the ground floor, with a small electric cooker hob on each floor. Within the main kitchen there was a large fridge-freezer and a combined cooker hob and oven, for communal use by over 300 nurses. Ultimately, some food needed to be kept refrigerated, but the worry had been not finding that food when you next went to retrieve it from the fridge. This was despite placing messages (in capitals), such as 'This food is the belonging of -----, please do not touch', on the fridge door. The only logical solution was not to leave food in the fridge. No use complaining, you learn to adapt … so we resorted to cooking and consuming meals on the same day. Frustrating behaviour, but surprisingly mirthful.

Boyfriends and Husbands   There were stringent rules in place, especially in regard to boyfriends and husbands entering the nurses' quarters. A rule that had raised the thought, 'If we were old enough to be responsible for a ward of 32 patients, surely we were old enough to be responsible for our own virginity'. Feeling affronted, we played certain pranks, the objective of which was to 'get one over' the warden, Mrs. Doland. These pranks included sneaking boyfriends and husbands to our rooms … not an easy task, but one which, if accomplished, was hugely satisfying. In executing the plan, one person would keep track of Mrs. Doland's movements, specifically where she was at any given time (i.e. which floor or wing, whether she was using the elevator or the stairs), and then skilfully manoeuvre the boyfriend or husband to the relevant room. It was even more satisfying if, in attempting this manoeuvre, the nurse was caught, as in the case of the nurse who resided on the fourth floor. Having successfully sneaked her boyfriend into her room, she was subsequently found out by Mrs. Doland, who promptly escorted the boyfriend to the lift that delivered him to the ground floor, and into the path of curious onlookers. How embarrassing! The lesson here was not to get caught. Thinking back, Mrs. Doland was only doing her job, but we resented her for doing so. Why? Perhaps because her approach to managing us was more geared towards that of managing children, rather than mature adults … a fact that, we felt, should be acknowledged and respected.

'Mischievous Wit'   Battersea Dogs Home is a prominent organisation in the UK that provides a safe haven for unwanted/stray dogs (and today, cats), with the objective being to find them a good home. Reflection, in this instance, is related to the phone in the hallway on the ground floor in the nurses' home that was accessible to all the residents. There were times when boredom necessitated an injection of fun, as in playing 'pranks' on the phone. I remember the phone would ring and someone would answer with the retort, 'Hello, Battersea Dogs Home, Mongrel section, how can I help you?'. The voice at the other end responded with, 'Oh, I'm sorry, I must have the wrong number', and then the subsequent click that resulted in an Ooops!

and a snigger! Phone rings again, and there is a repeat of the same retort and out-come. A little irresponsible perhaps, but you found enjoyment where you could.

Having Fun with the Split Shift My memory of working in the 1970s and 1980s is of the weekly rota that comprised 40 h (later reduced to 37.5 h), for both day and night shifts that included a variable shift pattern for day duties: early shift (07.30–4.00), late shift (12.30–9.00) and split shift (07.30–12.30 and 4.30–9.00). Night-shift timing was 20.00–0800 (12-h shifts = 4 nights on and 3 off). I remember having fun with the split shift. Usually, going out the previous night meant that I would not have acquired the allotted 8 h of sleep. In this instance, I would struggle to attend for the 07.30–12.30 parts of the shift, but would become quite sick for the latter half—an admission that was not far off from the truth, since I often did feel genuinely sick. Hey, we were young! Many nurses had worked predominantly night shifts, presumably for convenience, but over the years, all nurses were encouraged to alternate shifts (predominantly working day shifts, with intervening night shifts). The hours of work were long and fairly laborious, but we just got on with the job at hand and strived to make it as enjoyable as possible.

Less Fun memories There were also fewer fun moments, of sadness and under-standable confusion. There is the memory of a nursing colleague, who, for the purpose of simplification and confidentiality, is referred to as Melanie, who com-mitted suicide. The solemn vision of her plan re-enacted: preparing herself; bath-ing, the new nightgown, hair combed, everything clean and in its place. We were informed about the suicide, but it did not seem real, not until the coffin alighted from the lift. The sharp gasps and intakes of breath and looking surprised and fearful are still vivid in my memory, along with the question I had silently asked myself, 'What could have pushed Melanie to take her own life, and at such a young age?'

Thinking back on this memory, I can clearly visualise Melanie sitting in the hos-pital canteen, during coffee or lunch break, with a seemingly lack of interest in food; in fact, I had rarely seen her consume anything more substantial than a cup of black coffee. The parting in her hair was just above her forehead, with hair scooped back, either in a bun or in a pony tail that was held neatly at the nape of her neck. She suf-fered with psoriasis, a skin condition, that was clearly visible on her head, face and neck, which made her self-conscious. I remember the sad look in Melanie's eyes, who rarely smiled and seemed to have quite a weight on her shoulders. I suspected that there was something wrong, but at 18 years old, I was unsure of what to do. Melanie's death was a huge shock, and for her nursing colleagues, its effect was far reaching. We could not unsee her body alighting from the elevator, unhear explana-tions of how she planned her demise or visualise her in the final moments. As a result, we sought comfort by huddling together in each other's rooms. It was uncom-fortable and somewhat confusing for a while, but essentially, we needed to under-stand **WHY**? There was an explanation, but one we felt, in that instance, had not fully captured the sad loss of a life. Consequently, evaluation of the incident, and its ensuing impact on the students, had placed emphasis on management's awareness and of the importance which must be placed on the management of such situations. Specific focus was placed on how we were coping and whether there was adequate support in place (i.e. counselling) to counter the emotional impact. To this day, Melanie's suicide, and how she planned it to the very last detail, remains vivid in my mind. I now realise that her decision to take her own life was final. In exacting her plan, she had taken steps to ensure that she could not be saved.

Practical and Theoretical Skills My memory of performing these skills is based on Roper-Tierney-Logan Model for Nursing (Nursing Essay 2020). Originally published in 1980 and later revised in 2000, this is a holistic model that defines the activities of daily living (ADLs) as:

- Maintaining a safe environment.
- Communication.
- Breathing.
- Eating and drinking.
- Elimination.
- Washing and dressing.
- Controlling temperature.
- Mobilising.
- Working and playing.
- Sleeping.

The list also includes death and sexuality as activities of daily living, but these are often disregarded depending on the setting and situation for the individual patient.

For those patients who are less capable, nurses were required to assist them with their activities of daily living needs, and in doing so to adhere to available guidance, specific to which was the ability to perform effective pressure area care. Integral to the performance of this activity was an adequate supply of resources, which, as I remember, in the 1970s and 1980s could not be faulted. These resources included the sheep skin rug, rubber rings, sheets and draw sheets, incontinent pads, wash cloths, emollient and barrier creams. These resources, combined with the 2-hourly back rounds over a 24-h period, were beneficial in minimising the risk of a breakdown in a patient's pressure areas. The health professional was also expected to assist the patient with other ADL, such as eating and drinking, washing, dressing and mobilising.

The Pupil Nurse Practical Examination In the 1970s, great emphasis was placed on the individual's ability to correctly perform a full bed bath. Correctly, it had meant maintaining the patient's privacy and dignity (by pulling the curtains around the bed to ensure that there was no gaping) during the actual activity. Using the plastic bowl, you would make sure that the water was at the correct temperature, remembering to change this at the appropriate time during the task. If the patient is unable to turn themselves, providing the appropriate support (with arms). During this process, the patient's pressure areas were assessed, and if indicated, the appropriate barrier cream or dressing was applied. Mouth care was also performed, with specific focus placed on dentures. The patient was then helped to put on their nightgown if staying in bed, or if getting out of bed to get fully dressed, and aided to sit in the armchair by their bed. Reflection on my undertaking of this activity is still vivid in my mind. I remember being extremely nervous, as the assessor keenly observed my every move. As I did not want to fail, my approach to completing the task was quite anal. However, even then, I realised that conducting a patient bed bath was an important part of the nurse's role, an importance which over the years I have strived to be mindful of.

Bed Making In the 1970s and 1980s, my memory of the bed making protocol was of a ritualistic undertaking of the daily stripping and making of beds. In those days, the mattress was covered in a plastic sheet, which on removing or turning emitted a static electric shock to the nurse … an occurrence, which, when thinking back, brings a smile to my face, as I envisioned a picture of being electrified and my hair standing up in peaks. In my attempt to avoid further shocks, I remember kicking the bedframe (leather soles counteracting the effect of further shocks), an action that sometimes worked, and sometimes not. In making the bed, we were taught to focus on the mitring of sheets and boxing of the blankets, to achieve the perfect corners. This technique was so well ingrained in my mind that to this day (if using sheets and blankets), I still make my own bed in this way. Some years later, in the 1990s, I remember attempting to explain the concept of mitring and boxing of the corners to my students, and observing the confusion on their faces. Protocol had changed during this period to include the use of quilts, which, if memory serves me correctly, was not an effective change, since, in terms of temperature control, patients often stated that they were either too hot or too cold, and quilts would often slide off the bed. No surprise, then, that quilts were eventually phased out. Today, bed making is still a ritualistic undertaking, although mattresses are now enclosed in a durable plastic cover, and boxing and mitring are not stringently enforced.

2.2   Performance of the Wound Dressing Procedure

Even in the 1970s, strict policy and procedure guidelines were in place, the objective being to prevent or minimise the risk of infection. Specific in my memory is the wound dressing procedure, integral to which was the stringent handwashing protocol.

A Truly Aseptic Approach My memory of the undertaking of the wound dressing procedure in the 1970s is of a very strict protocol that comprised the sterile field, which included the cleaning of the dressing trolley from top to bottom, including the wheels, ensuring that all the necessary resources like dressings, wound dressing packs, masks, disposable apron and sterile gloves are available. The curtains were drawn to maintain privacy and to protect the patient's dignity. Those days, it was usual to have a second nurse to assist with the dressing procedure; therefore, she would open the wound dressing pack for the lead nurse, who would then arrange the various items on the sterile field. The second nurse would then open other relevant items, such as cleansing agent and sterile gloves, onto the sterile field. She would also make the patient comfortable, in readiness for the dressing procedure. As the lead nurse, you would explain the procedure to the patient and obtain their consent to proceed.

Handwashing   The memory of this activity is still vivid. This includes the sink and tall taps, and right (hot) water and left (cold) water, with the long nozzle. The handwashing protocol is as follows: first put on the disposable apron, wet the palm of hands, soap generously with Hibisol scrub (Hibiscrub) and massage fully including back of hands, in between fingers and up to elbows. To rinse, use elbows to manoeuvre taps, with elbows bent and holding both arms in the upright position; use green paper towels (seen as the more sterile approach to the towel on a roller); and use downward strokes to dry hands thoroughly.

The Dressing Procedure—Non-Touch Technique   After performing handwashing, you would then put on your mask and sterile gloves, and following a strict aseptic technique (utilising the plastic forceps), proceed to do dressing. This is a protocol that has survived over the years, although, admittedly, the use of masks, in certain situations, is not so rigid.

2.3   Poignant Reflections

Reflections on my training between 1973 and 1976 highlight some uncomfortable moments, some of which are depicted in the following accounts:

1974—First Experience of Poor Communication   Many authors (Bramhall 2014; Barber 2016; Ali 2017; Doyle 2020) allude to the positive impact of effective communication and its importance in the way we, as individuals, interact with each other, and similarly the negative impact of poor communication (Pincock 2004) during these interactions. My first experience of poor communication as a pupil nurse occurred on the ward office, where the ward sister, two staff nurses and myself were having a discussion. The ward sister asked me to get her some water for injection from the clinical room, and I promptly returned with a 500 ml container of water, which, unbeknown to me at the time, was used for irrigation and washouts. The water I should have got was the one in the glass vial, which was used to reconstitute drugs for intravenous use. The ward sister looked at me, and with a smirk on her face, and a derogatory tone of voice, said, 'You silly girl, that's not the water I meant'. Feeling stupid, I ran to the clinical room with tears running down my cheeks. Hot on my heels was the staff nurse, who, in her attempt to reassure me, berated me for crying and told me that I should never allow anyone to speak to me like that. She went on to explain that the ward sister was wrong to speak to me in that manner. I was there to learn, and it was their responsibility to ensure that I did. That day, I listened well, and going forward, the staff nurse's words have been a constant reminder of why I must never allow anyone to speak to me in that way again, but more importantly, why we should *all* strive to communicate well with the people we interact with in life. Admittedly, as a result of this experience, I became very defensive. Whenever I encountered poor communication, my initial reaction was to lash out with a response that was normally devoid of any tact. However, over the years, I believe that I have learned to listen and to think about what I would like to say before saying it, and consequently, my approach to dealing with issues around poor communication was more tactful and diplomatic (Anderson 2019).

Death is a natural passage of life, but for the young, it is an enigma that is often rarely experienced and may thus be poorly understood. For most people, it is an enigma that often incites fear and irrational behaviour, but it can incite humour too.

As I reflect on my childhood in Jamaica, I realise that there have been many deaths, although I can only relate my first real memory and experience of death, and of seeing a dead body, back to when I was about 6 years old. A family friend, Miss Morgan (which as a mark of respect was how we children addressed her), was a lady in her late 70s. She was a shopkeeper, who had lived in the Parish of Westmoreland in the local community all her life. Sadly, Miss Morgan had died while visiting her children in the capital, Kingston. Due to the heat, and to preserve the body, she was kept on ice for around 3 weeks, before transferring her back to her home Parish for the subsequent funeral. In the church, on the day of the funeral, the coffin was left open to allow the congregation to view the body. Miss Morgan looked as if she was sleeping—with her face made up, face powder and pink lipstick, she did not look scary. I remember thinking that Miss Morgan did not look like Miss Morgan. Her body was remarkably slim (considering she had been not fat, but somewhat over-weight). As it was later explained to me, her insides had been removed to ensure that freezing of the body would be more effective. I remember the grave, very deep and dark, and we, the children, were dressed in black and white (skirts, dresses, tunics, white socks), who had laughed, skipped and jumped, seemingly unaffected by the occasion and what it represents.

As I embarked on my nursing journey at the tender age of 18 years old, a journey in which I encountered numerous deaths, while some of the experiences from these were sobering, on recollection, there were some jovial moments too.

'Last Office Duties' Last office duties are the act of performing the final care for a patient; as such, dignity and respect are paramount. In the 1970s and 1980s, the last office duty task included the laying out of the body, during which any intravenous lines or urinary catheters were removed. The patient was given a full bed bath, all orifices (anus, nostrils, ears, vagina for women and tying of the penis for men) were plugged and men were shaved as appropriate. The body was then dressed in the white shroud, and openings were secured with pink tape. The shrouded body was then wrapped in the white sheet which was then folded as per protocol, taped to hold folds in place (which gave the body a mummified appearance) and then covered loosely with the white sheet, the one with the purple cross down the centre. Purple, a colour from that point forward, had been a permanent reminder of death. Part of this duty included accompanying the porter with the gurney to take the body to the mortuary, a task that was especially scary, if it was raining. My memory of the mortuary is a stark reminder of a cold and foreboding place …, of silence and the dimmed fluorescent lighting and of placing the body in that dark, desolate refrigerator. Fortunately, today's performance of the last office duty is far less onerous. Today, intravenous lines and urinary catheters are left in situ and capped off. The body is not washed, unless it is deemed necessary (as in the event of soiling). The patient is left wearing their gown or nightdress, and is wrapped in a plain white sheet. The body is then collected from the ward in a gurney, and is then accompanied to the mortuary by two porters, where the mortician performs a more detailed preparation. Thank goodness! I have often wondered why as human beings we fear the dead and not the living. After all, as the saying goes, the dead cannot harm you!

'Deathly Humour' I am not certain if humour is the best description of the events for this experience, not then anyway, but today, reflecting on the memory does incite a degree of mirth.

First Experience of Death as a Pupil Nurse I had been in training for approximately 10 weeks into my first placement, in the geriatric hospital, and was still very inexperienced. I was on duty, at around 7.30 pm, and the ward was quiet. The dimmed lights in the four-bed cubicle portrayed a gloomy ambience. The weather was disquieting—the heavy rain, accompanied by thunder and lightning, instilled a sense of fear in me. In those days, patients were allocated to specific nursing teams, which included either a staff nurse or an enrolled nurse, auxiliary nurse (healthcare assistant) and trainee nurses, who were *expected to* be hands-on from the beginning, to learn the job; there was no standing and observing, as is arguably the case today. This was an expectation that was much more so for the pupil nurse.

2.3.1 Case Study

Mrs. Dees, an 83-year-old lady, had died approximately 2 h earlier.

Unfortunately, for me, I was the only one available to assist the staff nurse, with whom I was working to perform Mrs. Dees' 'last office duty of care', prior to which the staff nurse had fully explained the protocol. Standing on the opposite side of the bed to me, the staff nurse commenced washing Mrs. Dees. First, she washed the right arm, then the left and then the remaining frontal areas with me drying in between. The staff nurse then explained that she needed to turn Mrs. Dees' body on her left side, towards me. On executing this action, an unexpected gush of air escaped from the body, which made it seem to come alive, a natural occurrence, as I had later found. Without thinking, I had let go of the body and attempted to run. The staff nurse, still holding on to Mrs. Dees' body, called out to me, urging me to return. I turned and looked at her with dread. I was so scared that all I wanted to do was to get out of there. The intermittent sounds of thunder and flashes of lightning did not help; however, still shaking, I walked sheepishly back to the bed. The staff nurse, with a sly smile at the corner of her mouth, attempted to reassure me. She explained that she understood that this situation was quite frightening, but there was no one else to assist her. I was still extremely nervous, but feeling that I had no choice, I managed to help the staff nurse to complete Mrs. Dees' last office duty of care. The memory of this experience remained vivid in my mind throughout my nursing career, albeit less frightening. Over the years, I have performed many last office duties of care, and while it was not a duty I was overly fond of, in its performance I was most proficient.

First Experience of Cancer and Subsequent Death My first experience of cancer and subsequent death occurred 6 months into my training while working at my second placement hospital, in a surgical ward.

2.3.2 Case Study

Mr. Young was a lovely gentleman in his early 50s married with two children. He was of medium build and 6′3″ tall. Following his receipt of a diagnosis of stomach cancer, he was admitted for surgery, a partial gastrectomy. Mr. Young's recovery from his surgery was fairly uneventful, and he was discharged home with an appropriate plan of care and subsequent follow-up in place.

Nine months later, on my fourth placement, and my second visit to this surgical hospital, I was surprised to see Mr. Young again, this time in a deteriorated state. His eyes were closed and he had not spoken. In fact, he was barely breathing. Being tasked with Mr. Young's care, I assisted him to his bed and closed the curtains around him. As I proceeded to give him a bed bath (including a shave), I was surprised how much weight he had lost and how weak he was. In fact, he was unable to raise himself up the bed (a movement that I was able to perform quite easily by myself). Unfortunately, during this manoeuvre, Mr. Young took his final breath. I remember feeling sad, a reaction, which at 19 years old I could not explain, but one that the mature version of me, and knowing what I now know, surmises as sadness for a very nice gentleman, who, in his early 50s, still had a lot of living to do. I had taken care to ensure that Mr. Young looked presentable for his wife, who had been waiting in the relative's room. She was upset, but the outcome was not unexpected. She thanked me for my help, and feeling genuinely sad for her, I gave her a hug.

Mr. Young was the first of my many early experiences of cancer and dealing with the subsequent death of a patient, experiences that contributed greatly to how I dealt with future incidences of cancer and death, as will be illustrated as appropriate throughout the book.

Hospice Visit I had been in training for about 7 months, when as part of the training program, my group undertook a planned visit to the local hospice. I remember clearly the environment—the silence, an acceptance of finality and yet a sense of peace. The nurse manager's voice was calm and reassuring. Her eyes were knowing and sympathetic. The poised manner emanated her expertise and competency. The group was silent, as she described and explained the service provided by the hospice. The emphasis was clearly on end of life, but with the inference of a laying down of life's burdens and transference to a better existence. The visit to the open plan ward laid bare its somber existence. There were curtains around each bed, but as previously explained by the manager, these were often left open, even at the point of death, a natural transition that made no attempt to hide the fact that a fellow patient had passed on. Apparently, each patient would have spoken about their situations, would have shared their fears and anxieties and would have been enabled to come to terms with death and to accept its inevitability. The visit was daunting, but also comforting, because it instilled in me the vision of a place where individuals could peacefully spend the last few weeks or days of their life, admittedly a very humane way to exit this world.

Revisit Years later, I revisited this environment, this time to visit the son of a close family friend, a young boy of only 12 years old (Aaron), a sobering experience in light of his age. It was also the same environment in which, years later, another family friend (Glenn) completed his final journey (refer to Chap. 8).

2.4   Changes to Practice and Associated Implications

Arguably, there have been numerous changes to nursing over the years that have impacted practice either positively or negatively. My recollection of some of these changes is described in the following accounts:

Wards, Capacity and Skill Mix In the 1970s and 1980s, wards were fairly large, mostly accommodating a mixed-sex capacity of 30-plus patients. Initially, men and women patients had occupied beds in the same area, with males on one side of the ward and females on the other, and finally with wards becoming single-sex wards. These wards were adequately resourced, with nurses of varying skill mix (enrolled and registered nurses, pupil and student nurses, auxiliaries) all working in unison to provide specified care to patients (Anderson 2010). Nowadays in hospitals, the wards are not gender mixed, although nurses are gender mixed between wards (UKEssays 2018).

Underlining the Importance of Good Nutrition in the Hospital Setting Good diet and nutrition are an important part of leading a healthy lifestyle. Combined with physical activity, it protects us from major health risks (such as heart disease and cancer) and promotes overall health. In terms of promoting health within the hospital setting, good nutrition is crucial to building health and resilience in patients, but also visitors and staff (Button 2020). Addressing poor nutrition is of key importance, since the evidence has shown that unhealthy meals have often resulted in malnourishment. A failure to recognise and treat malnourishment has vast implications for hospital trusts and patients, specifically slower patient recovery, and consequently prolonged hospital stays and increased costs (Carrell 2005). The evidence has further shown that patients were unhappy to eat hospital meals and that many relied on their relatives to bring them food during their stay in hospital (Button 2020).

My Early Memories of Patients' Meals   My early memory of patients' meals in the 1970s includes tapioca pudding, offal and jellied Eels. For patients who were unable to take solids, there was a choice of pureed meals (minced beef, lamb, chicken), pureed vegetables and other accompaniments that were not aesthetically pleasing to the eye nor to the palate. Admittedly, meals were a little more appealing for those patients who could have solids. One such meal had been the breakfast menu—the 'full English'—eggs (boiled, fried or scrambled), bacon, sausage, baked beans, tomatoes and even mushrooms … Wow! The lunch and supper menu was also quite decent. In the late 1990s/2000s, the patient's menu and the choice of meals had changed significantly. Choice of meals included individually, pre-wrapped, hot and cold meals, which included the sandwich. There was a time when the evening supper consisted only of a choice of soup, sandwiches, yoghurts, fruit salad or cheese and biscuits.

Efforts to Improve the Quality and Standard of Hospital Food   The increased scrutiny on the nutritional status of the meals being prepared for patients in the hospital setting, and whether these were fit for purpose, resulted in the instigation of several initiatives over the years, one of which was *the Better Hospital Food programme* which was launched by the NHS England in 2001. This initiative looked at the need for high standards in hospital food so that more meals were freshly cooked with care. Making meals tastier and more nutritious was, and still is, beneficial to improving the patient's experience of hospital food (Button 2020). Additional help and advice were sought from various celebrity chefs, including Jamie Oliver, who, based on his previous success with improving the nutritional status of school meals, was recruited by the health minister to liaise with relevant hospital catering staff to improve the current status of hospital meals (BBC News 2005; Ford 2005; Carrell 2005), a working partnership that had borne some fruit.

Protected Time and Space   One of the ideas promoted in the Better Hospital Food programme was protected mealtimes. There are obviously many reasons why patients do not or cannot eat in hospital; however one particular reason cited by patients is that their mealtimes were frequently interrupted by ward activity such as cleaning, ward rounds and medicine rounds and by having to leave the ward for diagnostic investigations (Button 2020). Ensuring that patients are able to eat their meals is the responsibility of the whole healthcare team, but typically nurses. In this context, protected mealtimes allow nurses to devote time to the meal service and to assist those patients needing help to eat, and it should be ensured that this occurred in a calm and peaceful environment (Ford 2005). My memory of this concept in the 1970s and 1980s is congruent with the current protocol. I clearly remember the ward settings, with no cubicles, which was just an open space that was divided into two sections, with the long dinner table and chairs down the middle. At mealtimes, ambulant patients would sit around the table to have their meals, those less mobile would sit in their armchairs by their beds and utilise the bedside table to eat their meals, while those who were bed-bound would sat upright in their beds and the nurses would assist them to eat their meals. Of course, in the 1970s and 1980s, teams were much larger, a fact that enabled staff to provide this very essential care. Today, mealtimes are still protected, with emphasis focused on ensuring that the patient's nutritional needs are adequately met. However, with the evident reductions in manpower, achieving the end goal is perhaps more difficult. Diet and nutrition have always been an important part of the care provided to hospital patients, an importance that has been championed by the nursing profession for many years. Even so, it is still a neglected branch of nursing, one that continues to attract scrutiny to this day (Button 2020). The role of good nutrition and its importance to improving patient outcomes are underlined in Anderson (Anderson 2010, 2005).

Interactive Time   While interactive time included mealtimes, it was also the time that had been set aside in the afternoons to enable nurses to interact with those patients who did not have any visitors. It was a time to stimulate—to talk, and taking the time to listen, hear and reflect. This activity had instilled in me a real sense of purpose from which I derived a tangible feeling of job satisfaction.

A Reassuring Memory of Feeling Valued   Thinking back on my placement at one of the Trust's hospitals evokes memories of appreciation and of feeling valued, during one specific Christmas period, while working on a medical ward in my second year of training. In this instance, teamwork (in which skill mix of staff and specifically the ward manager) was key. For me, Christmas was an especially nice time to be at work. I remember working as a team and sharing the load: preparing the patients for the day … washing, dressing and making those remaining in bed comfortable; helping others out of bed to sit in armchairs by their bed or around the large dinner table; putting on the Christmas hats; and helping those who could not feed themselves. After this, we ensured that individuals were comfortable, before focusing on the staff's needs.

At Christmas in the 1970s, nurse's meals were provided free by the hospital and were eaten on the relevant wards. I remember resetting the table after the patients had eaten, and the ward sister telling us to sit around the table and then serving us our Christmas meal. I remember pulling Christmas crackers and putting on our hats, the laughter and the sense of belonging. In that moment, nursing was the best job, ever! The ward sister had ensured that the nurses who worked the early shift (07.30–15.30) would go off duty at 2.30 p.m., with the late-shift nurses starting at 2 p.m. Also, if you worked on Christmas Day, you would be off on Boxing Day—the same for New Year's Eve and New Year's Day. In those days, things seemed simpler and less tedious. The main Christmas event was quite a spread that comprised a function that was laid out in the main restaurant. I remember the long table impressively decorated and adorned with a variety of foods that included whole dressed salmons and various roasts—chicken, pork, beef and lamb, plus accompaniments. For many of us, this was a magical time, and we felt valued and appreciated. Do not get me wrong, nursing was no picnic. We worked hard. The work was stressful and at times daunting, but by working as a team, we managed to make the experience less so. Another observation in the 1970s had been the importance placed on nurses taking their entitled breaks, which in comparison to today's nursing, where nurses are often hard-pushed to take their breaks, was well enforced.

Early Memories of Pain and its Management My early memories of pain and its management pertain to the second year of my training.

Scenario 2.1
This memory relates to one particular patient, a lady in her 60s, with end-stage cancer. Her pain was being managed with morphine analgesia, with two-hourly intervals or as needed for breakthrough pain. I clearly remember the emaciated state, emphasised by the distinct lack of muscle or fat on her bones, and the physical display of pain evidenced in her body language. She had taut physique, with bones clear to see, and the laboured breathing was evident in the rise and fall of her chest. The closed eyes scrunched up along with her face as the pain washed over her. Pain relief had comprised 1–2-hourly intramuscular injections of morphine. As there was not much flesh on her bones, the green injection needle had found its way into saggy skin, where it had met a hard, bony prominence. As a young nurse, I had wondered what it must be like to endure such pain and discomfort, and while you were so close to dying. Even at that early stage of my training, this was a distressing observation; hence, I was pleased when the morphine pump was introduced into practice. For me, this was a more humane approach to pain management, especially for those patients with end-stage diseases, such as cancer.

Over the years, pain management has progressed extensively to becoming a specialist field, where the objective is in ensuring that the individual's pain is effectively managed; that is, patients are kept comfortable and relatively pain free, with the onus being on preventing breakthrough pain and alleviating unnecessary discomfort. Today, effective pain management is integral to holistic care planning. This is especially important in managing patients' post-surgical procedures, where the utilisation of resources, such as patient-controlled analgesia (PCA), has secured huge improvements in both patient outcomes and their experiences.

End-of-Life Care (Previously the Liverpool Care Pathway) Effective pain management is crucial to end-of-life care planning (typically for cancer patients). The LCP was recommended as a model of good care by the Department of Health's End of Life Care Strategy in 2008, by the General Medical Council in 2010 and by the National Institute for Health and Care Excellence in 2011. It was designed to be used as a means to manage a patient's pain and distress when clinicians considered that they were in their last hours or days of life, and there was no appropriate reversible treatment for their condition (Department of Health and Social Care 2013). However, due to arising issues and concerns, e.g. when patients were wrongly being denied nutrition and hydration while being placed on the Pathway, the recommendation was made to phase out the LCP over the next 6–12 months, and that it be replaced by a personalised end-of-life care plan, backed up by good practice guidance specific to disease groups, in 2013 (Department of Health and Social Care 2013). The main objective of the end-of-life care plan is in ensuring that the patient experiences a 'good death' (Weston 2015).

2.5   1973–1975, Early Experience of Smoking and its Implications

In this context, I have chosen to emphasise the impact of compromised breathing. My understanding of compromised breathing is of a state where the individual is unable to breathe effectively as a result of reduced cardiorespiratory efficiency. Arguably, the ability to breathe effectively is something we all take for granted; hence, it is difficult to appreciate how not being able to do so will affect us. Over the years I have observed many episodes of compromised breathing, personal and professional. These will be explained as appropriate in the various case studies and scenarios in this chapter.

Compromised Breathing (1)—Severe Asthmatic The implications of smoking on peoples' health have been a long-standing problem. My first observation and experience of compromised breathing relate back to the 1970s, when I was a pupil nurse, in my first year of training, and during my placement in a medical ward.

2.5.1   Case Study

Mr. Eaves was a gentleman in his mid-70s. He was a known asthmatic, for which the prescribed treatment had been oxygen, regular nebulisers and inhalers. He was a smoker of approximately 20 cigarettes per day, which as an asthmatic was extremely counterproductive in attempts to restore effective respiratory function. My memory of the scenario of Mr. Eaves' smoking habit (taking a puff on his cigarette, the ensuing coughing and spluttering, and in an attempt to counter this, the usual puff on his inhaler) is surreal. I could not understand why he had chosen to smoke, when his breathing was so obviously compromised. This is a behaviour that I frequently observed over the years. While I acquired a better understanding of why people would choose to smoke in such situations, it is still a puzzling behaviour, considering the impact on their health and quality of life.

Fire Issues In the 1970s and well into the 1990s, smoking was visualised as a sociable pastime; hence, patients, relatives and visitors frequenting the health establishment were able to smoke freely within the hospital, in the wards (including in bed for patients) and within its grounds. Thinking back on this memory, I am strangely spooked. In light of the health and safety implications, such as cigarette causing a fire in beds, inflammatory effect of smoking and oxygen and risks of causing fires elsewhere, this was an extremely dangerous behaviour, which thankfully was eventually phased out.

Over the years, the impetus on fire and its implication placed the topic high on the health and safety radar. As a result, attempts to instigate changes in practice were reinforced with mandatory fire training updates for all employees working in the healthcare sector. My memory of these updates is of long and difficult-to-watch sessions. The manner in which the presentation was delivered (the fire officer talked through salient issues) was often quite mundane. So mundane in fact that you were often hard-pushed to stay focused, and not giving in to the temptation to fall asleep. I believe that this lack of focus was noted by the various presenters, because not only are today's sessions more animated and up-to-date on salient issues, but they are also more targeted to capturing and maintaining the individual's attention. There are still vocal explanations, but these are supported with slides and video presentations to aid both visual acuity and understanding.

2.6   Thought-Provoking Reflections

Reflecting back on the 2 years of my pupil nurse training and what this involved, I am reminded of some thought-provoking moments, as detailed in the following accounts, and how, as a young nurse, I had dealt with these:

Sputum My memory of this task is of collecting and emptying sputum pots—the slimy, sticky and frothy consistency … Aaagh, quite disgusting! Later on, my career witnessed suctioning sputum via tracheostomies and mouths to relieve the build-up of sputum and accordingly improve the patient's breathing. Still it was a disgusting task, but extremely beneficial for the patient.

Vomit I remember providing the patient with the vomit bowl and supporting their head with one hand, allowing them to vomit and trying to stop myself from retching. Sometimes, the vomit had only contained bile, which was not so bad, and other times food, which was quite bad. The sickly smell was quite nauseating, as was the subsequent disposal. The feeling of nausea that resulted in my inability to eat for hours later is still vivid in my mind, as are my thoughts at that time, which were 'what a job' and 'please, get me out of here'. However, despite the unpleasantness of the task, I realised that I needed to deal with it, if I wanted to continue down the nursing path. On a more cynical note, I guess, the short abstinence of dietary intake on my part, following these episodes, had been helpful in maintaining my weight … Smile!!

Manual evacuation is the manual removal of faeces from the rectum using nothing more than gloves and lubricant. In the 1970s, manual evacuation was a task that was necessitated more often than not for patients who were unable to perform this activity in the natural way. Working in the geriatric ward (now care of the elderly), many patients had required weekly assistance with this activity, which was carried out by the ward sister, with assistance from one of the nurses, in this case me, the trainee pupil nurse. Obviously, as the trainee, I was not expected to perform the task at this point; however, I was expected to observe the task being done, whether I wanted to or not. However, while this was an unpleasant task … oh my Lord, the smell … I do remember the evident relief for the patients, following its undertaking, and for that reason, the benefits had outweighed the unpleasantness.

Scenario 2.2

One such patient for whom this activity was necessitated was a young man, who, as a result of a serious bike accident, was a quadriplegic. He was trapped in a body that no longer functioned as it should from the neck down, although he could see, hear and speak. At 18 years old, I could think of nothing worse, and yet, I was unable to voice my fears. I remember looking at him, and thinking quietly inside what must it be like not having any control over your limbs, and being reliant on another person to maintain your activities of daily living needs: eating and drinking, and hygiene needs—bathing, brushing your teeth and urinary and bowel functions. I remember the team's concerted efforts to prevent bed sores while keeping him as comfortable as possible.

Scenario 2.3

I also remember patients in other ward settings, who were entirely reliant on the health professional, to fulfil their daily emotional and physical needs. These included patients whose cognitive status had been impaired by dementia and Alzheimer's disease, and who, in my opinion, were existing rather than living: every day, the same environment and a ritualistic routine that consisted of eating and drinking, washing, bathing and dressing, and either remaining in bed or sitting out in the armchair. Thinking back, I realise that these patients may not have had an awareness of their situation (you do not really know), but at 18 years old, it seemed a sad existence, like a life sentence, for which the only reprieve was death. However, as I progressed in my career and obtained some valuable life experiences (even though I strongly believe in quality rather than quantity of life), I fully understand that life is precious, and that for some people, regardless of the circumstances, it must be cherished.

A 'Fashionable Health Trend' This title emerged as a result of my memory of undertaking of a high colonic washout (HCW). This is a procedure that was used 'to wash out the contents of the large bowel, by means of copious enemas using water or other medication' (WebMD 2020). During an enema, water is retained in the colon for approximately 15 min.

During the 1970s, HCW was extremely useful for providing relief to those patients with faeces high up in the rectum, and who were unable to pass content naturally by themselves. In the performance of this procedure, I remember being kitted out with the appropriate attire: green apron and water boots and having the required resources—plastic sheet, bucket, funnel and hose, water for irrigation, lubricant and plastic sheeting for the floor—at hand. The procedure included placing the patient on their left side, legs drawn up towards their abdomen, lubricating the tube attached to the hose and funnel, inserting into the anus, regimentally pouring the water into the funnel, holding this upward so that the water is instilled into the anus and lowering at a downward angle, allowing the content to be expelled into the bucket. This process would be repeated several times until the content ran clear. As I reflect on this procedure, I am amused that such a mundane procedure had evolved to becoming not only a fashionable but also a profitable health trend. The remedial cleansing of the bowels that also doubles as a slimming technique? Who knew!

End of Training I completed my enrolled nurse training in March 1975, but even in those days, attrition had played its part. Of the 23 pupils who started, only 10 proceeded to graduate as enrolled nurses in 1975. This is an issue that continues to this day, to be a problem for the NHS. More than a third of nurses in training fail to complete the training course, and this has been the case for more than a century (UKEssays 2018).

Near the end of my training, I was working on a 32-bedded orthopaedic ward in the main training hospital, and continued to do so after I graduated, until 1976. Working on this ward was hugely enlightening in terms of my learning, especially my experience of working as part of a team and the benefits it afforded. However, there were moments when I questioned certain behaviours, as in the case of one particular patient, a lady in her early 40s, who had seemingly contemplated taking her own life. She suffered with the degenerative disease multiple sclerosis (MS) and consequently was paralysed from the waist down. This meant that she required almost total assistance with her activities of daily living needs. In an attempt to minimise the risk to her pressure areas, she was nursed on a water bed, the wave-like movements of which she described as a feeling of seasickness. I remember my colleague and I trying to assist this lady with her hygiene needs; turning her from side to side, and finally sitting her up in bed, supported by pillows, was not an easy task on a water bed. I remember the day the incident occurred. Unbeknown to the staff, this lady had been saving up her daily allowance of tablets, which she wrapped in tissue and stored in her locker draw, where I found them while looking for an item of clothing. Worried, I went to inform the ward manager, but was surprised by the manner in which she dealt with the situation. She seemed angry, and on approaching the patient (without closing the curtains) told her in an extremely harsh tone that she would not tolerate her committing suicide in her ward. The patient's response to this dressing down had been tears and embarrassment. Admittedly, I felt sorry for her, but at the time, I could not understand how she felt, or why she wanted to end her life. However, years later, after I acquired a better understanding of the physical and emotional impact of MS on the individual's life and quality of life, I did, and had concluded that the ward sister could have managed the situation more sensitively. Instead of being angry with this lady, she should have tried to understand why she felt her life was not worth living, and accordingly attempted to provide her with the support she required. The ward sister had made a very sad situation more so, and even though I did not realise this at the time, the incidence emphasised the importance of showing compassion at times when it is most needed.

There were also memories of this ward that included my colleagues. The completion of the daily rituals of care was a strongly team-orientated task that strived to evenly distribute the workload. For those nurses working on the early and late shifts, the aim was to complete the workload for that shift within the allotted time-frame, so that the next shift would not be overloaded. For the early shift, this was usually by lunch time, when after handing over to the late shift we all went for lunch. During this break, we often indulged in having a 'nap', but were also mindful to return to the ward on time. However, there was one nurse (a conscientious, but not the most confident, worker, who had always gone to her room in the nurse's quarters for her lunch breaks), who on one occasion failed to return to the ward. Unfortunately, we had failed to hide the nurse's absence from the ward sister, who suggested that we contact and advise her to return to work, and that she would have to work later to make up the lost time. On the nurse's return to the ward, she was quite embarrassed, but had readily accepted her punishment, so to speak. I am not quite sure what happened to her, but I do remember her moving on from the Trust. Overall, the knowledge, experience and learning gained during my time on this orthopaedic ward were hugely enlightening, in terms of orthopaedic nursing and in my transition to an enrolled nurse.

Hospital Closures within the Group and the Wider Context This title has incited memories of geriatric nursing (later care of the elderly (COTE)). In the 1970s to 1980s, patients who met the criteria for geriatric care were nursed separately in specific geriatric hospitals (as they were known then), but due to changes in policies and greater emphasis on funding and saving money, many patients were later integrated into the secondary care sectors on relevant COTE wards, as many of these hospitals closed. Over the years I have observed the closure of many of these geriatric hospitals (one of which had been a part of my training hospital group) that have resulted in either private residential homes or supermarkets being built on these sites. Another of the group's hospitals was a women's-only hospital. This had been a welcomed service for women who had wished to be treated in a woman-only space, but, as with most things, one that was eventually discontinued, with the hospital and site being sold, and which now accommodates a supermarket store. The main training hospital was closed and the services were relocated to a specifically built wing within another Secondary Care NHS Trust. Closure of the two remaining hospitals had rendered my training hospital group obsolete. Some years later, when driving past some of these sites, I was reminded of the memories and the experiences, and of how they contributed to my professional development, going forward.

Of course, there were further closures over the years. As reported by Triggle and Schraer (Triggle and Schraer 2017), the initial proposals for cuts in hospital services were part of a programme to transform the health service and save money across 44 different areas, even though reductions in the number of hospital beds, as a result of these cuts, could destabilise services. One way of compensating for these cuts was the movement of patients out of hospital into the community. In light of an ageing population, and growth in long-term conditions, such as dementia and heart disease, it was felt that such a strategy was more likely to benefit people in the community to stay well, rather than in hospital, when their health deteriorated. A major concern, however, was that community services were already feeling the strain and that many would be unable to cope with the additional increase in workload. Today, issues around hospital closures are still a cause for concern. This, combined with an ageing society and increases in longevity, raises questions as to whether the current availability of hospitals and beds is proportionate to facilitating a more robust approach to care delivery. Consequently, the focus has been placed on a new hospital building programme to ensure that the NHS's hospital estate supports the provision of world-class healthcare services for patients (Department of Health and Social Care 2019).

1976, Moving on As previously stated, I worked as an enrolled nurse in the orthopaedic ward until 1976, and had then sought employment at a small hospital, within another Trust, one that consisted of three wards, two of which provided care to orthopaedic patients and one to medical patients. While it could be construed as bias, I truly believe that as a small hospital, the delivery of care to patients was exemplary. The ward environment was also very conducive to enhancing the individual's learning, and increasing their self-esteem and morale, and accordingly a sense of job satisfaction. During this period, there were also moments of mirth that resonated with my early experiences of stealing food, when I resided in the nurses' home (1974–1975) in my training hospital. This moment of mirth was based on a nursing colleague's account of her experience of living in the nursing home at this hospital. Apparently, she had been having problems for some time with colleagues continually helping themselves to food that she placed in the communal fridge, a frustrating situation that had prompted her to react. Having bought several tomatoes, she urinated into a jug and had drawn up several mils of urine into a syringe, which she injected into tomatoes, and placed them back into the fridge. Unsurprisingly, on the next day, tomatoes were gone. I asked her how she felt. She shook her head, and stated that she had quietly hoped that whoever took them would have a very bad stomach ache. I remember thinking gross, but quite funny. Hey, we do what we have to do when we are desperate!

1978–1980s, Agency Nursing   After 2 years of working as an enrolled nurse at this hospital, I had decided to move on again, this time to work as an agency nurse, a role I maintained for 2 years (1978–1980), and intermittently, thereafter, until 1987. This period of working enabled me to work in various healthcare establishments and across various fields of practice that included A&E, high dependency unit, surgery, medicine, care of the elderly and neurosurgery, and to fully appreciate the many benefits, such as extension of my knowledge, experience and competency to perform my nursing role. Surprisingly, it was also during this period that I decided to make a career change. The reason for this decision was based on various changes to nursing and the realisation that I had become a little disillusioned with the profession. As a result (as illustrated in Chap. 4) I decided to undertake a secretarial course, and on completion proceeded to work as a secretary. During this time, I continued to work occasionally as an agency nurse, until I had my first child in 1983, and subsequently up to 1987, when I had my third child.

Compromised Breathing (2)   The second example of compromised breathing occurred while I was working a night shift as an agency nurse in a medical ward in a secondary care hospital.

2.6.1   Case Study

Mrs. Farley, a lady in her mid-40s, was diagnosed with chronic obstructive airway disease (COAD) (later changed to chronic obstructive pulmonary disease (COPD)). The time was approximately 20.45, the beginning of the night shift. I clearly remember Mrs. Farley in bed, with pillows stacked to facilitate an upright position; although with the oxygen mask over face, and its evident lack of effect, she was leaning forward and clutching the side of the bed. The tension in her body language and the laboured rise and fall of her chest had clearly indicated her struggle to breathe. This, combined with the paleness of her skin, bluish lips and wide, watery and fearful eyes, was a further indication of how unwell she actually was. I remember Mrs. Farley's husband, his look of dismay and the apparent uncertainty, in terms of how he could help his wife. After a while, he had stepped out …, only for about 10 min, but surprisingly, 10 min in which his wife had chosen to let go. As I observed Mrs. Farley, she appeared to have looked directly at me, as she took her final breaths. No longer experiencing pain or discomfort, her body was less rigid. Facial features were now relaxed and she looked much younger. A sense of calm had ensued.

Husband returned, seemingly, surprised, yet relieved. His wife was no longer in pain, and he would no longer have to observe her distress. As I progressed in my career, I have observed similar cases of compromised breathing, and have often thought of Mrs. Farley, and wondered why she had chosen that particular moment to make her exit from this life. In my attempt to make sense of this, I have chosen to believe that this was an opportunistic moment that enabled her to end the struggle and spare her husband any further distress.

Compromised Breathing (3) The following scenario is a personal reflection of compromised breathing that included my son and me.

Scenario 2.4

I finally came close to understanding what it was like not to be able to breathe effectively. It was a Saturday morning; the time was approximately 09:30, and I had just returned home after a 12-h night shift. The temperature outside was below freezing, and the burst pipes in the loft 2 days earlier had caused a flood. We hired machines to attempt drying out the carpets, a slow process, but there were some improvements. After a 12-h shift, I was extremely tired, but as I prepared to get some sleep, I felt decidedly uneasy, as I observed my 18-month-old son pacing up and down the room and struggling to breathe. He reached out to me and started to cry. I picked him up, and tried to comfort him, but he continued to cry as his discomfort persisted. I remember thinking he is not ok, but at that time had not connected this sudden onset of breathing difficulty to the burst pipes. I voiced my concerns to his father, and even though he is an asthmatic, it did not occur to me that my son was having an asthma attack. Due to my son's increasing distress, I contacted my GP, who clarified that he was having an asthma attack and advised me to take him to the local hospital A&E department, where he was examined and assessed by the doctor. By this time, my son's breathing was more laboured, as he paced around the room, holding on to the chair, and catching his breath. His crying was also more persistent—a fact that was later explained to me as his way of getting more oxygen into his lungs. Following the initial assessment, the doctor prescribed a Ventolin nebuliser which secured an almost immediate relief of symptoms. My son had stopped crying, his breathing was much improved and he looked and sounded much better. A diagnosis of asthma was made and he was admitted to hospital overnight and into the late afternoon the next day, for further treatment and monitoring. During this stay, my son clung to me. He remained in some discomfort with his breathing, but with regular nebulisers, ensuing relief was quickly forthcoming. Following this episode, we did experience further flare-ups, but we learned to appropriately manage those, in which the Ventolin inhaler had been a godsend.

My Personal Experience My personal experience of compromised breathing some years later gave me an up close and personal understanding of what it was like not to be able to breathe effectively. In this instance, I had a very bad cold, which meant my nostrils were blocked and I had to breathe via my mouth, an action that impacted my attempts to eat. The experience of trying to breathe and eat at the same time was frighteningly suffocating, and in this moment, I had thought about my son and my patients, and their experience of not being able to breathe effectively.

Status asthmaticus is a medical term used for the most severe form of an asthma attack that can lead to hypoxemia (abnormally low level of oxygen in the blood … notably, arterial blood), hypercarbia (abnormally elevated carbon dioxide (CO_2) levels in the blood) and secondary respiratory failure (Saadeh 2020). Status asthmaticus is severe asthma that does not respond well to immediate care and is a life-threatening medical emergency (Tidy 2016).

Advanced Technology   Over time, more advanced technology, in the form of continuous positive airway pressure (CPAP), is a method of positive-pressure ventilation used with patients who are breathing spontaneously, done to keep the alveoli open at the end of exhalation and thus increase oxygenation and reduce the work of breathing. CPAP is a mode of respiratory ventilation which is commonly used in the treatment of sleep apnoea, congestive cardiac failure and obstructive airway disease, most notably exacerbations of chronic obstructive pulmonary disease (COPD) and asthma (Dameron 2008).

Scenario 2.5

Compromised Breathing (4): This scenario is based on my memory from working as a bank nurse; on a night shift in the A&E department, I observed a wife and husband, in their 50s, both of whom suffered with asthma and mental health issues. As frequent attenders to the A&E department, they were well known to the team. Unfortunately, poor management of the wife's asthma (due to poor compliance) often resulted in frequent episodes of status asthmaticus. On this admission, the wife's status asthmaticus episode lasted well over 10 min, and at one point, I did wonder if her body would ever stop shaking. This was a new experience for me, and admittedly, I was intrigued. More intriguing was that when the wife eventually recovered from this attack neither she nor her husband seemed unduly worried. I suppose they were reassured by the fact that help was always available in their local A&E. However, in speaking to the A&E staff later, it was revealed that while they were quite adept at treating a status asthmaticus episode, in regard to this lady, managing the condition long-term was challenging.

Getting Tough on Smoking   For a long time, the emphasis has been placed on smoking, smoking-related illnesses and quality-of-life issues (Babjuk et al. 2015; National institute for Health and Care Excellence [NICE] 2015; Steinberg et al. 2017). Acknowledgement of the effect of smoking on the general population's health had resulted in the devising of health promotional measures to increase people's awareness of the dangers of smoking, and therefore encouraging them to stop. However, I have come to understand that smoking is an addictive habit, one that is perceived by many who smoke to be a sociable and enjoyable pastime, and that convincing these individuals to change lifestyle behaviours is a difficult task. My memory of smoking within the NHS began in the wards (after this pastime was discontinued in the hospital setting for patients, relatives and other visitors), to outside the hospital and into its grounds. I remember patients, some with intravenous infusion still in progress, standing outside the main entrance doors smoking, and the increasing number of cigarette butts in the sand pit sited just outside the main door. Encouraging people to stop smoking has been an uphill struggle, but there are noted successes such as stopping smoking in certain areas within the community settings, and the phasing out of smoking in all NHS establishments, apart from the mental health sector in 2005. No smoking meant no smoking anywhere on hospital grounds, and with signs clearly stating this message, strategically placed around the grounds, it was expected that people would be compliant with this ruling. However, as is later shown in Chap. 9, for some people, the opposite is true.

2.7   Conclusion and Lessons Learnt

This period in my nursing journey has highlighted key issues such as change, and the many implications of their impact on nursing and its practices; memories of the early years, and of colleagues, some of whom have long since departed the profession, and this world; memories that have raised a smile, as I remember the thought-provoking issues, and marvel at how I ever coped with the challenges posed; memories of the good old days—a time when nursing was intense, but fun, and yearning for elements of practices that have long since passed; and memories of smoking, and of how ongoing campaigns have contributed, and continues to contribute, to securing improvements in this area. Overall, this chapter reminds me of both positive and negative memories, and how they benefitted my professional growth over the years and my development into the nurse I became.

Chapter 3 underlines change, changing dynamics of nursing, nurse training and nurse's role, and highlights how these changes have influenced practice over the past 50 years.

References

Ali M (2017) Communication skills 1: benefits of effective communication for patients. Nurs Times 113(12):18–19
Anderson B (2005) Nutrition and wound healing: the necessity of assessment. Br J Nurs 14(Sup5):S30–S38. [Internet]. https://doi.org/10.12968/bjon.2005.14.Sup5.19955
Anderson B (2010) A perspective on changing dynamics in nursing over the past 20 years. Br J Nurs 19(18):1190–1191. [Internet]. http://tinyurl
Anderson B (2019) Reflecting on the communication process in health care. Part 1: clinical practice—breaking bad news. Br J Nurs 28(13):858–863. [Internet]. https://doi.org/10.12968/bjon.2019.28.13.858

Babjuk M, Burger M, Zigeuner R, Shariat S, Van Rhijn BWG, Compérat E, et al. (2015) Guidelines on Non-muscle-invasive Bladder Cancer (Ta, T1 and CIS [Internet]. uroweb.org. 1–42. https://uroweb.org/guideline/non-muscle-invasive-bladder-cancer/

Barber C (2016) Communication, ethics and healthcare assistants. Br J Healthcare Assistant 10(7):332–335

BBC News (2005) NHS food "needs Oliver treatment" [Internet]. news.bbc.co.uk. [cited 2020 Aug 21]. http://news.bbc.co.uk/1/hi/health/4521681.stm

Bramhall E (2014) Effective communication skills in nursing practice. Nurs Stand 29(14):53–59. [Internet]. https://doi.org/10.7748/ns.29.14.53.e9355

Button K (2020) Campaigning for better hospital food [Internet]. healthbusinessuk.net. [cited 2020 Oct 24]. https://healthbusinessuk.net/features/campaigning-better-hospital-food

Carrell S (2005) Senior medics call for celebrity chef to improve inedible hospital fare [Internet]. The Independent. [cited 2020 Aug 21]. https://www.independent.co.uk/life-style/health-and-families/health-news/jamies-hospital-dinners-are-just-the-remedy-for-britains-awful-nhs-food-say-doctors-752255.html

Dameron AL (2008) Continuous positive airway pressure [Internet]. empowher.com. [cited 2020 Feb 25]. https://www.empowher.com/media/reference/continuous-positive-airway-pressure

Department of Health and Social Care (2013) Review of Liverpool Care Pathway outlined [Internet]. Gov.uk. [cited 2020 Feb 25]. https://www.gov.uk/government/news/review-of-liverpool-care-pathway-outlined

Department of Health and Social Care (2019) New hospital building programme announced [Internet]. GOV.UK. [cited 2020 Oct 23]. https://www.gov.uk/government/news/new-hospital-building-programme-announced

Doyle A (2020) Communication skills for workplace success [Internet]. thebalancereers.com. [cited 2020 Oct 13]. https://www.thebalance.com/communication-skills-list-2063779

Ford S (2005) Improving the nutritional care of patients in hospital [Internet]. nursingtimes.net. [cited 2020 Oct 24]. https://www.nursingtimes.net/clinical-archive/nutrition/improving-the-nutritional-care-of-patients-in-hospital-09-08-2005/

National institute for Health and Care Excellence [NICE] (2015) Bladder cancer: diagnosis and management NICE guideline [NG2] [Internet]. [cited 2020 Feb 11]. www.nice.org.uk/guidance/ng2

Nursing Essay (2020) Roper Logan Tierney model activities of daily living [Internet]. nursinganswers.net. [cited 2020 Oct 13]. https://nursinganswers.net/essays/using-roper-logan-tierney-model-essay.php?vref=1

Patterson C (2012) Reforms in the 1990s were supposed to make nursing care better. Instead, there's a widely shared sense that this was how today's compassion deficit began. How did we come to this? [Internet]. The Independent. [cited 2020 Oct 24]. https://www.independent.co.uk/voices/commentators/christina-patterson/reforms-1990s-were-supposed-make-nursing-care-better-instead-there-s-widely-shared-sense-was-how-today-s-compassion-deficit-began-how-did-we-come-7631273.html

Pincock S (2004) Poor communication lies at heart of NHS complaints, says ombudsman. BMJ 328(7430):10-d-0. [Internet]. https://doi.org/10.1136/bmj.328.7430.10-d

Saadeh CK (2020) Status asthmaticus [Internet]. Medscape. [cited 2020 Oct 13]. https://emedicine.medscape.com/article/2129484-overview

Steinberg GD, Sachdeva K, Jana BRP (2017) Bladder cancer treatment and management. [Internet]. Medscape. [cited 2020 Oct 13]. https://emedicine.medscape.com/article/438262-overview

Tidy C (2016) Acute severe asthma and status asthmaticus [Internet]. patient.info. [cited 2020 Feb 25]. https://patient.info/doctor/Acute-Severe-Asthma-and-Status-Asthmaticus

Triggle N, Schraer R (2017) Hospital cuts planned in most of England [Internet]. news.bbc.co.uk. [cited 2020 Aug 18]. https://www.bbc.co.uk/news/health-39031546

UKEssays (2018) Changes in roles and responsibilities of nurses in the moder [Internet]. ukessays.com. [cited 2019 Oct 19]. https://www.ukessays.com/essays/nursing/changes-in-roles-and-responsibilities-of-nurses-in-the-modernisation-of-nhs-nursing-essay.php?vref=1

WebMD (2020) Natural colon cleansing and detox: Is it necessary? [Internet]. webmd.com. [cited 2020 Oct 13]. https://www.webmd.com/balance/guide/natural-colon-cleansing-is-it-necessary#2-4

Weston C (2015) An answer to the question of what is a good death? [Internet]. mariecurie.org.uk/blog. [cited 2020 Oct 13]. https://www.mariecurie.org.uk/blog/what-is-a-good-death/48655

The Changing Dynamics of Nursing: A Personal and Professional Experience of Nearly 50 Years

3

The Nursing Journey: How Had it all Began? As verified by the evidence, the nursing journey began with Florence Nightingale in the 1800s. Hospitals during the Victorian era were in pretty awful condition, and nurses at that time received no formal training, a situation which Florence was desperate to change. As a result of the subsequent outbreak of the Crimean War, Florence was asked to bring together a team of 38 nurses who would go to support soldiers at the Scutari military hospital in Turkey, where the conditions pertaining to basic hygiene and infection control were considered way below a level acceptable to meeting the needs of the soldiers. Consequently, increases in death rates (more than 4000 soldiers died during the nurse's first 4 months) triggered further investigation by the British Government which resulted in the implementation of measures to improve the situation at the hospital and reduce the level of deaths. This was the first time women were allowed to serve in the army. Florence was known as the 'Lady with the Lamp', because she carried a lamp during the night to see how the patients were doing (Klainberg 2010). The Nightingale School of Nursing, which was founded by Florence Nightingale, was the first facility of its kind. Those who trained at this school were sent to hospitals all over the UK. Florence Nightingale had made nursing a profession for respectable women. Until that time, nursing was not considered appropriate for women, and men played the major role in treating the sick. Florence Nightingale's achievements changed the NHS forever (Klainberg 2010), and her research contributions are considered a great legacy and a tribute to the nursing profession (BBC Newsround 2020).

The National Health Service Integral to the nursing journey is the National Health Service (NHS) which was launched by the Health Secretary Aneurin Bevan in 1948. The concept of the NHS was based on the premise that this health service would be available to everyone in the UK and that they should be able to access healthcare, despite how much or how little they had. Before the NHS, people would usually have to pay for their healthcare, similar to health services in other countries, such as the USA, where healthcare is paid for at the point of delivery through insurance. In

© Springer Nature Switzerland AG 2022
B. Anderson, *A Uro-Oncology Nurse Specialist's Reflection on her Practice Journey*, https://doi.org/10.1007/978-3-030-94199-4_3

the UK, NHS treatment is 'free at the point of delivery', as it is paid for through the taxes. Access to care is contingent on the individual being a UK European Union (EU) citizen. Non-UK citizens are expected to pay for their care, and would normally be charged following the receipt of such care. The NHS is made up of various individuals (doctors, nurses, radiologists, paramedics, ambulance service, occupational therapists, physiotherapists, social workers, etc.), who together work in unison to deliver high-quality standards of care to the general public. Integral to this objective is the continual advancement of technology, which is more sophisticated than that which was available in the past (BBC Newsround 2020).

The 1990s saw a fundamental organisational change made to the NHS, with the introduction of the 'internal market', under the NHS and Community Care Act 1990. NHS trusts were created in 1991 as part of a restructuring that made them independent bodies, encouraged to compete to raise standards. Health authorities stopped running hospitals directly and 'purchased' care for their population from providers such as hospitals. 'When Trust status was introduced, this led to financial problems. There were hospital closures, redundancies and job freeze. This was partly due to the internal market, but also due to the NHS not receiving sufficient funding from the government' (O'Dowd 2008).

Notable Abuse of the NHS Admittedly, the NHS has accrued many successes since its launch in 1948, but as I have witnessed over the years, there is also ongoing abuse of the institution. A typical example of abuse of NHS services is by non-resident pregnant women, who travel to the UK in the eighth month of their pregnancy, supposedly for a holiday. They subsequently go into labour, have their baby during this 'holiday' and then fly home. Normally, this would not have been a problem, but because in this example, and other similar cases, the appropriate funds were not collected upfront, and due to the difficulties in doing so retrospectively, there was ultimately a significant deficit in recouped funds. As a result of the spotlight being placed on this particular issue, the rules with regard to travel and pregnancy were reconfigured—women are no longer allowed to travel to the UK in the latter months of their pregnancy. Other examples of abuse of the NHS include fraud (which according to recent reports is mostly committed by NHS employees), inappropriate attendance at A&E departments (Toulson 1996) and an ageing society that significantly increases the pressures, in terms of healthcare, and the ensuing impact of costs in its delivery (Anderson 2010).

Arguably, much of this abuse is equated to the misdirected belief that healthcare within the UK NHS is 'free' at the point of use, which is technically untrue, since it is paid for through peoples' taxes. This belief that the treatment is free is further compounded by the fact that not everyone contributes equally to the 'pot', and the perception that the people who contribute the least are the very people who use the service most. Indeed, for a long time, the NHS was seen as a money pit or a black hole, to which no amount of funding was ever sufficient to fill the bottomless void. It is evidently a soft touch, and an easy target for abuse. I believe that these are fair points that accurately contain elements of truth. As I have stated in Anderson

(Anderson 2010), a person's health is their most valuable asset, and the NHS is one of our greatest legacies, one which we should be proud of, and accordingly nurture. However, considering the challenges faced by the NHS annually to fund the services they deliver, I have often wondered if the current method of funding NHS healthcare is realistically sustainable, under existing budgetary methodology. What I am trying to say is how does one effectively predict the unpredictable, when the onset, and spread, of illness or sickness within the populace is unknown? Or indeed, budget for the ensuing financial impact? A challenging task, indeed.

3.1 The Changing Dynamics of Nursing

In exploring the available literature, it is evident that not only has nursing evolved extensively, but the process has also been transformed from the previously conceived notion of it being a vocation to the status of a respected profession, a profession that has become more complex in ways that could not have been imagined a generation ago (Tiffin 2012). Today's healthcare system is described as dynamic and changing, and is more sophisticated than that of previous generations, primarily due to care delivery being based on technology and science (Johnson 2015). However, due to the increasing prevalence in the number of complex illnesses, such as diabetes, obesity and other conditions, combined with other issues, such as reduced resources and funding, caring for the sick today is much more complicated (Tiffin 2012). This is a situation that is further compounded by the fact that the nursing profession has always been highly dependent on migration, and that is still the case today. The latest figures from the National Audit Office show that 17.9% of NHS nurses were born abroad (NHS Digital 2017; Department of Health and Social Care 2020) making the UK one of the highest importers of nurses in Europe. Conversely, more than 50,000 British nurses were found to be working in the Organisation for Economic Co-operation and Development (OECD) nations (UKEssays 2018). When there are an estimated 44,000 nursing vacancies across the NHS (12% of the nursing workforce, which could hit 1,000,000 in a decade) (The Guardian 2019), my question is why are so many British nurses working in the OECD. Is it due to better pay and conditions, or a better work-life balance? Perhaps, this is a situation that requires further exploration.

Support for Nurses Over the past 50 years, the nursing profession and its practitioners have been supported by a number of organisations and unions. Two such organisations are the Nursing Midwifery Council (NMC) (previously the GNC, UKCC) and the Royal College of Nursing (RCN). The NMC's core function is to establish and improve standards of nursing and midwifery care to protect the public. The RCN's role is to stand up for nurses (and healthcare support workers), and work to improve terms and conditions and the working environment for its members, and it has been championing nurses and nursing since 1916. An important element of this support is the role of the modern matron. As discussed in Chap. 2, nursing matrons are an integral part to nursing, and to steering the profession's image (UKEssays 2018). The modern matron's role was developed in response to some patients' perception of the detachment of nursing from its vocational history; they are responsible for overseeing all nursing within a department or directorate. Unfortunately, their role had been poorly received by the majority of nursing staff, seemingly because its imposition was not called for by any professional group within the health service, and many have argued that there are too many modern matrons in comparison to nurses (UKEssays 2018).

Issues Impacting the Nursing Image Negatively Over the years I have observed issues that have impacted negatively the nursing image and the NHS efforts to deliver optimal care to the public. These have included whistleblowing, an initiative that was designed to encourage health professionals, specifically nurses and doctors, to report any worrying observations within their area of practice, an action for which they would not be penalised, or berated by their colleagues or the organisation for whom they worked (Patterson 2012). However, while there is evidence to show that many nurses and doctors had observed worrying practice, many had elected not to speak out, partly because of the potential ramifications, and partly because they did not feel confident that they would receive the promised support from the organisation. Seemingly, the real conditions in which we work and the way people are treated are vastly underreported (Patterson 2012).

An example of where whistleblowing had been shown to be beneficial relates to the Mid-Staffordshire NHS Trust, where in March 2009 a report from the Healthcare Commission (HCC) found the standard of care at the Trust 'appalling'. Consequently, the Trust actions were stringently scrutinised and some extremely worrying revelations were uncovered. Revelations included dirty wards, long waits for medical attention, safety and funding cuts, poor practice and poor patient care, leading to needless deaths and dignity issues. The HCC finding led to an independent enquiry, chaired by Robert Francis, who reported in February 2010 that the failures in patient safety and care were caused by inadequate training of staff, staff cutbacks and overemphasis on government targets (Dyer 2013).

Even though I was aware of the Mid-Staffordshire Inquiry, and had subsequently read the Francis Report, I had not fully appreciated the full implications of this report, until I watched a televised drama of the actual events. I must admit that seeing the actual display of poor practice, up close and personal, was extremely upsetting. This incident had shown the NHS in very poor light, in terms of the organisation's ability to deliver compassionate care, of the highest quality and standard, to patients. One of the issues that had been highlighted in this dramatised version had been whistleblowing, and the difficulty faced by those individuals, who, while conflicted by their loyalty to the Trust, had made the very difficult decision to speak out, despite the potential ramifications. Whistleblowing is an important consideration in terms of protecting vulnerable patients within the NHS, and as such it should not be discouraged (Patterson 2012). Based on my observations and experiences on practice, there needs to be a significant boost in the individual's confidence, one that is founded on the reassurance that if they choose to report poor practice, they will have the support of management and will not be penalised for their efforts.

Nursing Values: The 6Cs   The 6Cs comprise care, compassion, competence, communication, courage and commitment. Their purpose is to ensure that patients are looked after with *care* and *compassion,* by *competent* workers who *communicate* well, and dare to make changes—*courage* that improves care and can **commit** to delivering this all day, every day (NHS England 2021). The 6Cs, the concept of 'energise for excellence for nurses, midwives and other care staff', began with Jane Cummings and Katherine Fenton and was rolled out in December 2012 (NHS England 2021). These nursing values were a recommendation from the Francis Report, in which compassion within nursing was revisited and 'compassion in practice' became a key phrase which helped to introduce and formalise the idea of the 6Cs.

#Hellomynameis   'Hello, my name is …' was started by Kate Granger after an experience in a hospital where a member of staff did not introduce themselves; the 'Hello my name is ...' campaign became part of the 6Cs which encourages staff to introduce themselves by name (Anon 2020). I believe that this is a valuable campaign, and having attended a key speech by the founder, Kate Granger, in my Local Trust, I was reassured that I had been meeting this requirement, and in fact had always done so.

Nurse's Pay   The issues around nurses' pay are long-standing, and as illustrated in the following accounts consistently attract scrutiny during the annual pay reviews. One of the identified issues relates to clinical grading, whose introduction in 1988 was considered one of the most controversial changes to nursing and one that caused chaos before Project 2000 revolutionised nurse training (O'Dowd 2020). This system moved all nurses on to grades such as D, E and F, and worked on the basic idea that pay should be dictated by the tasks performed, rather than by rigid job titles. Its introduction saw an overwhelming majority of nurses appealing, as they believed that they had been wrongly graded. The grading system was not properly funded, and there was no agreement between staff and management on the criteria for different levels of seniority. Its introduction resulted in divisions between staff, as some nurses doing the same job were put on a higher grade than their colleagues. Consequently, there was industrial unrest, as some individuals took the decision to go on strike. Around 6000 nurses took part in a protest (with just 600 actually going on strike), clashing with Prime Minister Margaret Thatcher, who said that strike action was 'hitting out' deliberately at patients. This initial action was followed by a wave of strikes and protests from nurses who feared that the NHS would collapse because of low pay, staff shortages and a lack of investment. It took until 2003 for all appeals and concerns to be dealt with (O'Dowd 2020).

Funnily enough, as I think back on my time in the urology ward, and of working as a Band 5, Grade 'D' RN, I clearly remember when they introduced into practice the incentive of an additional 1–2% boost to pay for those nurses who had excelled during a specified period of working. I must confess that I was thrilled with this incentive, as it had continually motivated me to excel. Admittedly, the Trust was not as thrilled. After a while, they had questioned the legitimacy of my claim to receive this incentive, with my line manager, who had promptly verified that it was. As a result, the Trust concluded that if I was continually excelling, then it was obvious that I was on the wrong grade. I remember smiling at this conclusion, since it had been beneficial in supporting my later application for promotion.

I still remember my first month's pay, *£37.51*, a sum that has remained indelible in my mind, and one at which I am often amazed, when remembering how creative I had been with this paltry sum. The fact that I was able to pay the monthly sum for the nurses' home residency and to buy the essentials, most importantly clothes, and had managed to save was a feat short of genius. In the 1970s, and probably more so now, for the average 18- and 19-year-olds, fashion was key, in terms of how we were perceived by those in our social circle. Wearing the same attire twice? Perish the thought! What if someone from the social network were to acknowledge this fact? Ultimately, not wearing the same attire twice was a rule that had seen many (myself included) spending a significant part of their pay each month on clothes, which, admittedly, may never be worn again. In terms of nurses' pay today, the evidence has shown that there is a large variation in pay scales, which range between £13,000 and £67,000 (UKEssays 2018). In comparison to nurses' pay in the 1970s, it could be argued that nurses' pay is better than it used to be, although it could be further argued that in view of the changes to the nurse's role and scope of practice, and of course inflation, it may still not be reflective of the individual's role, status or worth (Patterson 2012).

Recruitment and Retention and Staff Shortages The fact that our citizens are living longer (longevity) has become a real issue for the NHS, an issue that, combined with the ever-increasing pressures of work and staff shortages, has increased the pressure on healthcare organisations, and accordingly their workforce, to meet this challenge. Increasing staff shortage has been a major 'bugbear' for the NHS, and evidently one that directly impacts recruitment and retention efforts (UKEssays 2018). The issue of how to recruit and retain staff is a problem that has garnered increased attention over the years, and one that is directly linked to retirement. This was a topic that I had addressed in Anderson (Anderson 2010) article, '*A Perspective on Changing Dynamics in Nursing over the Past 20 Years*', in which O'Brien-Pallas et al.'s (O'Brien-Pallas et al. 2004) study had noted that the workforce was ageing, and that the potential loss of experienced nurses through retirement at the age of 65 years was likely to exacerbate nursing shortages. However, nurses in this age spectrum could potentially be retained, if measures were in place to delay impending retirement. Delaying the retirement of these nurses was perceived as a significant boost to human resources, not only in terms of absolute numbers, but more importantly in terms of the individual's experience and expertise in supporting nurses who are still in training, as well as newly qualified RNs, who are adjusting to their role. Other issues in regard to staff shortages are attributed to hospitals having to cut staff amid a spiralling NHS cash crisis (Campbell 2016).

Increasing Workloads Another issue to consider in terms of staff shortages is increasing workloads. The evidence has shown that nurses are working harder and for longer hours, and that this, combined with significant reductions in manpower, has led to increased tension, stress, burnout and a considerable reduction in job satisfaction. Consequently, to redress the 'work-life' balance, nurses are taking more sick days (UKEssays 2018). To many, the fun factor, once experienced in practice years ago, is now a distant memory.

Other Long-Standing Issues Over the years, I have observed many issues that have impacted the patient throughput and the organisation's efforts to deliver optimal care to the public. One such issue was bed blocking, a significant problem for hospital trusts, that contributed to increases in length of stays, and therefore in bed shortages. The issue of bed blocking had been highlighted when I worked in the Nursing Bank. This is a problem that arose due to the difficulties faced in transferring patients back to the community, as illustrated in the following scenario:

In this particular situation, the patient, a lady in her 60s, had been an inpatient in a side-room cubicle in a medical ward for 1 year plus. Numerous attempts had been made to discharge her from hospital, attempts that were *unsuccessful* because she had no home to return to. This situation had led to increasing frustration in terms of the rising cost to the Trust. The difficulty in discharging patients back to the community had become evident during my time in the urology ward. While there were discharge coordinators to oversee the patients' impending exit, the task was often compounded by the lack of vacancies in the community, whether it be to the patient's own home, nursing home or residential homes. The most recent high-profile incident highlighting bed shortages was in 2019, pertaining to a 4-year-old boy with suspected pneumonia, who had been forced to sleep in a hospital treatment room floor because there were no available beds (BBC News 2019). Sadly, this is an issue that I believe will burden the NHS for the foreseeable future.

Creating Space The need to create more space is a long-standing problem that continues to impact services today, specifically making admissions and discharges of patients more streamlined, and at the same time attempting to meet the targeted specifications while keeping a strict reign on funding, as verified in the following accounts:

Day Rooms Up until the late 1990s, the day room was seen as an important part of creating an interactive space within the ward setting. A television, radio, magazines and books were available; it was a place where patients and visitors could relax and interact with each other away from the main ward area. Sadly, the shortage of beds significantly impacted ward capacity, and increased the pressure on health establishments to deliver care within the stipulated target specifications. As a result, the day room had become expendable, and in many cases, it was reconfigured to accommodate the secretaries (as they were then) who were moved out of the side rooms. These side rooms were then reconfigured to accommodate patients. After some time in the day room, the secretaries were again moved, this time to a more appropriate venue within the hospitals. The day room space was then reconfigured again to create more beds to accommodate the overspill of patients from chiefly the A&E department. To my knowledge the day room, as it was in the past, has never returned.

The Outlier Ward The outlier ward has been in existence since the 1990s, and in fact, as a bank nurse, I have worked in some of these wards. The main objective of these wards was to cope with the yearly winter pressure of accommodating the over-spillage of unplanned and emergency patients. However, because the running of this additional service necessitated recruitment of extra nurses from the nursing bank and nursing agencies, it has proven to be a costly exercise for the NHS.

Changes to Nurse Training As illustrated in Table 3.1, nurse training has changed significantly over the years (Patterson 2012; Cipriano 2010; Francis and Humphreys 1999; Glasper 2018), specifically the discontinuation of the EN training—where the arguments for its discontinuation were based on the claims that ENs were 'misused and abused', in that employers had often expected ENs to perform the jobs of RNs, but with lesser remuneration and career prospects (Francis and Humphreys 1999). Apparently, the phasing out of the EN role had left a skill gap in the UK nursing care, one that raised some questions. Seemingly, in filling this gap, it was seen as unrealistic to expect the more highly qualified Project 2000 nurses to carry out the more menial tasks that had been performed by the EN (Francis and Humphreys 1999), a revelation, which to anyone who was previously an EN is quite demeaning. As an EN, performing these more menial tasks was not perceived to be a less important role to that of an RN. In some ways, I suppose academia had created a form of snobbery and hierarchical misgivings. I believe that a nurse is first and foremost a nurse, and that despite their academic status, in terms of delivering care, from the most menial to the most skilled duties, the patient must be kept squarely in the forefront.

The Nursing Bursary The nursing bursary was originally instigated on the first September 2012 as an added support to enable student nurses to at least meet the challenges of day-to-day living expenses while striving to conform to the nurse training rituals (Department of Health and Social Care 2020). I have personally observed the importance of the bursary. Casual communication between myself and a Project 2000 student nurse (Maria) had revealed that despite the bursary, she had struggled to cope with the monthly finances as well as to feed herself. Apparently, in most weeks, she had survived on 'Rice Krispies', for breakfast, lunch and dinner, as she did not have any money left over to afford more nourishing meals. Thinking back to my EN training, my colleagues and I appear to have had a much easier time,

Table 3.1 The evolving nature of nursing and changes to nurse training

1850–1854	Florence Nightingale goes to Turkey to lead a team of nurses caring for soldiers in the Crimean War
1855	Mary Seacole establishes the British hotel, a convalescent home for soldiers in the Crimean War
1860	Nightingale Training School opens at St Thomas Hospital in London. One of the first institutions to teach nursing and midwifery as a formal profession, the training school was dedicated to communicating the philosophy and practice of its founder and patron, Florence Nightingale
1860 onwards	From the 1860s onwards, a series of nurses' training schools began to produce fairly large numbers of educated women … This description sets the scene for the rise of professional nursing that has gained in status and scope since the late nineteenth century
Before 1880	Before 1880, the hospital treatment of illness was fairly rare. Where home services were adequate, a sick person was attended by the family doctor and nursed either by female family members or by servants. … However, from the middle of the nineteenth century, the discovery and application of anaesthetics and antiseptic surgery advanced medical technique and allowed all classes to seek treatment in hospitals
1900s	More hospitals establishing their own training schools for nurses; in exchange for lectures and clinical instruction, students provided the hospital with 2 or 3 years of skilled free nursing care …
Mid-1900s	Until the mid-nineteenth century, nursing was not an activity which was thought to demand either skill or training. Nor did it command respect. As Florence Nightingale was to put it, nursing was left to 'those who were too old, too weak, too drunken, too dirty, too stupid or too bad to do anything else'
1916	Royal College of Nursing was founded with 34 members
1919	Nurses Act established the first professional register help by the General Nursing Council …. The early British Nurses Association led to the General Nursing Council being established in 1919; the role of registering members of the nursing profession was passed to the United Kingdom Central Council in 1979 and then to the Nursing and Midwifery Council in 2002 and these bodies also defined the scope of practice and codes of ethics
1940	The state enrolled nurse is formally recognised with 2 years of training
1950–1951	Male nurses allowed to join the professional register
1972	Briggs Committee suggests a move to degree preparation of nurses and that practice be based on research
1983	The United Kingdom Central Council for Nursing, Midwifery and Health Visiting sets up a new professional register with four branches (mental health, children, learning disability and adult) reflecting former types of training and qualifications: Registered General Nurse, Enrolled Nurse (General), Registered Mental Nurse, Enrolled Nurse (Mental), Registered Nurse for the Mentally Handicapped, Enrolled Nurse (Mental Handicap), Enrolled Nurse, Registered Sick Children's Nurse, Fever Nurse, Registered Midwife and Registered Health Visitor
1986	The introduction of Project 2000, a new type of nurse training (which was conducted by higher education institutions—colleges and universities, rather than hospital-based schools), replaced the old apprenticeship style of training and elevated the academic status of most newly registered nurses to that of a higher education diploma. This was a prelude to the introduction of the all-graduate curriculum in 2010

(continued)

Table 3.1 (continued)

1989	The apprenticeship style of training was seen as outdated and ill-equipped to preparing the nurse trainees for the demands of rapidly changing and expanding healthcare systems. Consequently, calls to elevate the status of most newly registered nurses to that of a higher academic level (diploma level) had seen the phasing out of the 2-year enrolled nurse training in the UK, despite its popularity. Phasing out of the EN role had resulted in a skill gap that had led to the nursing associate's role, and for them to be registered with the Nursing and Midwifery Council (NMC), the successor of the UKCC
2002	Nurses are able to prescribe medication
2004	RCN votes for degree-only preparation
2008	Nursing research demonstrated on the world stage
2009	All nursing courses in the UK become degree-level professionalisation of nursing …. Therefore, it can be seen that medical treatments and both professional nursing practice and education progressed considerably through the nineteenth and twentieth centuries
2010	Elevating the academic status of most newly registered nurses to that of a higher education diploma was a prelude to the introduction of the all-graduate curriculum
2013	All nurse training programmes must be at degree level, with no option to study instead for a diploma
2015	Nursing bursary phased out
2016	Nurse revalidation is a new requirement for all NMC-registered members to revalidate every 3 years in order to ensure that their registration can be renewed. Revalidation, introduced from April 2016, replaced the previous PREP (Post-Registration Education Practice)
2019	A £5000.00 grant is offered to nursing students by the government to help with training

Source: Patterson (Patterson 2012), Cipriano (Cipriano 2010), Francis and Humphries (Francis and Humphreys 1999), Glasper (Glasper 2018), Mullaly (Mullally 2002), NMC (Nursing Midwifery Council 2021)

since the meals cooked by the group were certainly more nourishing than Rice Krispies. In the November 2015 spending review, it was revealed that student bursary would be removed from the first August 2017, and hence new nursing, midwifery and most allied health students were no longer able to receive NHS bursaries. Instead, they were given access to the same student loan system as other students (UKEssays 2018). The cancellation of the nursing bursary and issues relating to the fact that nurses are often in debt long after they have completed their training make me realise that as a pupil nurse, I was quite fortunate, since I did not have to pay for my training, although, in my attempt to supplement my wages, 6 months into my training I registered with a nursing agency, where I had worked as an auxiliary nurse. The money was not great but the added learning was beneficial. I suppose that in the later years of my academic journey (apart from the EN Conversion course), I was also fortunate, since all funds had been duly paid by the Trust. Personally, I did not believe that the bursary should have been cancelled.

However, there has been some success in this area. As a result of the Conservative Party winning the 2019 election, and with ongoing campaigns to reinstate the bursary, Boris Johnson had intervened with the offer of a **£5000.00** loan to students to support their nurse training. On the back of this has been the launch of a new television campaign in March 2020, the purpose of which is to encourage new recruits to the nursing profession. However, while this loan may be quite a relief for those intending to embark on nurse training, for those already in the system, this is quite a blow, since the previous removal of the bursary has left them with financial debts. There has been some discussion in regard to writing off this debt for relative individuals; however, we will have to wait and see how this is finally resolved.

Nurse Revalidation As a nurse, there are specific requirements of the role, of which keeping yourself up-to-date on current trends in nursing is crucial.

Integral to this is the previously introduced Post-Registration Education and Practice Project (PREPP) in 2002 (Mullally 2002). This exercise necessitated the completion of 5 study days relevant to the individual's areas of clinical practice, and is a mandatory requirement prior to the Nursing Midwifery Council (NMC) personal identification number (PIN) renewal (Nursing Midwifery Council 2021) which ratifies the individual's right to practice. The PIN renewal fee has increased over the years from £30 for 3 years to £76.00, £100.00 and £120.00 per year, respectively.

Revalidation for nurses and midwives (Nursing Midwifery Council 2021) was introduced in April 2016 and replaced the previous PREP (Mullally 2002). In addition to increases in the PIN renewal fees, the previous requirement of 5 study days had evolved into the completion of a lengthy reflection on the individual's practice over the intervening 3 years, plus an assessment to ascertain whether the learning gained had contributed positively to their personal and professional development, and accordingly to improving patient care and clinical practice outcomes. I completed my first and only nurse revalidation in 2017. It was a worthwhile activity that improved my knowledge and understanding of my patients' problems and accordingly my ability to provide them with the necessary support.

The Role of Academia The rise of professional nursing has gained in status and scope since the late nineteenth century, a rise in which academia has played and continues to play a vital role (Cipriano 2010). The expansion of practice and the discovery of new treatments had squarely placed the emphasis on the acquisition of specialised knowledge, and advanced professional decision-making skills, that ultimately verifies the individual's ability to practice competently (Cipriano 2010). The belief is that obtaining an advanced nursing degree prepares the individual for a changing world of possibility. With the right skills and knowledge, the next generation of nurses can make a bigger difference for patients, communities and our national healthcare environment (Tiffin 2012). However, in a report by Patterson (Patterson 2012), questions were raised by a number of individuals (including doctors) in regard to this increased emphasis on academia, and whether these highly qualified nurses were, in fact, 'too posh to wash'. Moreover, did they see themselves as nurses or at a level more fitting to that of a doctor? Apparently, nurses were being told by nursing lecturers from 'day one' that as student nurses, they are not the handmaidens of the patients or doctors, but that they are 'equal professionals', only to find that in the wards, nobody cares about their scientific pretensions (Patterson 2012). The report had also shown that some nurses had questioned the real benefit of having a degree in that, as highly trained profession- als, they should not be expected to deal with the more menial jobs (such as giving a bedpan) that are perceived to be better suited to the less qualified practitioner. This is a conclusion that is congruent with the question previously posed for Project 2000 nurses, in terms of being overqualified to carry out the most menial of tasks (Cipriano 2010), to which my response remains the same, i.e. despite academic status, in delivering care from the most menial to the most skilled duties, the patient must be kept squarely in the forefront. There is however some agree- ment that a degree is a necessary requirement in certain specialised areas of prac- tice (where one requires a brain), but for those nurses working at ward level, this is just overkill (Patterson 2012).

These comments had given me pause for thought as I reflect on past practice and on my interaction with two Project 2000 nurses. After the launch of this training in 1986, and while working as an EN, with a student in the ward, I remember asking her how she was getting on, and what her future plans were, following the comple- tion of her training. Not only was her answer surprising, it had led me to deduce that she was not truly impassioned about a career in nursing. The student told me that she was only doing the nurse training as a backup to support her finances. Apparently, after qualifying as an RN, she had no intention of actually working as a full-time nurse in the wards. Her focus was on management, in or outside nursing. I must admit that I was a little taken aback by her honesty, and at that moment had thought about training, and of how funding was being unfairly exploited by those who had no intention of transferring the learning and the skills gained back to the nursing profession.

In contrast, some years later, in the late 1990s, I remember speaking to another Project 2000 student nurse (Tom, for clarity), with whom I had worked in the last 6 weeks prior to the completion of his training. I remember congratulating him and asking him how he was feeling, now that he had completed his training and was an RN. His answer to my question gave me pause for thought. 'Beverley', he had said, 'I am glad that I have passed my exams, and am now an RN', although, as an RN, I have mixed feelings'. 'If I am honest, I am scared, since I have come to realise that whilst my theoretical knowledge is adequate, practically, I feel that I am lacking the skills to deliver optimal care to my patients', a fact he attributed, in part, to not spending sufficient time in the ward, and therefore not acquiring the necessary hands-on experience and learning on the job. I could see that he was really troubled by this admission. It was clear that changes were needed to the training protocol, specifically changes to ensure that an appropriate balance between time spent in the classroom and in the clinical area was important to ensuring the appropriate learn- ing outcomes. I took on Tom's concerns, and in the hope that these would be addressed passed them on to the powers that be—the university representative. Thinking back on this account and on the issue of hands-on experience, it was interesting to note the claim in Patterson (Patterson 2012) report that students are now taught less nursing, and less about the elements of fundamental care. It is further suggested that as universities push out cohorts of practitioners who are, in some respects, less prepared, the expertise in practice is also more diluted (Patterson 2012).

As a cancer nurse specialist, my decision to complete my master's degree had been partly based on the Nursing Midwifery Council (NMC) requirement, partly to gain a greater physical and emotional understanding of my patients and partly as a personal accomplishment. Of course, people, colleagues and those in the wider circle asked if I would now be paid more money, or if I would now be seeking promotion. These were reasonable questions, and because I understood why they were posed, my answer was always honest. As the MUCNS, I greatly enjoyed my role, specifically my interaction with my patients; hence the motivation to complete this higher level of learning was not inspired by my desire to seek promotion or indeed an increased salary, but by my desire to extend my role, and accordingly improve the care delivered to my patients. Admittedly, I could have sought promotion (there were certainly opportunities), but since my desire was to continue interactions with my patients, I was happy with where I was on the professional ladder, and was thus content to remain there. Even so, I believe that questions and concerns in regard to academia and the benefits it affords should be addressed.

Today's nurses are paid according to their grades not by academic status. For instance, a Band 7, ward manager, without a degree receives the same pay as a Band 7 Clinical Nurse Specialist, with a master's degree, which, based on anecdotal conversations with various colleagues, poses the question of why individuals should have to study to degree level, if this additional study makes no significant improvement to either their status or pay? In terms of the ward manager, some feel that a degree is an over-qualification, and for others, that knowledge and experience should suffice. While I had not consciously considered this question before, it is an anomaly that deserves further scrutiny. I believe that a reconfiguration of pay that acknowledges academic achievements (especially if they are mandatory to the role) could be the added incentive that would encourage those practicing at an advanced level to undertake the relevant studies befitting that role, and accordingly remain in said positions. In my experience, not everyone is academically driven. There are those who demonstrate impeccable knowledge and expertise of their chosen field; while they may not have the required academic qualifications, they are excellent nurses, nonetheless. However, I believe that if we accept that nursing has evolved, and has elevated its status to that of a respected profession, then the NMC's requirement for all practitioners who are practicing at an advanced level to have the academia befitting that level is not unreasonable.

In regard to the question of whether highly qualified nurses are too posh to wash, as a cancer nurse specialist with a master's degree, I certainly do not think I am too posh to wash. I firmly believe that at the heart of nursing is the nurse, who despite their rank or academic status should be willing to address the needs of the patient, and do so in the most menial of circumstances. In this context, I believe that academia is hugely beneficial, in that it has enabled me a greater understanding of my patients and the problems they encounter, physically and emotionally, following the receipt of a cancer diagnosis, and for that reason, I am better equipped to support them at this time.

The Beneficial Role of Science and Technology in Nursing Clearly, the world has changed, and so has the work nurses do. Today's nursing is more fast-paced and technology dependent, and because caregiving has become far more complex, and often involves large amount of paperwork and endless lists, a more robust approach to recording key information is necessitated (Johnson 2015; UKEssays 2018; Patterson 2012). Integral to this objective is science and technology, and the associated high-tech equipment that is developed to be more user friendly (UKEssays 2018). In the past half-century, the advances in computing technology have driven many of the changes that now dictate the way the NHS functions: from the humble desktop PC to MRI, CT, nuclear bone scan and position emission tomography (PET) scans (as later explained in Chap. 6) to the latest cutting-edge computing 'med-tech' that miniaturises monitoring devices, enabling them to be worn unobtrusively, and deliver accurate patient information.

Today, the most common technology used in both the nursing and medical profession is the computer. Nurses and doctors use them every day as a way to document the care given to a patient, and they are also widely used for online access to other activities, such as mandatory and statutory training. This training can be accessed via the internet, although it has to be approved by the NHS (in fact several of my colleagues have completed their degrees via this route). In attempting to maintain standards, all nurses have to attend and complete regular education courses to keep up-to-date with the new trends and information used in the current day. However, while new technology is advantageous for improved healthcare, in that it saves lives, there are also disadvantages, in that training staff to use it is a costly exercise (UKEssays 2018).

The Role of Social Media The evidence has shown that social media is a concept that has saturated every industry, and that nursing is no exception. Limited evidence has shown that *social* media can be incredibly positive in promoting health, and in engaging with others, in terms of nursing and medical practice (Paton 2020). The creative use of social media has limitless potential in nursing education, nursing management and healthcare (Paton 2020). For nurses, social media allows them to connect their personal and professional lives, facilitating conversations with colleagues about healthcare advances, current best practices and more (Paton 2020). Social media is also hugely integrated in how practitioners interact with their patients, and in how they practice (Johnson 2015). While some think that the internet is destroying the paternalism that used to be at the heart of healthcare, there are those who embrace the benefits it affords. For instance, there are huge opportunities for nurses to assist patients to self-manage long-term conditions and create new avenues for peer support (Johnson 2015). It is recognised that there are some obvious risks; however, with good guidelines and governance, they can be managed (Johnson 2015; Paton 2020). In today's healthcare climate, patients are more empowered to take control of their own care and voice their health needs—a development that has attributed to changing the patient-provider dynamic in a very positive way (Johnson 2015). As I have personally observed in practice, social media (Twitter, Facebook, WhatsApp, etc.) had been extensively utilised by many of my colleagues (nurses and doctors), specifically to enhance communication within the multidisciplinary team.

3.2   Changes to the Nurse's Role

Types and Roles of Nurses   In the UK, there are over 300,000 nurses working in a variety of settings, such as hospitals, health centres, nursing homes, hospices, communities and academia, with the majority working for the NHS (NHS Digital 2017). There are many different types of nurses—these can range across adult nurses, mental health nurses, children's nurses, learning disability nurses, district nurses, neonatal nursing, health visitors, practice nurses, prison nurses, school nurses and healthcare assistants. These nurses work in a range of specialties from the broad areas of medicine, surgery, theatres and investigative sciences such as imaging. Nurses also work in a large area of sub-specialities such as respiratory, diabetes, neurology, infectious diseases, liver, research, cardiac and stoma (UKEssays 2018). There are also many different levels to being a nurse. These include the ward manager (sister), staff nurse, healthcare assistant, lead nurse and matrons, respectively, who, all in all, make up our NHS and work as a team to provide the best possible care for the patient (Tiffin 2012; UKEssays 2018; Patterson 2012).

Male Nurses   The stereotypical roles of a nurse in the UK have changed significantly, since the 1990s, but it still remains that the majority of the nursing profession includes women, equating to around 90% of the total workforce. While male nurses were allowed to join the professional register in 1950, during the 1970s and 1980s, numbers were far less than that of female nurses, although admittedly numbers were more concentrated in the mental health sector. However, due to changes in society, and the evolving image of the nurse, men are now more involved in nursing and in various fields of nursing such as midwifery (Johnson 2015; UKEssays 2018). More male nurses have meant more choices for patients, who, in terms of dignity issues, have the opportunity to decide whether to be treated by a male or a female nurse (UKEssays 2018).

Over the past 50 years, the nurse's role, and the scope of practice for nurses, has changed significantly, and perceptions of the role have changed from being seen as helpers or assistants for doctors to healthcare professionals in their own right (Johnson 2015; UKEssays 2018; Patterson 2012; Cipriano 2010). Today's nurses are advanced nurse practitioners (ANPs), the first of which is the clinical nurse specialist (CNS). These ANPs are nurses, doctors, consultants, prescribers, nurse educators, nurse-anaesthetists and nurse researchers (Tiffin 2012; UKEssays 2018). They are critical thinkers, who are able to make complex clinical decisions that

50 years ago would almost certainly have been made by doctors (UKEssays 2018). This improved scope of practice has been seen as beneficial in terms of patients being seen quicker, but on the other hand the care provided to patients and attending to their needs and wishes may be less (UKEssays 2018). However, in terms of credibility, the requirement from the NMC is that these nurses are highly trained and well educated, and as such, emphasis is placed on achieving the level of academia befitting an ANP's role—usually at master's degree level (Tiffin 2012; UKEssays 2018).

Key Responsibilities of the Nurse For nurses, the completion of mandatory and statutory training ensures that the care they give to patients is in line with the guidance, one that is based on current evidence. As a healthcare practitioner, in this case doctors and nurses, you have a responsibility to ensure that you are up-to-date with your mandatory and statutory training, and that these are completed within the specified time frames (i.e. on a 1–2-yearly basis). Not only is this important to the performance of the practitioner's role, but it also provides the NHS organisation with a safety net and protection against ensuing complaints from both patients and health professionals, and accordingly reduces the likelihood of the Trust being fined for negligent practice. To improve the efficacy of said training, increased emphasis has been placed on online training. During my years of nursing (even though the task could be difficult), I was always mindful to ensure that I completed training updates in line with the Trust's requirements. Updates included basic life support, intermediate life support and advanced life support training; moving and handling; safeguarding adults; health and safety; child protection; and many others. In the case of moving and handling, training protocol had changed significantly since the early years. As I reflect on moving and handling training (previously patient or manual handling), I clearly remember the lifts that had been outed over the years. These include the Australian lift (a most uncomfortable lift as I recall), the bear hug and the rocking manoeuvre. The main reason for the discontinuation of these lifts was attributed to health and safety issues in regard to staffs and patients and protecting the NHS from incurred fines.

Information Governance Training For years, increased emphasis has been placed on information governance training, now *'Data Security Awareness Training (DSAT)'* since 25th May 2018 (LDC 2019). Recent issues around the loss of patient's notes, and accordingly confidentiality, have placed greater focus on the maintenance of contemporaneous patient records, chiefly accurate documentation. This scrutiny is a result of the society we now live in, and the increased impetus on having someone to blame when things go wrong. As healthcare professionals working within the NHS, nurses and doctors encounter many issues in the performance of their daily activities. These issues are compounded by the fact that we interact with many emotional people, in most cases relatives who are looking for someone to blame when a loved one has passed away, or a patient who feels that their treatment has gone wrong, and consequently in seeking compensation for their perceived grievances, they will sue the *organisation* (NHS), nurse or doctor, who may find themselves in court, regardless of whether the patient's claim is valid or not, since all allegations must be investigated (UKEssays 2018).

Documentation   In today's nursing, documentation is much more sophisticated (Elrick 2021). The maintenance of contemporaneous records is deemed crucial to support or refute incoming allegations against the health professional and validate the care they deliver to patients. Basically, it is their way of accounting, in writing, every action undertaken (UKEssays 2018). Nonetheless, documentation has acquired some justifiable scrutiny over the years. This scrutiny has been compounded by the fact that *nurses* are now expected to manage a larger patient load, and since this incurs more time to complete relevant documentation, there is consequently less time for patients (UKEssays 2018; Patterson 2012). Certainly, reflection on my years in the wards has triggered memories of increased pressures of work in terms of delivering optimal care to patients, but, specifically, a lack of time to complete documentation at the end of the shift which often resulted in me, and other nurses, working unpaid overtime. Thinking back on my experience with documentation, and how the process has changed since the 1970s, I am reminded of the traditional Kardex, whose description by a previous EN of 'a folded card-stock roadmap' to all things for the patient that had been completed in pencil and continuously crossed out or erased and updated (O'Dowd 2008) is an accurate description of my own memory of the Kardex. I remember when the Kardex was subsequently replaced with a system where notes were held in individual folders, and stored at the foot of the patient's bed. This was a practice that gave easy access to visitors (family and friends), and one that had given pause for concern in regard to confidentiality and issues around its violation. Such concern has resulted in notes being stored in a secure unit, within the ward area, which can only be accessed by authorised health professionals.

Evolving Technology   The evidence confirms that there are a number of nursing, technology and information systems being used in the NHS today, all, seemingly, extremely beneficial to increasing efficiency in practice and improving patient outcomes (Elrick 2021).

However, for the purpose of this book, I will focus on the InfoFlex information system in terms of its use in streamlining patient information and the documentation process in local practice.

InfoFlex, defined as a comprehensive digital healthcare from a single solution, is quite simply the most efficient way to manage patient pathways. InfoFlex has grown to support more clinical specialities and to be used in more NHS Trusts than clinical systems from any other provider. It serves over 40,000 users of clinical systems and millions of patients (Chameleon Information Management Services (CIMS) 2020). This system increases efficiency by allowing members of the multidisciplinary teams greater access to patient information, and accordingly helping to streamline documentation and making the process more user friendly. In my local area of practice, InfoFlex has been an integral part of the documentation process in cancer care for some time. In terms of the weekly urology multidisciplinary team (UMDT) meetings, InfoFlex makes the documentation process more user friendly, in that relevant patient information is more easily accessible to all members of the multi-disciplinary team. InfoFlex also enables nurses to maintain their own patient records in which the documentation of key information can be accessed by the MUCNS team and other members of the multidisciplinary team. To date, InfoFlex has proven to be extremely constructive in enhancing and expediting both patient and practice outcomes.

Infection Prevention and Control Infection control plays a big part in the NHS every day, so new technology is being developed all the time (UKEssays 2018). As a result of the rising trend in infection rates, and accordingly in increased scrutiny on health organisations to minimise the risks to patients and the public, emphasis had been placed on research in this area and for the findings to be stringently applied to improving both patient and practice outcomes. As I have observed in local prac-tice, the basic handwashing procedures remain much the same, although increased emphasis was placed on the appropriate use of hand disinfectant, and as such, these were strategically placed both within the clinical area and at the various ports of entry to wards and departments.

The Bed Making Ritual In terms of completing this task, I am sure that many of us will remember times when gloves were used inappropriately—as in when nurses had worn gloves to make a bed, even though its use was only indicated in situations where bed linen was soiled with urine, excrement or blood. Another issue had been the inappropriate use of the skip, when instead of having it in the clinical area it was left in the sluice room, with nurses travelling with dirty linen down the length of the ward to put it in the skip. Infection control has been regimental over the years, not only in terms of bed making, but also in other areas, such as handwashing, wound management, methicillin-resistant *Staphylococcus aureus* (MRSA) and other healthcare-associated infections (HCAIs). Over the last decade, my memory of infection prevention and control is of the yearly training updates, the objective of which is in ensuring that the guidance was being stringently adhered to in practice, and accordingly enabling the NHS to avoid incurred fines.

3.3   Conclusion and Lessons Learnt

According to Cipriano (Cipriano 2010), the scope and status of nursing have changed since the days of Florence Nightingale and Mary Seacole, days in which the apprenticeship model of training had reaped little power or reward. Nursing today is dynamic and changing, and because it is driven by science and technology, there have been some exceptional achievements and advancements in both manage-ment and treatments. While some might perceive the increased requirement for nurses to attain higher levels of academia a little unrealistic, for others, it is a very necessary requirement, in terms of advancing their professional development. As such, it is one that necessitates some reconfiguration, in terms of acknowledging the individual's status, practically, theoretically and figuratively. Reflecting back on practice over the years, perhaps the transition taken place in nursing was not always positive; however, I do believe that many from this era would agree that the standards of care delivered to patients should be remembered with a sense of pride, and that such pride should continue to drive practice going forward.

Chap. 4 reports on my decision to take a sabbatical from nursing, and highlights the opportunities, experiences and learning gained, my return to nursing and subsequent progression in my career.

References

Anderson B (2010) A perspective on changing dynamics in nursing over the past 20 years. Br J Nurs 19(18):1190–1191. [Internet]. http://tinyurl

Anon (2020) Hello my name is. Hello My Name Is: a campaign for more compassionate care [Internet]. hellomynameis.org.uk. [cited 2020 Oct 24]. https://www.hellomynameis.org.uk/

BBC News (2019) Boy slept on hospital floor due to lack of beds [Internet]. bbc.co.uk. [cited 2020 Oct 1]. https://www.bbc.co.uk/news/uk-england-leeds-50713236

BBC Newsround (2020) Florence nightingale: Where did modern nursing first begin? [Internet]. BBCnewsround. [cited 2020 Sep 20]. https://www.bbc.co.uk/newsround/52397246

Campbell D (2016) Hospitals told to cut staff amid spiralling NHS cash crisis [internet]. The Guardian. [cited 2020 Oct 20]. https://www.theguardian.com/society/2016/jan/29/hospitals-told-cut-staff-nhs-cash-crisis

Chameleon Information Management Services (CIMS) (2020) Infloflex, better data, better health [Internet]. infoflex.co.uk. [cited 2020 Oct 13]. https://infoflex.co.uk/

Cipriano PF (2010) The world of nursing—then and now—American Nurse [Internet]. americannurse.com. [cited 2020 Oct 24]. https://www.myamericannurse.com/the-world-of-nursing-then-and-now/

Department of Health & Social Care (2020) The. The NHS nursing workforce [Internet]. [cited 2020 Oct 24]. https://www.nao.org.uk/wp-content/uploads/2020/03/The-NHS-nursing-workforce.pdf

Elrick L (2021) Technology in nursing: How electronics are changing the field [Internet]. [cited 2021 Feb 23] https://www.rasmussen.edu/degrees/nursing/blog/technology-in-nursing/

Francis B, Humphreys J (1999) Enrolled nurses and the professionalisation of nursing: a comparison of nurse education and skill-mix in Australia and the UK [internet]. Int J Nurs Stud 36:127–135. [cited 2020 Oct 2] https://www.myamericannurse.com/the-world-of-nursing-then-and-now/

Glasper A (2018) The regulation of the nursing associate profession: an overview. Br J Healthcare Assist [Internet] 12(1):38–41. https://doi.org/10.12968/bjha.2018.12.1.38

Dyer C (2013) Mid staffs trust is to face criminal charges over patient's death. BMJ 347(aug30 3):f5375–f5375. [cited 2020 Oct 5] [Internet]. https://doi.org/10.1136/bmj.f5375

Johnson S (2015) How has nursing changed and what does the future hold? [internet]. The Guardian. [cited 2020 Oct 12]. https://www.theguardian.com/healthcare-network/2015/mar/17/how-has-nursing-changed-and-what-does-the-future-hold

Klainberg M (2010) An historical overview of nursing. In: Klainberg M, Dirschel KM (eds) Today's nursing leader [internet]. Jones & Bartlett, Burlington, MA. https://publish.jblearning.com/index.php?mod=jbbrowse&act=book_details&id=737

LDC (2019) New information governance toolkit (IGT) and the GDPR [Internet]. [cited 2019 Dec 28]. https://ldc.org.uk/new-information-governance-toolkit-igt-and-the-gdpr/

Mullally S. Nursing times, VOL: 98, ISSUE: 10, PAGE NO: 40 2002. Introducing 'PREP and The NHS Plan' [cited: 2021 March 02]. https://www.nursingtimes.net/archive/introducing-prep-and-the-nhs-plan-07-03-2002/

NHS Digital (2017) The number of nurses and midwives in the UK—Full Fact. [cited: 2021 March 09]. Source: NHS Digital, Hospital and Community Health Service (HCHS) Monthly Workforce Statistics – Provisional Statistics, Oct 2017. https://fullfact.org/health/number-nurses-midwife-uk/

NHS England, Introducing the 6Cs, Values essential to compassionate care [Internet], [Cited 2021 February 08]. https://www.england.nhs.uk/6cs/wp-content/uploads/sites/25/2015/03/introducing-the-6cs.pdf

Nursing Midwifery Council. We've introduced revalidation for nurses and midwives [Intranet] [cited 2021 March 02]. https://www.nmc.org.uk/news/news-and-updates/weve-introduced-revalidation-for-nurses-and-midwives/

O'Brien-Pallas L, Duffield C, Alksnis C (2004) Who will be there to nurse? JONA J Nurs Administration 34(6):298–302. [Internet]. http://journals.lww.com/00005110-200406000-00009

O'Dowd A (2008) Nursing in the 1970's: 'You are here to do the work, so get on with it'" [Internet]. nursingtimes.net. [cited 2020 Jun 9]. https://www.nursingtimes.net/archive/nursing-in-the-1970s-you-are-here-to-do-the-work-so-get-on-with-it-03-03-2008/

O'Dowd A. Nursing in the 1990s [Internet]. nursingtimes.net. 2008 [cited 2020 Oct 24]. https://www.nursingtimes.net/archive/nursing-in-the-1990s-12-05-2008/

Paton F (2020) 4 positive uses of social media in nursing [Internet]. [cited 2020 Oct 1]. https://nurseslabs.com/4-positive-uses-social-media-nursing/

Patterson C (2012) Reforms in the 1990s were supposed to make nursing care better. Instead, there's a widely shared sense that this was how today's compassion deficit began. How did we come to this? [Internet] The Independent. [cited 2020 Oct 24]. https://www.independent.co.uk/voices/commentators/christina-patterson/reforms-1990s-were-supposed-make-nursing-care-better-instead-there-s-widely-shared-sense-was-how-today-s-compassion-deficit-began-how-did-we-come-7631273.html

The Guardian (2019) Nursing shortages forcing NHS to rely on less qualified staff—report [Internet]. The Guardian. [cited 2020 Oct 24]. https://www.theguardian.com/society/2019/nov/28/nursing-shortages-forcing-nhs-england-wales-to-rely-on-less-qualified-staff-report

Tiffin C (2012) Beyond the bedside: The changing role of today's nurses [Internet]. Huffpost. [cited 2020 Oct 13]. https://www.huffpost.com/entry/nursing-school_b_1384285?guccounter=1&guce_referrer=aHR0cHM6Ly93d3cuZ29vZ2xlLmNvVsLw&guce_referrer_sig=AQAAANOokjavdXXf61ajp2zrJ22jZ1XZpF_TiOS4Dg-k6VqecK76mjS8AfPW4p_eHRToxml8m0MXlqRPr9CkWvyawu4bgOGNiKRR9Loj8F2ki6h4_x4spH4

Toulson S (1996) Inappropriate attenders: a quality issue in A&E. Prof Nurse [Internet] 11(5):299–300. http://www.ncbi.nlm.nih.gov/pubmed/8604423

UKEssays (2018) Changes in roles and responsibilities of nurses in the moder [Internet]. ukessays.com. [cited 2019 Oct 19]. https://www.ukessays.com/essays/nursing/changes-in-roles-and-responsibilities-of-nurses-in-the-modernisation-of-nhs-nursing-essay.php?vref=1

A Constructive Interlude in my Career Path

4

4.1 1979–1992

Valuable Time out I believe that as we go through life, changes in the normal status quo may force us to question our choices and our path in life, and accordingly in making decisions to effect change. Such questions emerged in 1979, at a time when I thought a change in my career path was warranted.

Secretarial Work While I was still in secondary school, I had taken the opportunity to undertake additional study in the form of typing and shorthand, at evening classes. I remember struggling with the shorthand—it was like an alien language to me. In successfully completing the course I acquired the basic principles of typing and shorthand, but had not seriously considered this as a career path, since my focus was always to become a nurse. However, in 1978, while working as an agency nurse, I was somewhat disillusioned with nursing and believed that I needed a change in career path. After considering my options, I decided on secretarial work, and accordingly completed a secretarial course, at the local polytechnic college. On completion of this course, I went on to secure work as a secretary, within the commercial sector—firstly, working for an amusement games company, and secondly, with a fashion catalogue. The 2 years that I worked within the commercial sector provided me with some useful learning that contributed to the acquisition of skills, i.e. typing, which, on my return to nursing, had proven useful in subsequent academic undertakings. I continued working as an agency nurse during this period (approximately one shift per week), as I believed that it was important to keep my nursing skills up-to-date. I worked as a secretary until 1983, when I had my first son. However, leading up to the time when I should have returned to work, and even though I had embarked on the task of finding a suitable childminder, the thought of leaving my son was too difficult. Fortunately, it was a difficulty that was simplified with the pregnancy of my second son. I did not return to work.

© Springer Nature Switzerland AG 2022
B. Anderson, *A Uro-Oncology Nurse Specialist's Reflection on her Practice Journey*, https://doi.org/10.1007/978-3-030-94199-4_4

In 1984, 7 months after having my second son, I felt that it was important to continue working as an agency nurse, but that these hours should be centred around my family. Having made this decision, and with the full support of my husband, I returned to work, initially working in evenings, 2 days/week, from 4 to 9 p.m. In some ways, this time out enabled me to accomplish certain goals, such as learning to drive and having a certain degree of financial independence, while being a full-time mum. I continued to work as an agency nurse until March 1987, 3 months before having my daughter in June 1987. I did not return to working as an agency nurse during this time, since my priority was to be available for my children. The flexibility afforded by my not working enabled me to interact with and be involved in activities such as taking them to school and picking them up; attending school activities such as concerts, parents' evening and excursions; and taking them to swimming and to indulge in other social activities.

4.2   'Bev's Hot Kitchen'

Running my own business was a venture that developed on the back of my cookery skills. As a young girl in Jamaica, being able to cook was a non-negotiable expectation that resulted in my preparation of quite a few meals that were keenly examined by my grandmother. After joining my parents years later in the UK, this expectation continued until I left home. I guess having cooked so much in my young years, it was nice not having to do so, and instead enjoying someone else's cooking. However, getting married, having a family and not having much money, you quickly learn to do things for yourself. Having catered for my friends on numerous social gatherings, one in particular, Bea, was convinced that my catering expertise should be marketed—albeit a conviction that I was initially reluctant to consider. However, sensing my reluctance, Bea devised a cunning plan. She telephoned me and asked if I could prepare a variation of cakes for her. At this point, I had no reason to believe that she had an alternative agenda, so I agreed to her request, and proceeded to bake a large variety of cakes. On delivering the order to Bea, she looked at me, smiled and said that the cakes looked lovely, but that I would have to take them home again, unless I charged her for them. Surprised at this remark, I told her that she was a friend, and that I could not charge her. Still smiling, her response was that in that case, she did not want them.

I had no idea of how to price my products, but seeing that she was serious, I came up with the sum of £5.00 for the lot. Feigning frustration, Bea laughed, and told me that I was impossible. She went on to reiterate her previous advice that I should seriously consider running my own business, and that this should be from my own home. Apparently, having spoken about my cooking skills with family, friends and colleagues, many were eager to utilise this service. I told her that I would think about it, and I did.

'The Enterprise Allowance Scheme' I thought that if I was going to do this business, I should do it properly. To enable me to get on the right path, I visited the local

Job Centre, who advised me about the *Enterprise Allowance Scheme*—a government scheme that provided a short training and guidance course for individuals who wanted to run a small business from their own home. I subsequently enrolled on this course, which was surprisingly enlightening in terms of pricing my products and running a viable business.

I subsequently developed my own business, *Bev's Hot Kitchen'*, an event organisation venture, in 1988, that provided authentic Afro-Caribbean and English cuisines. As owner/manager, I provided catered service to a wide range of clients. Services included private functions like weddings and birthday parties, school teachers' meetings and a take-away service option that included authentic Afro-Caribbean and English hot meals. The business also provided the options of a selection of home-cooked, frozen, ready-made meals; orders for cakes for weddings, birthdays and Christmas; and many other items, selected from an itemised price list. I was able to effectively manage a small business, through the planning and prioritisation of work. I achieved improved economic skills through dealing first hand with accountants and bank managers. In many ways, working from home was advantageous, but there were also drawbacks. Often, my attempts to please both my clients and my children resulted in the conflicting decision of whose needs should come first, and consequently a sense of guilt. Nonetheless, I managed to survive the inherent struggles, and ran this business for 4 years, 1988–1992.

Work Experience An added achievement to running my own business was my appointment as a tutor of 'Authentic Afro-Caribbean Cookery', in 1990, at the local Adult College. This was an immensely enjoyable undertaking that had often necessitated a demonstration of how to make various dishes using a previously prepared dish to support demonstration. This activity had made me think back on previous television cookery programmes, where the presenters had used this technique and the quote, 'This is one I made/prepared earlier'. Needless to say, the fact that I was able to use this technique and quote in my cookery class was quite refreshing.

A necessary undertaking for this appointment was the completion of the *'ACSET' Teacher Training Course,* which I proceeded to utilise during the 2 years of running this course. This opportunity greatly enhanced my organisational, planning and presentation skills, as well as extended my communication skills—skills that had proven useful on my return to nursing in 1992.

Surprising Truth I remember soon after starting this business the look of surprise and shock on my girlfriend Lor's face, and with mouth ajar, and eyes wide, her exclamation, *'Bev, you can cook!'*. Thinking back, I guess her shock was justified. You see, living in the nursing home during the pupil nurse training stage, everyone in our group was able to cook, and for the most part was able to 'rustle up' a simple but nourishing meal. I guess having to cook in my early years in Jamaica, and subsequently when I came to the UK, cooking had lost its appeal. So yes, I had hidden the fact that I could cook, and accordingly had gotten away with not having to do my fair share for a long time. For Lor, the fact that I can cook still evokes a degree of surprise.

Working as secretary in the commercial sector enabled new skills, such as typing, shorthand and word processing, and the opportunity to continue working intermittently as an agency nurse during this period and between having my children. By working in this manner, I was able to maintain my nursing skills and to earn my own money. Arguably, to some, the need to earn my own money may seem unimportant, although for me it was important to maintain a degree of financial independence, one that allowed me to buy the essentials and to contribute to the 'household pot'.

However, in 1992, the country was in recession, and although I only ran a small business, its impact was felt. After 4 years of running *Bev's Hot Kitchen'*, while the business had not completely folded, sales had tailed off, and as a result, I needed to reconsider my options, going forward. I conducted discussions with my husband, who felt that since our youngest child had started nursery, perhaps it was time to re-enter the outside world—meaning nursing. While I tended to agree with him, because I had deliberated doing something entirely different, I was a little reluctant. However, after fully considering all my options, returning to nursing seemed the most prudent decision. It was, after all, something I was good at. Yes, it would be challenging, but hopefully fulfilling, in terms of progressing my career and still being there for my family.

4.3   Returning to the Fold

Once the decision was made to return to nursing, I applied to the local hospital to seek work in the Nursing Bank. My application was accepted; however, as an enrolled nurse (EN), who had not actually worked as a nurse for 4 years, this had been incumbent on the undertaking of the Back to Nursing Course, the objective of which was to bring me up-to-date with current nursing practices, before allowing me to work as an EN on the Trust's Nursing Bank.

The Back to Nursing Course in 1992 comprised training in school for nurses who had children and who were either now in nursery or school to work around them. The course was designed to update the individual on all fields of practice and on the basic principles of delivering care within each field. Once I completed this course, I proceeded to work in the Nursing Bank. Working in this context increased my knowledge and experience, and extended my learning in terms of these practices. I was allowed to choose my hours to fit around my children and their routine. In those days, I was able to work the 09.30 shift (the latest am start time) and finish at 13.30, prior to picking up my children from school. Shift patterns had extended to working weekends, and later on to working nights. I had worked across various fields of practice, which included surgery, medicine, renal, accident and emergency (A&E), high dependency unit (HDU), care of the elderly (COTE) and outpatient department (OPD), between 1992 and 1996, across which I gained some invaluable knowledge and experience that contributed to my learning and improving my skills.

The Accident and Emergency (A&E) Department Based on my experience of working in the A&E department for 3 years, I concluded that while this environment was a stressful and at times a violent place of work, it presented me with many opportunities to learn about the different aspects of emergency nursing, as gleaned from the many patients who had passed through the department's doors. It was also a lucrative learning environment, one that significantly contributed to my knowledge and experience and my competency to perform various procedures, such as electrocardiogram (ECG), venous cannulation and venepuncture, skills that had proven beneficial on my return to working in the wards. However, in regard to nursing students, I was aware that the A&E department was often not as conducive to fulfilling their learning needs. Many struggled to find their niche within the team and their opportunity to learn was often obscured by a lack of support, the consequence of increased workloads and inadequate staffing levels.

During the 3 years that I had spent in the A&E department, working both day and night shifts, l had learnt how to deal with difficult patients and their relatives, typically in dealing with the Friday nights' drunken (inebriated) binges and the resulting outcomes. Thinking back on these times, I am reminded of an earlier episode in the 1980s, while working as an agency, EN, in another A&E department. This was my first experience with the inebriated patient. It was Friday night and the time was around 01.30 in the morning. I can clearly remember being assigned to this inebriated gentleman who presented to the department, and clearly not for the first time. Apparently, he attempted to find his way home via the British Rail train, but while attempting to alight from the carriage, he missed his footing and fell to the ground, knocking his head. I remember the vomiting, the incoherent ramblings … calling for his wife and asking me to call her, even though he was worried that she would be angry with him. On calling his wife, it was clear that she was not amused. After relaying the news that her husband was in the A&E department, she promptly suggested that we should keep him there, since she had no intention of travelling to the hospital at that time of night. In reporting the wife's response to the patient, his response of 'Oh, dear', 'I've done it this time', indicated his lack of surprise to this. While the situation was quite funny, it was also a little sad, since as a result of too much alcohol, his behaviour had been more akin to that of a naughty school boy rather than a grown man. Even more sad was that this was a recurring behaviour, one that would most likely be repeated the following week.

My later experiences in the A&E department were acquired as a bank nurse in the 1990s, while working on a Friday night shift. I had to deal with not only the inebriated patient, but also the consequent knife stabbings, and verbal and attempted physical abuse of staffs, as illustrated in the following:

On this particular shift, I was working in one of the four-bedded cubicles, when my nursing colleague, who was working in the main assessment area (Majors), entered my cubicle with face flushed and eyes full of dismay. Surprised to see him in this state, I asked what the matter was. Apparently, an inebriated gentleman, whom he attempted to assess, sat up suddenly on the trolley, punched him in the head and consequently knocked him to the floor. I had correctly deduced that he was upset and shaken by the incidence. A deduction that was verified by his remarks … 'I am f…..g fed up with this s..t'. Because he was a smoker, I suggested that he go and have a cigarette, to try and calm himself down. He did, but the effect was minimal. In fact, he remained upset for the remainder of the shift, and to my knowledge did not return to work in the A&E after that.

It is another Friday night, and another drunken early-morning episode. A young man, in his 30s, the victim of a knife stabbing, following a fight outside the pub he had been drinking, was accompanied to the A&E department by a police officer. His behaviour was intriguing. Although he was covered from his head to his waist with dried blood, he seemed not to be unduly worried or concerned. Surprised by the patient's lack of concern, the police officer asked him if he realised how close he came to losing his life? A question to which his response of 'you should see the other guy' was even more surprising. Seemingly, getting drunk was an enjoyable pastime, and hence the ensuing ramifications were inconsequential. This patient was one of many (over 30 patients) who visited the department that night. With reflection on this figure and on the nights so far, the A&E on-call doctor had questioned the rationale for treating these patients, when most seemed unconcerned about their life/health/safety, and moreover were likely to repeat the same process the following week. It was a question that had given me pause for thought, and one for which I did not have the answer.

The next reflection is based on a senior RN's personal account of her experience following the attempted assault by an inebriated patient. Fortunately, for the RN, she was a brown belt karate student, but unfortunate for the patient, since during their altercation, she had 'knocked him out cold'. Of course, the incident had raised questions in regard to whether the RN used excessive force to restrain the patient. The RN had in turn questioned the rules around the abuse and assault of health professionals, and why they should have to tolerate abusive behaviour from patients, when all they are trying to do is help them. The RN was understandably unapologetic for her actions. In fact, she was adamant that if a similar situation were to occur again, her response would be the same.

In this instance, the question posed was when will patients take responsibility for their behaviour and their actions, evidently a question that has received consideration from the Health and Safety Executive (HSE). Violence against staff is a long-standing problem that has gained impetus over the years, and one to which the NHS has committed their support since 1999, with the instigation of a zero-tolerance attitude towards such violence, and consequently there has been a significant increase in the numbers of offenders being prosecuted since 2003. The zero-tolerance rule comprises abuse and assault of staff, both verbal and physical, with emphasis placed on respect, and that this should work both ways (NHS Employers 2019).

The Impact of Targets Working in the A&E department provided me with an upfront and personal experience of the impact of targets on care delivery. The implication of the 4-h waits on decisions and subsequent patient throughput was clearly focused on avoiding a breach and subsequent fine. Another impacting issue on the

4-h waits was capacity, a lack of which had resulted in extending the waiting areas to corridors, and indeed any spare area within the A&E department. I am acutely reminded of patients on trolleys, head to head, in the A&E corridors, and the challenging task of attempting to deliver care (such as giving a bedpan to a patient on a trolley in an open corridor), with only a blanket to provide a modicum of privacy and dignity. Sadly, the issue of nursing patients on trolleys, in corridors, is a practice that still exists today (BBC News 2019), and one that continues to raise significant concerns.

Acute Urinary Retention (AUR) During my time in the A&E department, I personally observed AUR patients presenting to the department with symptoms of increasing pain and discomfort, symptoms which necessitated expedient action in the form of assessment and accordingly catheterisation. Although my knowledge and experience of AUR were lacking at this time, I was aware of the apparent need for clarity on its management, clarity that I had later provided during my time in the urology ward (*refer to Chap. 5*).

4.4   Personal Insight from the Patient's Perspective (1)

As a nurse, many of us will experience being a patient at some point during our career. My experiences of being a patient were extremely enlightening in terms of gaining an insight and understanding of the patient's mindset.

Urinary Tract Infections (UTIs) My experiences of UTIs as a patient relate back to 1972 when I was 17 years old, one year before I started my nurse training. I remember the excruciating pain during the weekly visit to the local club, usually an activity that I enjoyed immensely. However, on this particular night, I was feeling a little unwell, even before arriving at the club, a feeling that intensified as I stood outside, talking to my friends. I was now experiencing a great deal of pain and discomfort on my left side, and accordingly I was bending over and clutching my arms under my chest. At the time, I was uncertain as to what could be causing such pain. Seeing my evident distress, one of my friends offered to drive me to the local hospital A&E.

By the time I arrived in the A&E, I was feeling sick, hot and sweaty, and the pain was so bad that I could hardly speak. The doctor took one look at me, and after an initial assessment of my symptoms determined that I had a urinary tract infection (UTI), for which he prescribed oral antibiotics and an antipyretic (paracetamol), and 4 h later, my symptoms improved significantly. However, despite the pain being reduced to a dull ache, and my temperature nearly within normal range, my thought at this time was that I did not wish to experience such pain again. Unbeknown to me at the time, this had been wishful thinking, since during my second year of training (1974), the same symptoms manifested again, this time while I was in the nurse's home, watching television. Knowing instantly what these symptoms meant, I contacted the on-call sister, who arranged for me to be admitted to a bed in the ward, where I was cared for by my colleagues overnight, and was later transferred to the nurse's sick bay ward at the main hospital the next day. After spending 4 days in the sick bay, I was allowed to return to the nurses' home, and later to my parents' home, until I fully recovered. Once again, this was an experience that incited much pain and discomfort, and an ensuing paranoia of toilets, particularly public toilets.

1976—Wisdom Teeth Extractions This was my first real experience of being anaesthetised. There is the memory of the morphine-based Omnopon and Scopolamine (sickness drug) (Om and Scop for short), and the floating feeling thereafter. Aaaah, such bliss. Honestly, in that moment, I had wondered if that is how a drug addict might feel following the habitual fix. Not so blissful, however, was the ensuing pain, once the effect of the drug had worn off.

1993, Surgery One year back to nursing and working in the bank, a long history of gynaecological problems had led to the decision to have a hysterectomy. I guess the saying that too much knowledge is not always a good thing is very true. Being overly cautious, on my admission to receive this surgery, I had taken into hospital my own drinking glass and cup, knife and fork and a pillow case, having observed patients who had been nil by mouth from 12 midnight, but were left until the afternoon for their procedure; concerned that this should not happen to me I had voiced my concerns to the nurses who ensured that my surgery went ahead in the morning as planned. I remember being in theatre, lying on the table, prior to being anaesthetised, counting back from ten and remembering nothing after seven. Wow! That was fast. On my return to the ward from theatre, I remember the nurse who was looking after me asking how I was feeling, as she recorded my vital signs. In terms of pain, I was fairly comfortable; the morphine-based patient-controlled analgesia (PCA) machine had worked its magic.

Appeasing Thirst I remember the incredible thirst, the dry mouth and the licking of my lips to encourage some moisture. I also remember saying to the nurse, may I please have a drink, and her response, sorry Beverley, you cannot have a drink yet. In my determination to gratify my thirst, I reiterated my request for a drink a few minutes later, and promptly promised not to be sick. I asked for a cup of tea, but to my surprise received a pot. I drank it all, and to prove a point that I was not sick.

Reflecting on my surgery and the subsequent experience of thirst reminded me of caring for those patients who had undergone surgery, and who, having returned to the ward, had complained of thirst, and me casually saying, 'I am sorry, you cannot have a drink', without giving much thought or understanding of how they actually felt. However, now that I understood this feeling of thirst and its need for gratification, I did not casually say, 'I am sorry, you cannot have a drink'. Instead, I explained why they could not have a drink at that time (in case they were sick, or they could aspirate), and then offered them an ice cube wrapped in gauze to suck on, or a pink mouth swab, dipped in cold water, to moisten their lips and mouth— actions that provided some relief for the persistent thirst.

The Catheter and the Commode Experience   There is the embarrassing memory of being catheterised, the tube inside my bladder draining urine into the catheter bag, and upon its removal, the fear of developing a urinary tract infection (UTI) verified by the symptoms of discomfort, burning, stinging, frequency and the ensuing interrupted sleep. The use of the commode was also embarrassing. Based on clinical experience, while I would normally clean the commode's seat before offering to a patient, I know that this action may not be carried out by all nurses, a knowledge which in this instance had heightened my concerns regarding my hygiene needs. I remember establishing eye contact with the nurse looking after me, and noting her unspoken acknowledgement of my concerns, by the winking of her eye and the cleaning of the commode seat with the disinfectant wipe, and my countered acknowledgement of a thank you, with the nodding of my head. This was an insightful experience, one that on my return to work I was mindful not to forget.

Overall, the care I received was excellent. The nurses and doctors acknowledged and respected my concerns and ensured that they were addressed. Admittedly, being a nurse had played its part. My personal experience of being a patient was hugely enlightening in terms of my learning and seeing things from the patient's perspective. Based on this experience, I had concluded that every doctor and nurse should experience being a patient, a conclusion that I shared with my GP, following my discharge from hospital, and his subsequent visit to my home, and surprisingly one with which he fully concurred.

4.5   1992–1998, Bank Nursing

I was a bank nurse for 6 years and during this time I worked across various fields of nursing practice. This was a period of working from which I acquired some extremely valuable knowledge and experience that contributed to enhancing my learning and boosting my confidence. Working independently, and as part of a team, enabled me to be more assertive, in that I was not afraid to challenge concerns or ask questions to quell my curiosity. In a world of harsh realities, I learnt that people are very intolerant of individuals who, in the performance of their duties, are unable to do so competently. As a result, I resorted to undertaking relevant study activities to ensure that I was up-to-date with my practical and theoretical knowledge, and that I acquired the necessary skills to enhance my performance as a nurse. These skills included intravenous cannulation (IVC), intravenous venepuncture (IV), electrocardiogram (ECG) recording and completing the IV drug calculation course (for the administration of intravenous drugs).

The Enrolled Nurse Conversion Course   The Enrolled Nurse (EN) Conversion course became necessary following the decision to phase out the enrolled nurse role in 1989. At this time, the jobs of current ENs were safeguarded; hence they could either continue as ENs until retirement or upgrade to the registered nurse (RN) level via specially designed 'conversion courses'. The English National Board for Nurses expected a relatively low number of ENs to take up these courses, but in fact, the numbers of ENs who took the opportunity to enhance their careers significantly exceeded their expectation (Francis and Humphreys 1999). I completed this course between 1995 and 1996, while working as a bank enrolled nurse. Thinking back, I am reminded of several key areas of learning, and experiences that provided me with laughter, pause for thought and new knowledge. These areas of learning were as follows.

A Baffling Experience   This learning was acquired during one of the several teaching sessions, in which the lecturer recounted her baffling patient experience of the recording of her own vital signs. At the time, the mercury thermometer, placed in the patient's mouth, was the instrument widely used to record an individual's temperature, unlike today where the temperature is recorded by placing a digital thermometer in the individual's ear. Blood pressure was recorded manually, using the sphygmomanometer and a stethoscope, with the onus on the practitioner's ability to accurately interpret the results. Today, blood pressure is electronically recorded by the Dinamap machine, which also interprets the results. According to the lecturer, the nurse had placed the thermometer upside down in her mouth (mercury tip outside mouth), and in recording her blood pressure had incorrectly interpreted the result as systolic 60 and diastolic 140, which equates to 60/140 mmHg. This was an intriguing observation that had clearly highlighted the nurse's lack of knowledge and experience, but even more intriguing, and very worrying, was that the nurse did not seem to acknowledge these mistakes.

Interestingly, a few years later, I observed a nurse making the same mistake of placing the thermometer upside down in a patient's mouth. However, remembering the lecturer's report of her experience, I tactfully pointed out her mistake, and explained how she should correctly perform the task. Over the years, I was always mindful that the recording of a patient's vital signs (temperature, pulse, respirations, oxygen levels and blood pressure) is an integral and important part of providing patients with effective nursing care, and that in performing the task, healthcare practitioners have a responsibility to ensure that they have the appropriate training to do so effectively.

A Gratifying Experience   In another lecture, students were required to deliver a demonstration, in which their communication and presentation skills were keenly observed. For my presentation, I decided to take advantage of my cookery skills and elected to demonstrate how to make 'Jamaican Rum Punch'. As the weather was extremely hot, it seemed to be the perfect choice. This recipe comprised a number of ingredients, of which the alcohol, in this case Wray and Nephew

Overproof rum (over 70% alcohol), was key to achieving the authentic taste. Ensuring that I had all the ingredients in place (including ice), I proceeded to perform the demonstration in front of 12 students and 3 lecturers, who closely observed my every move. During the demonstration, I explained each step of the recipe, and proudly linked the drinks' origin to my Jamaican roots. Having made up the fruit component of the punch, and being mindful of the alcohol content, I held up the rum flask and asked the audience if they wanted me to add it in—a question that received a resounding 'YES!' The smell of the rum was intoxicating. Without further ado, I filled plastic cups with ice, poured over the vibrant deep pink liquid, added a slice of lime and gave it to the eagerly awaited audience. The sounds of Hmmmmh! verified their approval as the smooth liquid caressed the welcoming taste buds. The previously prepared copies of the rum punch recipe were well received by both students and lecturers.

Inspirational Placements In completing this course, I was fortunate to have accessed some inspirational placements that included mental health, maternity and district nursing. On the mental health placement, I found the patient dynamics intriguing. Patients were from various classes, ethnic backgrounds and professions. Their ages ranged between early teens and late 70s, while professions comprised students, teachers, accountants, lawyers and doctors (psychologists, psychiatrists, general practitioners). Thinking back, perhaps my perception of mental health nursing had been clouded by my naivety and an element of unconscious bias. It was evident that I had placed certain patients (i.e. doctors, lawyers) into certain boxes, an action I attributed to my difficulty in associating them with having mental health issues. However, as I later learnt, mental health problems are not discriminatory of age, profession, class or race, and at the end of the day, receiving the right support is crucial to helping individuals to understand the emerging emotions and to deal with the ensuing fallout. As mental health nursing was not a part of my original EN nurse training, in undertaking this placement, I initially could not appreciate its relevance to my nursing role, in supporting patients with mental health issues. However, by the end of this placement, I came to better understand my relevance in treating this illness.

The maternity placement was extremely rewarding. I was initially worried that I would be squeamish to observe the birth of a baby, but the opposite was true—seeing a new life enter into the world was mesmerising.

My first experience on this placement was of a mother of three, who was admitted to the unit in labour with her fourth baby … a baby who was clearly inpatient to be born as his delivery, which took less than 5 min, had occurred while his mother was being transferred from the trolley to the bed in the middle of the reception area. I remember thinking, Wow! That was fast!

The second experience was of a mother who, having lost her first baby boy to cot death, was understandably apprehensive. While her apprehension was assuaged by the safe delivery of a beautiful baby girl, it was nevertheless a poignant reminder of the loss of her son.

The third experience was of a lady from a Black, Asian and Minority Ethnic (BAME) background. Having had a spinal anaesthetic administered, she did not have the strength to push her baby out; hence, delivery was vacuum assisted. Her husband was not in attendance at the birth but her mother-in-law was. Thinking of my own experience of giving birth and the therapeutic benefit of having my husband present, what intrigued me the most about this situation was the mother-in-law's detachment from her daughter-in-law, in that she did not show any emotion or attempt to comfort her at any time during the birth. In reflecting on this experience, and on the daughter-in-law's seemingly lack of concern at this behaviour, perhaps the mother-in-law's behaviour was simply one that was consistent with a cultural norm.

This placement was an amazing learning curve, one that validated my own experiences of pregnancy and of becoming a mother.

The district nursing placement provided me with an understanding and an appreciation of how the principles of working in the community setting differed to those in the hospital setting, and enabled me to appreciate how a change in dynamics, in terms of the environment and a shift in power/control, could impact the individual's confidence, comfort level and ensuing behaviour. This relates to patients and healthcare professionals. In terms of patients, I had learnt that a patient may feel uncomfortable and less empowered in hospital, but more so in their own homes, while a reverse scenario was likely to be true for the healthcare professional. In fact, reflecting on the memory of visiting patients in their own homes, I can attest to feeling less confident and a little out of my comfort zone. This was an extremely useful placement.

Recording and Interpreting Blood Pressure An important duty of the healthcare professional is the ability to perform accurate vital sign monitoring, and more importantly to be able to interpret the results of said undertakings. One such vital sign is the recording of the blood pressure. Traditionally, the measuring of the blood pressure was undertaken with a sphygmomanometer (also known as a blood pressure meter, blood pressure monitor or blood pressure gauge). The sphygmomanometer is composed of an inflatable cuff, to collapse and then release the artery under the cuff in a controlled manner, and a mercury or mechanical manometer to measure the pressure. This is used in conjunction with a stethoscope, to enable the practitioner to listen to the readings between the systolic and diastolic points, noting any changes, and having the knowledge and expertise to correctly interpret these results.

Auscultatory Gap in Hypertension Of specific note should be the practitioner's ability to identify the auscultatory gap, also called a silent gap/interval. This is the interval of pressure where Korotkoff sounds (believed to be caused mainly by blood jetting through the partly occluded vessel), indicating true systolic pressure, fade away and reappear at a lower pressure point during the manual measurement of blood pressure by auscultatory method. The auscultatory gap occurs when the first Korotkoff sound fades out for about 20–50 mmHg only to return at the diastolic point. It can result in various erroneous blood pressure reading (Shrestha 2011).

Having an understanding of the auscultatory gap or silent interval, a topic that I had been made aware of in 1995, while undertaking the Enrolled Nurse Conversion course, had proven to be a valuable learning curve. Blood pressure monitoring today is performed by using the portable digital Dinamap machine, which enables the user to record the blood pressure, heart rate, respirations and O_2 levels. It increases efficiency when performing the various patient observations, but is unable to pick up abnormal readings or to identify the silent interval. For this reason, practitioners must be able to conduct a manual blood pressure reading to avoid missing any red flags. However, since most nurses are not taught how to perform a manual recording of the blood pressure, they would not be able to accurately interpret the result. Technology is a good thing, but I am a great believer in practical skills. As such, in the undertaking of a blood pressure recording, individuals must be able to apply a common-sense approach, one that is based on knowledge and experience, to interpreting the results, identifying any red flags and accordingly raising the alarm, if so indicated. It should be noted that in the manual recording of the pulse and respiration, it is just as important to identify worrying irregularities, such as erratic speed and rates—irregularities that would be difficult to interpret if performed by the Dinamap machine.

Teaching and Assessing in Clinical Practice (998)   This accomplishment was a part of the conversion course and was hugely beneficial to enhancing my mentoring and teaching skills. Since obtaining this qualification in 1996, I have mentored many students. This is a rewarding experience, because not only was I able to pass on knowledge to these students, but I had also learnt from them. More importantly, my mentoring and teaching skills have enabled me to help students and my colleagues to realise their learning objectives.

A Puzzling Remark   Thinking back on the EN Conversion course, I am reminded of the discussions around changes to nurse training, and one nursing tutor's reference to these changes, which she contextualised with the remark that she would not want any of the new Project 2000 nurses to 'wash her backside'. This was a puzzling remark that prompted me to ask the tutor why she felt this way, seeing that she was responsible for training these nurses. Her answer was surprisingly honest. Based on her experience, she believed that while nurse training had evolved, in essence, training was now more theoretical and less practical. Consequently, a lack of hands-on experience had resulted in a more basic approach to delivering patient care. As an EN, thinking back on how in-depth my training was, perhaps I was correct in thinking that the tutor's remark was an indirect compliment to the EN training.

Having completed the Enrolled Nurse Flexible Training course and becoming an RN, I continued to work in the surgical field. This comprised working on a very busy, 30-bedded surgical ward, caring for colorectal (cancer of the colon) patients, for nearly 3 years. The staff included an impressive mix of skills—from the nurses to the doctors to other allied health professionals, and even though I was a bank nurse, I was made to feel that I was an important part of the team. The work, while interesting, was equally stressful, and many of the patient experiences were quite profound, as illustrated in the following scenarios:

Scenario 4.1
I remember a lovely lady, who was in her late 80s. Despite an extremely poor prognosis, she received multiple treatments, but with little evidence of any significant improvements. One day (while giving her a bed bath), she looked at me straight in eye, and said, 'If I was a horse, you would shoot me, wouldn't you?' This was a pointed question that prompted me to ask why she felt this way. She had rightly deduced that the treatments were not working, since she continued to feel unwell. In any case, she had had enough, and did not wish to go on. For me, this was a sobering admission that posed the question of when it would be appropriate to ask the patient what they actually want, and accordingly listen to their answer and respect their decision.

Scenario 4.2
Another lovely lady, also in her 80s, was being nursed in a two-bedded cubicle. She had undergone an anterior resection plus the formation of a temporary colostomy, which was to be reversed 2 weeks later. Sitting in the armchair by her bed, wearing a pink dressing gown, her grey hair neatly styled and wearing a little make-up, she was very ladylike. It was evident that having a stoma was a change in her body image she did not want, since she refused to look at it, and attempts to encourage self-care were unsuccessful. Consequently, she was kept in hospital in the intervening period prior to the reversal of the stoma. I must admit that I was intrigued by this lady's behaviour, and in that instance was reminded that everyone is different, and as such will deal with upsetting issues very differently.

Scenario 4.3
There was a gentleman, in his early 40s, who had undergone an anterior resection and formation of a permanent colostomy. I remember him being back in the ward, with intravenous fluids, catheter, oxygen via the face mask and distinctive faecal smell that emitted from the colostomy. With his eyes closed, tears running down his cheek and looking very sad, he asked me if it was all over (it being the surgery). It was later revealed that he was unhappy about the surgery, but had had no choice in the decision. As a reasonably young man, it was clear that the thought of a permanent stoma was distressing. Once again, importance was placed on the emotional impact of a change in body image, and the implications thereof.

Based on my experience of nursing these patients and many others, I realised that for some patients, the emotional and physical impact of a diagnosis of colorectal cancer is devastating; thus, receiving the appropriate support was crucial. Nevertheless, I can clearly remember nurses (myself included) bypassing these patients in the ward. I suppose possible reasons for this could be that we were too busy, or we did not have the appropriate knowledge, experience or skill to provide the necessary support. These are feasible explanations, but to be honest, I was concerned. In an attempt to rectify the situation, I had undertaken conversations with my good friend (Lor), who was also a nurse. This conversation resulted in her suggesting my undertaking of a counselling course, for which, following application to the local college, I secured a place in the Foundation Certificate in Psychodynamic Counselling Course, a 1-year course, condensed into 4 months. The course was intensive, but hugely beneficial, in terms of understanding human behaviour and the importance of effective communication skills, such as questioning, prompting cues, hearing, listening and silence, when dealing with emotional issues. The course incorporated a weekly counselling session that enabled insight into myself, and being honest about my assessments of, and my understanding of, my feelings. A week after completing this course, I was given the opportunity to test the learning and experience gained with two patients, who were admitted for tests, which unfortunately resulted in a diagnosis of colorectal cancer. I believe that having undertaken this course, I was more confident in my approach to dealing with patients' emotions and providing them with the required support following their receipt of a cancer diagnosis, as evidenced in the subsequent Accreditation of Prior Experiential Learning (AP(E)L) assignment in 2003.

However, while my newly acquired skills were beneficial in supporting most patients, for a few, they were less successful. Approximately 3 weeks after completing the course, I can remember a specific gentleman, who was in his early 60s, being nursed in the single side-room cubicle. He was diagnosed with Dukes C carcinoma of the bowel, for which the predicted prognosis was poor. I could see that coming to terms with this news was difficult. In speaking to him, it was clear that he had perceived the diagnosis as a threat to his life. As such, he was not in a state of mind to appreciate any words of wisdom or reassurances. While I admit that I was disappointed that my attempt to reassure this gentleman was unsuccessful, disappointment was lessened by the realisation that in such situations, not everyone will be accepting of the offer of support.

4.6   Conclusion and Lessons Learnt

Having my children helped me to gain perspective on certain issues and to reassess my options. In terms of running my own business, this venture provided me with new experiences and skills as well as the time and flexibility to work around my children. I was able to be there for the important things, such as the many school activities, to honour other commitments and still managing to realise my own dreams. A popular item on the price list was my version of the English Christmas pudding, but for my family and friends, the yearly gift of my Jamaican Christmas pudding was equally popular. I continued to give these puddings as gifts after I had closed the business, and still do today.

My return to nursing in 1992, working as a bank nurse and the learning gained over this time, greatly contributed to extending my knowledge and developing my nursing skills. The learning gained during my time in the A&E department was especially enlightening in terms of dealing with salient issues and my understanding of human behaviour. I am aware that while I may have been a little biased against the discontinuation of the EN training, the subsequent EN conversion to RN status, and a one-degree status, gave nurses an equal opportunity to progress up the professional ladder. For me, the receipt of comments of genuine respect and admiration from senior colleagues for the converted EN was inspiring. Apparently, the converted EN's knowledge, experience and skills, and their ability to transfer these to enhancing patient care make them excellent RNs, a praise indeed, and one with wish I fully concur. I believe that my personal experience of being a patient, combined with the learning gained from the psychodynamic counselling course, enabled a greater insight into my patients, and as such, I was better placed to provide them with care that was more targeted to meeting their individual needs.

Chapter 5 provides an overview of urology nursing that highlights key elements of this field of practice, typically activities within the urology ward and how I contributed to developing practice within the clinical area.

References

BBC News (2019) Boy slept on hospital floor due to lack of beds [Internet]. bbc.co.uk. [cited 2020 Oct 1]. https://www.bbc.co.uk/news/uk-england-leeds-50713236

Francis B, Humphreys J (1999) Enrolled nurses and the professionalisation of nursing: a comparison of nurse education and skill-mix in Australia and the UK. Int J Nurs Stud 36(2):127–135. [cited 2020 Oct 2] [Internet] https://linkinghub.elsevier.com/retrieve/pii/S0020748999000061

NHS Employers (2019) Violence against staff [Internet]. nhsemployers.org. [cited 2019 Nov 2]. https://www.nhsemployers.org/~/media/Employers/Publications/Violence against staff.pdf

Shrestha S (2011) Auscultatory gap in hypertension [internet]. Medchrome. [cited 2020 Oct 20]. https://medchrome.com/basic-science/physiology/auscultatory-gap-hypertension/

Urology is defined as the branch of medicine concerned with the study of the anatomy, physiology and pathology of the urinary tract, and the care of diseases of the urinary tract of men and women (Nursing Explorer 2019). This field of practice is divided into two parts: management of diseases that are of the benign (noncancerous) pathology and diseases of malignant (cancerous) pathology (urooncology). This tumour site consists of five tumours, bladder, prostate, kidney, testicular and penile *(Fig. 5.1 … to be redrawn)*. Management of these cancers involves the members of the urology multidisciplinary team (UMDT), who work in accordance with standards of practice that aim to ensure quality of services across the UK (National Cancer Action Team et al. 2009).

Fortuitous Find Searching through some of my academic work, I found a diary (in which I detailed most of my journey in the urology ward between 1998 and 2005), a fortuitous find that contributed to a true and accurate recounting of some of the events and experiences during this time.

5.1   1997–2005: Urology Nursing

Having completed 3 years working as a bank EN in various fields of practice, general and cancer, I had more or less decided that urology was the field of practice I would like to specialise in. I commenced working in the urology ward in 1997, initially as a 'D' Grade, RN, bank nurse and then as a permanent member of staff, a role I commenced in September 1998 and following promotion to a senior 'E' Grade Staff Nurse held until July 2005. As illustrated in the following recounting of the events, my journey within this field of practice has been interesting and informative.

While performing my E Grade daily duties, I regularly took over management of the ward, in the absence of the F or G Grade, and provided the appropriate leadership that ensured that patients received the required standard of care and support. I

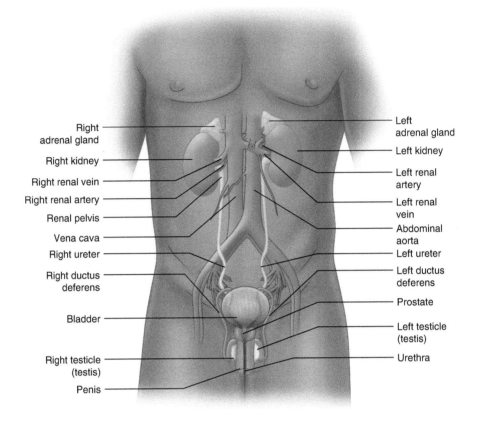

Right adrenal gland — Left adrenal gland

Right kidney — Left kidney

Right renal vein — Left renal artery

Right renal artery — Left renal vein

Renal pelvis — Abdominal aorta

Vena cava — Left ureter

Right ureter — Left ductus deferens

Right ductus deferens — Prostate

Bladder — Left testicle (testis)

Right testicle (testis) — Urethra

Penis

Fig. 5.1 Source: Image © 2003 Fairman Studios, LLC. Jennifer E. Fairman, MA, MPS, CMI, FAMI, Associate Professor. Art as applied to medicine, John Hopkins, School of Medicine. https://medicalart.johnshopkins.edu/fairman/ (Accessed 10 January 2020)

was also responsible for assessing patients, identifying problems and concerns and accordingly liaising with appropriate members of the multidisciplinary teams (MDTs), to secure the best patient outcomes. I believe the manner in which I was required to undertake management of the ward, often at short notice, demonstrated my capabilities and my ability to work with the MDT, under my own initiative.

The Urology Ward The urology ward was a unisex ward that comprised 13 cubicle beds, and a short-stay section that comprised 10 beds. Together, both sections delivered an effective and efficient service to meet the needs of urology patients, cancer and non-cancer. For the 13-bedded section, types of care included the following: for prostate patients: prostate surgeries, such as transurethral resection of the prostate (TURP) (coring out of the prostate) and prostatectomy (removal of the prostate); for bladder patients: transurethral resection of bladder tumour (TURBT) and cystectomies; for kidney patients: nephrectomies, extracorporeal shock wave lithotripsy (ESWL) and percutaneous nephrolithotomy (PCNL); for testicular patients: orchidectomies; and for penile patients: surgery or conservatory management. The short-stay section was meant to operate on 5 days per week, but due to increased patient demand often operated over a 7-day period. This section provided care to patients requiring urological procedures, such as trial without catheter (TWOC), flexible and GA cystoscopies, small TURBT, colonoscopy, endoscopy and endoscopic retrograde cholangiopancreatography (ERCP) (a procedure that combines endoscopy and fluoroscopy to diagnose and treat certain problems of the biliary or pancreatic ductal systems). In my (unbiased) opinion, the level of care provided to these patients, in both sections, was exemplary. The eventual closure of the short-stay section and its consolidation within the main ward had a huge impact (in terms of efficiency) on service delivery.

Our Returnees The title *'Our Returnees'* was the fondly used title to describe patients, who, over the years, had received multiple admissions to the main ward. Admissions usually commenced for tests to confirm a diagnosis or for treatments, or as readmissions, that often ended with their deaths. Based on the many patient feedbacks, it was evident that patients valued the care received during their various admissions. The urology ward was an environment in which long-term friendships and relationships were forged; hence the emotional impact, following a returnee's subsequent death, was upsetting for the family as well as the health professional.

Acknowledging Competency For me, the urology ward was a specialist field of practice, where patients received exemplary care from highly skilled practitioners. These included the ward manager, Bands 6 and 7, Grades F–G; staff nurses, B and 5, Grades D–E; and healthcare assistants, Bands 3–4, whose combined knowledge and experience spanned 20 years or more. In terms of doctors, these included urology consultants, specialist registrars, senior house officers (SHOs) and junior house officers. My memories of this time are of doctors joining the team as junior doctors, SHOs, registrars or consultants. Some SHOs left and then returned as registrars or consultants, while some left and took up posts at other Trusts. In terms of experience, some of the more senior consultants have been with the Trust for a number of years and are still in post today: such loyalty, or perhaps they genuinely enjoy the job!

Team members included other health professionals (HCPs) such as allied health professionals: physiotherapists, occupational therapists, speech therapists and discharge coordinators. Individual's knowledge and expertise were an integral part of supporting nursing staff within the clinical area. One such HCP was a member of the acute pain team, the pain CNS, who, through working closely with nurses in the urology ward, delivered weekly updates for staff on the efficacy of pain control and on how to use the machines. Other teaching sessions included catheterisation (mainly for female patients), which was delivered by the UCNS (JP) and other senior members of the nursing team. Male catheterisation is a specialist procedure, for which the appropriate training must be undertaken. In terms of acknowledging competency, I remember clearly the specific moment when recognition was given to the urology nurses by one of the senior consultants. In this moment, concerns were raised by a senior registrar, in regard to a senior nurse's decision for a urology patient. The consultant's response to this concern was refreshing. He told the registrar that he had full confidence in all the senior urology nurses, specifically in their competence, expertise and their decision-making skills. The consultant had further suggested that if a senior nurse raised concerns in regard to a patient's health, or their plan of care, then doctors should listen to these nurses, since, in his experience, their assessments are usually correct. Praise indeed, and quite a morale boost! It should be noted that as senior nurses, the decisions we made were incumbent on knowledge and experience of the urology field of practice that which had been supported by relevant guidance, including those that had been made by the consultants themselves.

Nevertheless, there were times when acknowledging competency required a subtle nudge. Having worked as a Band 5, 'D' Grade RN for over 2 years, and acquiring the necessary skills to support our role, my colleague (JC), another Band 5 RN, and I concluded that we were working above our pay grade. In fact, we frequently worked at Band 6/7 grades, but without the recognition or the pay to support this. At the very least, we deserved to be promoted to 'E' Grade status, and as such made the decision to raise this with the management. However, being a little nervous, JC suggested that I raised the issue and that she would support me. On approaching the lead manager at the time, and explaining our thoughts on promotion, she suggested that we take this up with our line manager, which I did. To our knowledge, there was only one 'E' Grade post available, a fact that I was unhappy about, as we both deserved promotions. On approaching the line manager, I stated my concern (about the 'E' Grade post), and suggested that if there was only one post, we should both share it—essentially, each working half as a Band 5, 'D' Grade and half as an 'E' Grade. At this suggestion, my line manager smiled, and said that she would keep it in mind. We were both subsequently offered interviews, following which we were both offered an 'E' Grade post. On further exploration, it was revealed that our line manager was aware that we were working above 'D' Grade status, and would have offered us both 'E' Grade posts. After that, JC and I were like 'Bim and Bam'. A few months after I obtained the MUCNS post, she was also promoted to a job share role on the benign side, working with the 'G' Grade Urology CNS, at Band 6 level—later upgraded to Band 7. We continued to work in urology, JC on the benign side and me on the cancer side, with our paths overlapping as necessary. As I was about to embark on my final journey, JC obtained her next promotion as an advanced nurse practitioner. Long may she continue to enjoy her work.

Complementary Learning Urology nursing is a field of practice that is highly committed to learning. During my time in the urology ward (1998–2003), this included the weekly teaching sessions that enabled urology doctors to present relevant topics of interest, and the 2-monthly audit seminars that were often supported by drug company representatives. These sessions were organised by the urology CNS (UCNS) (JP), and were attended by available members of the UMDT, including nurses, who were given the opportunity to present their own topics of interest. In my case, this was the presentation of the outcomes from various AUR audit undertakings, including the devising of the AUR Pathway and its implementation in the A&E department in 2003, as well as the presentation of the outcomes from the bladder cancer audit in 2006. As I remember, everyone valued these sessions and their contribution to enhancing urology practice and the care provided to these patients.

Mentoring and Preceptorship The completion of the ENB 998 course with the EN Flexible Conversion Course and the Preceptorship Package enabled me to honour my mentoring and preceptorship responsibilities within the clinical area to students and colleagues. My recollections of these sessions highlight positive interactions between students, colleagues and mentor (me). Students felt supported in an environment that was both non-threatening and conducive to achieving their learning objectives. Integral to this had been a conscious effort on my part in ensuring that I was respectful of the individual's feelings and concerns, and that their experiences were based not only on theory but also on practice; hence an appropriate balance between theory and hands-on activities was crucial. The completion of the EN Conversion Course placed emphasis on the recording of the patient's vital signs, and the activity's importance in raising the health professional's awareness of worrying red flags, specifically those related to the recording of the blood pressure, an importance I proceeded to share with my colleagues and students within the clinical area.

In this context, reflection is related to a student whom I was mentoring and her acquired learning during our interaction with one particular patient, a gentleman in his late 70s. After we assisted this gentleman to have a wash, we proceeded to transfer him into the armchair by his bed …, an action that resulted in him having a stroke, and consequently in his return to his bed. Needing to test the theory, and in an attempt to explain to the student what occurred, I proceeded to record his vital signs: blood pressure, pulse and respirations. From my interpretation of these, I was able to explain to the student where the change in the blood pressure (the exact time of the stroke) occurred, as well as explain changes in the pulse rate, oxygen levels and respiration rates and what these meant. In this instance, it was good to be able to link the theory to practice.

Providing the appropriate support for the newly qualified nurse, or a new member of the team, was, and still is, important to enabling a constructive period of adjustment within the clinical area. Crucial to this support is acknowledgement of the individual's competence and skills, and enabling them to practice in a way that boosts their confidence and self-esteem. The completion of the preceptorship training package enabled me to effectively deliver this support.

Evidence of Patients' Appreciation I remember that the Trust's effort to improve the care provided to cancer patients had resulted in the development of the oncology ward to accommodate those patients at the end stage of their cancer journey. One such patient was Mrs. M, an Italian lady in her early 80s, with end-stage renal cancer. However, while Mrs. M met the criteria for transfer to the oncology ward, convincing her to do so was difficult, since she had genuine fears, ones that had been borne out of acute anxiety, and of not knowing the ward, or the nurses, to whose care she would be entrusted. As a result, she strongly refused the transfer, and stated her wish to remain with us in the urology ward, a wish that was granted. However, during this period, Mrs. M became more fearful and anxious, and because she did not wish to be alone had frequently requested that a nurse stayed with her, which was not an easy task considering how busy the ward was. Sadly, Mrs. M's condition deteriorated quite rapidly, and she died a few days later. Of course, we had similar experiences with other patients, and while it was flattering that they wanted to stay with us, the fact that most would have been with us for a while (perhaps from the early stages of their diagnosis, and would have returned to the ward several times before the end stage of their illness), the emotional impact for those nurses involved in their care over this time was usually significant.

Another poignant memory is of a lady who, in her early 50s, was admitted to the ward for assessment and tests, which sadly confirmed a diagnosis of metastatic kidney cancer. She was in the ward only for a short time, but the suddenness and the severity of the diagnosis were alarming for her, and especially her husband, who understandably was devastated by the news, especially as she did not get the chance to return home again. The news was also extremely sad for the nurses and the doctors. In that moment, life, and the fear of losing it, was greatly heightened.

Kidney Stones Interestingly, as I reflect back on the early years in the urology ward, kidney cancer had been the most significant occurrence. However, there were other problems, such as kidney stones, for which the classic presentation is acute renal colic. The classic symptom of a patient presenting with acute renal colic is the sudden onset of severe pain, which comes in waves and usually lasts between 20 and 60 min. Pain normally originates in the flank and radiates along the side of the body, between the hips and ribs, or in lower abdomen and finally spreads to groin. At least 50% of patients will also have nausea and vomiting. The treatments of choice for kidney stones are percutaneous nephrolithotomy (PCNL), extracorporeal shock wave lithotripsy (ESWL) procedures and effective pain management (Persad 2021).

5.1.1 Case Study

Mr. Howard was a pleasant gentleman who was in his early 40s. He had suffered with kidney stones (of which he was apparently a frequent maker) for some years. He was married with two children, and had been employed during this time. Mr. Howard had been a regular admission over several years (a true returnee), with acute renal colic, a condition that not only impacted his quality of life, but also had a marked effect on his family and his work.

Reflection on Mr. Howard's numerous admissions vividly highlights moments of pain, distress and increasing discomfort that had been evident in his body language: the grimace of face and eyes tightly shut, tensed body, sweating, shaking and tears. There was also his wife's evident distress. I can still visualise her sitting by her husband's bed, holding his hand, tears in her eyes, as she openly stated her fears regarding the impact of this condition on both their and their children's lives. I remember Mr. and Mrs. Howard's many discussions with the urologists regarding surgery, and their ensuing reluctance in view of his age, but now, because of the increasing impact on his quality of life, whether removal of the kidney would be in his best interest. On Mr. Howard's final admission to the ward, his symptoms were more severe, and consequently more difficult to control. It was now apparent that removal of the kidney was the best way forward. Surgery was extremely successful. Mr. Howard's recovery was uneventful, and his quality of life much improved. He was discharged home with subsequent follow-up maintained on an outpatient's basis. I must admit that I was happy with this outcome; it was difficult seeing Mr. Howard in so much pain.

Developing and Extending Skills I realised very early on in my nursing career that to be an efficient and competent practitioner in today's nursing, I must take steps to ensure that my knowledge and skills kept pace with current policies, procedures and practice guidance. This included the acquisition of practical and theoretical skills that enabled me to function efficiently within the clinical area. In terms of urology nursing, these skills included:

- Intravenous (IV) drug administration.
- Venepuncture.
- Venous cannulation.
- Male catheterisation.
- Bladder scanning.
- Digital rectal examination.
- Intra-vesical (directly into the urinary bladder) administration of cytotoxic drugs, i.e. chemotherapy, mitomycin C and immunotherapy, Bacillus Calmette-Guérin (BCG), MUCNS role.

These skills, combined with the previously obtained recording of a 12-lead electrocardiogram, enabled me to operate in a wider role than described in my job description, and consequently in the performance of my nursing duties, I was a more effective and efficient practitioner.

Socialising Over the years, I had come to appreciate the team-building exercises, of which the social interactions had been hugely enjoyable. In the early years (1998–2005), my memory of the yearly Christmas socialising events (a thank you for all our hard work), aptly entitled the 'Grange years', was particularly enjoyable. With its relaxed ambience, music, dancing, interaction, laughter and evident sense of fun, this had been a hugely popular venue. Granted, the food could have been more exciting, a fact that had been highlighted by one particular team member, who described the roast beef as if 'eating leather'. Nonetheless (for some), the drinks and the atmosphere had been a reasonable recompense. These yearly socialising events had continued, and are still ongoing today, although, in my estimation, none had incited the same sense of fun or feelings of belonging as did the Grange years.

Implications of the Trust's Merger The chief objective of the merger of the Trust in 1999 was to deliver a more robust service within the hospital group and in the wider community. My memory of this merger highlights change that impacted services and nurses' working patterns. In terms of care delivery, the urology ward had been on the same level, and located directly opposite the urology theatres, a fact that had been instrumental in facilitating ease of access and improved efficiency in service delivery. However, following the Trust's merger, services within the surgical field were reconfigured. This included the urology ward being merged with the main surgical ward and becoming the main centre for the admission of all surgical patients (orthopaedic, general surgery and urology). This was a change that I believe had impacted the quality and standard of care delivered to urology patients. As previously noted, the urology teams provided exemplary care to patients that which had been based on competency and expertise.

It was soon evident that while the nurses from the surgical ward were highly skilled in this specific field of practice, in terms of urology practice and performance of certain procedures (e.g. caring for those patients who were having a bladder irrigation, following transurethral resection of bladder tumour (TURBT) or transurethral resection of prostate (TURP)), this was less evident. Admittedly, the team eventually acquired the necessary expertise, but I believe that in some ways, the quality and standard of care received by urology patients, prior to the wards being merged, were never the same again.

Changes to Practice As time went by, this practice changed again. Further reconfiguration of urology practice had seen the service being moved to various venues within the hospital, but with the elective part of the service being transferred to the Trust's second main hospital, from where all patients accessed care, regardless of where they lived. Over time, the remaining hospitals and outpatients' outlets within the group were closed, with services being integrated in the urology sections, within the two main hospitals. This resulted in a significant increase in cross-site working: a requirement of the MUCNS role, with which I gladly complied for 13 years. However, due to the aforementioned changes in ways of working and how services had been reconfigured, the decision was made to permanently move my base to the Trust's second main hospital, a change that incited some resentment on my part, since I had no choice in the decision.

Consolidation of Services The consolidation of services on specific sites resulted in changes in nurse-led services. For many years, the nurse-led delivery of cytotoxic treatments was made from a central location in one of the Trust's hospitals, but was later moved to another location and venue within the first main hospital, and finally to its current venue, in the urology centre in the second main hospital. It was felt that consolidating this service on the same site and location would provide a more robust service. Unfortunately, this change was not embraced by all patients. Most were opposed to the idea of travelling to yet another hospital (albeit in the same Trust), unless, of course, they lived in the area and locality. For some patients, the issue of a prior negative experience at this hospital (combined with the evident variations in travelling time and distance) clouded their judgement and hence their reluctance to move. In some respect, this merger was advantageous. However, based on my subsequent observations of practice, I would argue that in terms of patients and employees, the benefits were not equally distributed across hospitals. This merger incited some resistance from nurses, myself included, who felt that the change had been instigated without due consideration being given to their feelings, or indeed how this would impact their working life. Perhaps, I was resistant to these changes, because I missed the old ways of working.

Work-Based Learning (WBL) Exercises Since joining the urology team in 1998, as a senior staff nurse, I completed a number of WBL activities, which included the devising of supportive practice information, the first of which was the trial without catheter (TWOC) leaflet (*Appendix B*). This leaflet was devised to provide information to patients who were having their catheter-removed post-surgical outcomes or episodes of urinary retention. The leaflet explained what a TWOC was, why the procedure was necessary, the protocol following the TWOC and what would occur if the patient failed the TWOC. Between May 2001 and September 2001, I completed the urology course (ENB 978) which enabled me a greater understanding of the problems associated with catheterisation, catheters, urinary drainage systems, catheter valves, urinary tract infection (UTI) and healthcare professional's role in the overall management. From this course, I had written 'the management of patients with an indwelling urethral catheter' assignment. I also formulated the Catheter Valve (*just a useful device?*) (*Appendix II)* and the management of patients with an indwelling urethral catheter document, both of which were widely used within the clinical area, as a resource to complement both colleagues and student nurses' learning.

In July 2002, my mentor (JP) suggested that an evaluation of the proposals made in the Catheter Valve document and the findings from the management of patients with an indwelling urethral catheter assignment be carried out, but that this should provide a broader view to further assess the choice and use of catheters, drainage systems and catheter valve. An audit entitled '*are we providing patients who are admitted to the A&E department in urinary retention with the most appropriate drainage systems?*' was visualised. The audit was to be undertaken in two parts: the first audit to monitor how many patients presented to A&E with urinary retention and added complications, and determine whether change was needed in this area of practice. The second audit was to implement the findings from the first audit. Having established that a protocol was needed to manage patients who presented to the A&E department with acute urinary retention (AUR), the first audit commenced in August 2002 and ran until January 2003, with a total of 20 patients being admitted to the A&E department in AUR during this time. The audit outcomes had led to the development of the AUR Pathway (*refer to* Fig. 5.2, *page 116*).

Working in collaboration with members of the multidisciplinary teams, I led the development of a management pathway, of which a laminated A3 format was subsequently implemented in the A&E department on first September 2003. An audit following the Pathway's implementation was presented at the urology seminar on 19th September 2003, with subsequent monitoring and re-auditing occurring during this period. A re-audit of the Pathway and the results was presented at the Urology Audit Seminar in 2004. This was a completely new experience for me, and since I had not attended an audit before, or presented anything in front of a large audience, I was extremely nervous. In hindsight, I could have done better, but seemingly, what I did was okay. The consultants and doctors were very supportive. They felt that everyone did extremely well, and that we should all be very proud. Following this presentation, the A&E representatives requested a leaflet to provide information to patients on their presentation to the A&E department with AUR. As a result, I developed (in conjunction with the team) the AUR leaflet and contacted the Regional Manager at Bard Limited (now Bard Medical UK, a leader in urology and continence care), who agreed to print the leaflet.

Again, with the support of the UCNS (JP), I also devised a 'pocket-size' version of the AUR Pathway. This comprised 'the *Pathway*' on one side, and the words '*Acute Urinary Retention, Think Pathway*' on the other. The intention of this

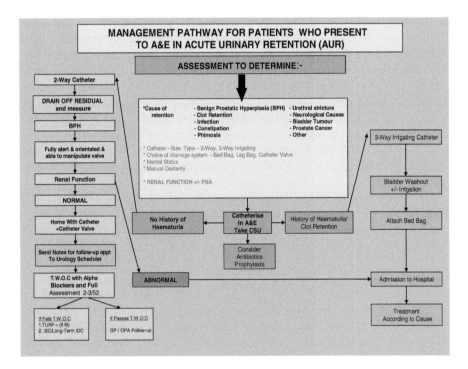

Fig. 5.2 The AUR pathway

pathway was to prompt junior doctors to utilise it, when assessing and treating patients who presented to the A&E department with AUR. For teaching purposes, the urology consultants requested A4 and pocket-size versions of the pathway, both of which were laminated for practicality. This pathway was used in the development of a poster by the clinical auditor, which was accepted for entry into the Clinical Institute of Excellence competition in 2004. Although it did not win, it did receive some encouraging feedback.

Lessons Learnt   Since I had not undertaken an audit before, I quickly realised that something which was meant to be a fairly straightforward exercise was actually quite intricate. I have learnt that in the undertaking and implementation of change into practice, to obtain successful outcomes, it is important to acknowledge all of the relevant individuals involved in the task and ensure that they are all consulted, but more importantly that their feelings and opinions are taken on board and respected.

Publication   In appreciation of my efforts with this audit, I was encouraged by one of the senior urology consultants to consider publishing my work. Flattered by another suggestion to publish my work, I proceeded to write, in conjunction with my colleague at the time, my second article and second publication, entitled Acute Urinary Retention: Developing an A&E Management Pathway (Anderson and Khadra 2006).

Accreditation of Prior Experiential Learning (AP(E)L) Study   In 2003, I was encouraged by my then line manager (YM) to AP(E)L my previously undertaken WBL studies to diploma level II. This involved getting in contact with the university's head of AP(E)L studies, the lecturer whom I had subsequently met to identify study options and their suitability for AP(E)L. From 1998 to 2005 I completed a number of WBL projects, modules and learning packages towards obtaining the Diploma of Higher Education Nursing (Dip. H.E. Nursing) in Development in Healthcare Practice, which was awarded in May 2005. These included the following:

Set modules:
- The promotion of continence and the management of incontinence (ENB 978).
- The management of patients with bladder and bowel dysfunctions.
- An introduction to the understanding of research methods in healthcare.

AP(E)L projects
- A reflection on the foundation and diploma in psychodynamic counselling.
- A reflection on a current practice and the issues relating to this practice—which included my reflection on assessment, catheterisation and use of urinary drainage systems in relation to the management of patients who presented to the A&E department with acute urinary retention (AUR).

- The role of patient-focused assessment in continence care.
- Urinary catheterisation: a reflective account.

5.1.2 First AP(E)L WBL Assignment

The first WBL activity to be in the AP(E)L was the psychodynamic counselling course, which was undertaken in 1996–1997. This was a reflective exercise that enabled me to update the course from certificate level to diploma level II status. The initial number of credits at diploma level was 15, but following submission and subsequent review of assignment (which included 1 case study), I was offered the opportunity to increase to 30 credits (if I increased the number of case studies to 2). This was a challenge that I fully embraced, and for which I received the promissory 30 credits. Professionally, the learning gained from this course has proven hugely beneficial to improving my future practice in terms of my patients and my colleagues, and personally in terms of my parents, my children and me. The following assignment is illustrated in full and in real time:

5.2   Reflective Essay on Foundation and Diploma in the Psychodynamic Counselling Course 1996–1997

My name is Beverley Anderson and I am a staff nurse currently working on a 13-bedded urology ward. The work is interesting, and on the whole rewarding, but very stressful at times. This essay is a reflective account of the entitled course, based on what motivated me to do the course, how knowledge and skills gained subsequently helped me to develop personally and professionally and whether counselling has changed since completion of the course.

In January 1996 I completed the Enrolled Nurse Flexible Conversion Course. I found the course intensive but challenging and the knowledge gained informative. My nursing skills and practice extended and developed, and the intense studying 'whetted' my appetite to acquire more knowledge. I had at this time been working nights for 2 years, in a very busy 20-bedded surgical ward. The work consisted mostly of patients with carcinoma of the bowel, requiring corrective colorectal surgery. Informing these patients that they had carcinoma could be devastating and psychologically overwhelming. I needed to understand or at least try to understand the impact such news had on these patients, for although I acknowledged their devastation, I was inexperienced in my attempts to offer them constructive support. I discussed my concerns with a friend, who suggested that counselling could be beneficial, so I enrolled on the Foundation and Diploma Course in Psychodynamic Counselling. The course was intended to help the student develop fundamental counselling skills and enhanced interpersonal skills, and in so doing develop an understanding of counselling theory and practice, and human growth and development from a psychodynamic perspective. The course enabled me to explore the dynamics of the individual's behaviour, in particular how experiences commencing from conception and ending with death affected coping abilities throughout their lives.

Psychoanalytic theory is the derivative of psychoanalysis, a theory of human behaviour. Sigmund Freud, the founder of psychoanalytic theory, based his findings upon the unconscious, specifically the role of unconscious processes as motivators of behaviour, hence the presumption that early experiences are the causes of later behaviours (Reber 1995). These early experiences are referred to as object relations (ORs), which Melanie Klein suggests are the drives and accompanying feelings which link the self to the object, in this situation, the mother and her baby. According to Noonan (Noonan 1983), early OR experiences denote a strong emotional bond between the mother and her baby and are formulated on the baby's need for food and safety. These are provided by the mother's breast and her arms and are the main source of his/her survival. The experiences gained from these relations are theoretically seen as either good or bad. Good object relations are supposedly formulated on the concept that when the baby cries, the mother responds by feeding him/her with milk from her breast to appease his/her hunger, while holding him/her lovingly in her arms, allowing him/her to feel safe, secure and loved. Such an experience is believed to enable the baby to relate to future experiences in later life with happy thoughts. If the opposite response were true, i.e. the baby cries, but there is no mother with breast/milk to appease his/her hunger, and no loving arms to hold him/her, then supposedly he/she would not feel safe, secure and loved, and referral back to this experience in later life would fill him/her with dread.

Various studies (Noonan 1983; Klein 1987; Winnicott 1991) have proven that the experiences gained from early OR relationships between the mother and her baby formed the foundation to all future experiences, and are essential to the baby's development. The more favourable these experiences are, the more effective will be the baby's ability to cope with changes that are presented throughout the stages of his/her development, i.e. adolescence, midlife, old age and death. Melanie Klein stated that successful working through experiences in the early years involved some negotiation between the paranoid-schizoid and depressive positions. These positions provide alternate ways of dealing with anxiety, and are likely to be used throughout life whenever stress arose. In the paranoid-schizoid position, the absence of the good breast/mother is experienced as the presence of a bad and frightening one, which is why feelings of paranoia and the defence 'splitting' (separating good and bad experiences) emerge (Noonan 1983). A person may use 'splitting' to avoid conflict, by separating good and bad feelings, which belong together within oneself and another.

Counselling is an alternative way of working through the problems that are presented throughout the individual's life. The process involves consultation and discussion between two individuals, one of whom (the counsellor) offers advice of guidance to the other (the client), helping to identify and clarify problems while providing support as the client makes adjustments to overcome or come to terms with them (Blackwell 1994). According to Noonan (Noonan 1983), each individual is the product and author of their own particular history and is therefore active in contributing to its shape and form. The psychodynamic approach to counselling therefore is to help the client to get in touch with their feelings and to make sense of their experiences (Cube 1997).

From a psychoanalytic perspective, and in terms of what was gained from the course, how has a knowledge and understanding of ORs helped in relation to myself, my parents, my children and my patients?

Myself The relationship with my parents during puberty and adolescence was turbulent in nature, and as such had continued well into adulthood. Up to the age of 12, I was fortunate to have had a happy relationship with my parents. Sadly, the relationship between us changed, and I went from feeling loved and nurtured to feeling bitter and unloved. My parents' change in behaviour was the cause of much confusion and distress, and consequently my indifference to them. I also came to believe that I did not need them in my life. To cope with my situation, I inadvertently instigated the defence 'splitting', which is where I changed my perception of my parents, recognising only the bad aspects in them. There were times, however, when my memory of our relationship brought back happy times, but was also too painful to deal with, in the realisation of what I had lost. To keep the pain away, I maintained a negative perception of my parents. This 'splitting' continued until we were reunited some years later. The course enabled me to work through early experiences of my childhood, and examine subsequent behaviours between my parents and myself. I was able to integrate the good as well as the bad memories and come to see my parents as 'more whole'. Eventually, I was able to resolve the conflict between us and return to having a more meaningful relationship. In fact, my relationship with my parents was one of the factors for acceptance on the course.

My Parents By becoming more open and honest in my understanding of past experiences with my parents I was able to work through my emotions. I finally understood that they were only humans, and as such were prone to make mistakes. I also realised that they were 'pretty' good parents, who had in fact provided me with good experiences from our early relationships. Perhaps, my turbulent and erratic behaviour was too much for them to handle, and changing their behaviour towards me was the only way they could cope. By allowing myself to remember the happy as well as the sad memories, and accepting that both perceptions should be integrated, I had worked through the turbulence of adolescence, and was finally ready to have a more adult and mature relationship with my parents. My current relationship with my parents is one of balance and mutual understanding.

My Children Adolescence covers the years between 12 and 13 for early adolescence and 20 and 21 for late adolescence. It is the period in which the adolescent is experiencing and resolving turbulence which is set into action by the biological process of puberty. When I started the course, my two eldest children, both boys aged 12 and 13, were entering the throws of puberty and adolescence, and changes in their behaviour had begun. According to Erickson (Erickson 1985), profound changes are manifested in adolescence. The adolescent's behaviour stems from the paranoid-schizoid position; hence his/her behaviour could reflect strong emotional upheaval and could quite often be irrational and unpredictable. In view of this, the adolescent's relationship between he/she and his/her parents could be stressful, because at this time it is a reflection of his/her emotional state and the confusion he/she feels inside. The adolescent's survival of this stage of his/her development would now be highly dependent on his/her initial OR experiences, and having the opportunity to freely express the turmoil he/she feels inside. Erickson (Erickson 1985) further suggested that although the adolescent's behaviour towards his/her parents may be irrational and unpredictable, what he/she needs at this time is reassurance that his/her parents will be able to withstand it, and continue to provide him/her with unfailing love and support. Erickson's comments were explicit, and had accurately depicted my children's behaviour. In addition, he had clearly defined my role in this situation to provide my children with love and support throughout this changeable time.

It is nearly 6 years on since I completed the course, and my children, now 19 and 20, are approaching the end of adolescence. I have noticed considerable changes in their behaviour, especially of a developing maturity and a regard for other people and their feelings. No doubt they will continue to change, and will do so for some time.

My Patients The knowledge I gained and the skills acquired helped me to develop a better understanding of my patients. I felt less uncomfortable with their grief and more able to offer them emotional support. I can remember soon after completing the course two patients in particular, whom I felt I was able to help.

As previously stated, early OR experiences are interrelated throughout the stages of human growth and development. The stage of life depicted in the following critical incidents is midlife. Midlife commences around the age of 35, the exact period varying among individuals. The process of transition runs for some years and is at full maturity around the age of 65. The stage is often called midlife crisis because death and mortality and a sense of running out of time are its main focus (Hildebrand 1995).

5.3   Case Studies

5.3.1   'Lady in the Dark'

Mrs. Quinn, a lady in her late 30s, had been admitted to the ward for investigations, which confirmed advanced carcinoma of the bowel. She was happily married and had a daughter, 3 years old. This lady had a full life, which included a responsible job she clearly enjoyed. She was informed of the results of her tests with her husband present, during the late afternoon. The results of her tests meant that Mrs. Quinn's life expectancy would suddenly be cut short. She was a lady nearing 40, and perhaps a little too young to be dealing with the crisis of midlife, in particular visions of her impending death and lack of time. The handover report suggested that she took the news well, but appeared to be 'a little quiet' thereafter. Receiving such traumatic news, how she would subsequently cope with the fallout would now depend on her early OR experiences. Instead of looking forward and planning her life, Mrs. Quinn was suddenly faced with viewing her life in terms of quality, rather than quantity, and having to decide how she would spend her remaining time with her family.

It was approximately 2:30 in the morning, and I was checking the patients when I noticed Mrs. Quinn sitting up in bed, awake and a little restless, and all alone in the dark with her 'fears' to keep her company. I went into Mrs. Quinn's cubicle and asked if she was okay. She stated that she was, but I could see that she was not. I asked her if she wanted to talk, which she did. I sat with Mrs. Quinn, and allowed her to talk. I listened while she spoke of her fears for her daughter, of the possibility of her not being there for her as she grows up, and of her feelings of loss of autonomy and her sense of helplessness. At this moment, Mrs. Quinn probably felt that she was a bad mother who was not able to provide her daughter with loving arms to hold her, so that she may feel safe, secure and loved and go on to enjoy good experiences in later life. Being a mother myself, I could empathise with Mrs. Quinn's dilemma, and placed in her position was able to understand the devastation she must have felt, having received such traumatic news, and then to be left alone to cope with the implications. My imagined sense of loss, and threatened loss, initiated deep sadness within me and I needed to reach out to her. Listening to Mrs. Quinn, and providing her with temporary respite from her feelings of loss and despair, was all that I had to offer. I could not reassure her that everything would be okay, because they would not be. Instead, I listened and allowed her to talk. By talking she externalised some of her fears and had taken a small step towards coming to terms with her situation. It would later appear that by listening, while allowing Mrs. Quinn to express herself, I had helped to reassure her in that moment. She wrote back a week later thanking the staff for their help, and especially me, for supporting her during what she described as *'a black moment'* during her time in hospital.

5.3.2 The Pacer'

Mrs. Rowan was a lady in her early 50s and happily married to her second husband. Her first husband, with whom she had two children, both girls, now 18 and 20 years old, had died 9 years earlier from leukaemia. She had lost a sister 2 years previously from carcinoma of the bowel. This lady was admitted for investigations scheduled for the following day into altered bowel habits.

We had just completed handover, the time was approximately 9:45 p.m. and the ward was as ever very busy. I was hurrying to commence the nursing duties when I observed Mrs. R pacing up and down the ward corridor, looking very anxious and fearful. There were only 3 nurses on duty and 20 patients, all needing a great deal of care and attention, so I needed to press on. My first instinct was to ignore Mrs. Rowan, and probably would have prior to the course, but from her given history, and the indicated fear in her eyes, I suspected the reason for her anxiety and needed to reassure her. I approached Mrs. Rowan, invited her to take a seat and asked what was troubling her. At first, she was reluctant to speak to me, and had suggested that I was busy and she did not want to disturb my work, but I insisted. As she began to speak, she slowly burst into tears as she professed her fears regarding her impending tests. Of most significance to her current state of mind were the previous deaths of her first husband and her sister. Mrs. Rowan had convinced herself that she too would be diagnosed with carcinoma of the bowel and that it would result in her death. An understandable assumption because, as Salzberger-Wittenberg (Salzberger-Wittenberg 1970) pointed out, any loss would evoke feelings connected with earlier losses and the threat of future ones. Feelings of paranoia and persecution, life and death experiences and loss of control, all characteristics of midlife and the paranoid-schizoid position, would also have contributed to Mrs. Rowan's state of mind. Such feelings, according to Josephine Klein, are instigated in an attempt to bring about an adequate appeasement to the present crisis of life (Segal 1992).

Mrs. Rowan was worried about leaving her husband, but her biggest worry focused on her daughters and their possible loss of another parent while they were still so young. Feelings of guilt, and the presumption that 'she was not quite the good enough mother', coupled with her sense of failing them, prevailed. As I listened to and observed Mrs. Rowan, it was obvious that her present problem stemmed from her underlying fear of dying and a situation which she felt powerless to overcome. Mrs. Rowan had obviously worked over the possible implications to her life if her tests were to prove positive for carcinoma and in her doing so had indicated her need to be reassured that those things could change. Prior experiences of death demanded that she faced up to her own death and its implication on her family. By incorporating questioning skills learnt in the course, and utilising specific 'open' and 'closed' questions, which included prompting and probing cues, I was able to make Mrs. Rowan see that her situation was not completely futile. I allowed her to identify the cause of her problem and possible ways in which it could be resolved, in her case coming to terms with her present situation. If she did have carcinoma, there was always a possibility that it would be operable. By interjecting hope, I allowed Mrs. Rowan to visualise an alternative outcome to her situation, extended time and a life with her family. Whatever the outcome, her family would survive and continue to live their lives.

I spent almost 30 min sitting and listening to Mrs. Rowan, and while her fears and anxieties may not have been entirely abated, she seemed less anxious and fearful. Mrs. Rowan later thanked me for listening to her; I had apparently helped to reassure her. She was however surprised, because past experiences of hospitals had led her to believe that nurses, because they were so busy, did not have the time to listen to their patients. Her statement made me more aware of why listening to patients was such an important part of my daily nursing duties.

5.3.3   How Has Counselling Changed since my Completion of the Course?

From recent discussions with two practicing counsellors, one of whom uses the humanistic approach and the other psychodynamic, it was agreed that from a Freudian perspective, counselling used to be very analytical in terms of it being geared more towards the middle classes, and can still be. In their view, counselling has become more accessible and is therefore more acceptable. They have also stated that with education, and the availability of more types of therapy and different schools of thought, people from different ethnic groups and classes over the last 10 years are more open to seek counselling. Some of the stigma has been broken down, and people realise that there is another way to resolve their ongoing problems and deal with the stresses and strains of modern-day living apart from 'popping pills'. Counsellors have further suggested that doctors (i.e. general practitioners) are aware that counselling, as an alternative form of therapy, can be effective. In appropriate situations, GPs see counselling as a first choice of treatment rather than a last resort, and are more likely to recommend its use instead of conventional treatments such as antidepressants or sleeping pills. In support of this statement, there is evidence to show that some GPs' surgeries are now employing counsellors as part of their team to provide alternative therapy for their patients (Waterlow 2001). When I asked for their views regarding counselling in relation to other cultures/countries, counsellors agree that counselling is more likely to be regarded as an acceptable and constructive alternative; moreover, such an approach would greatly reduce the level of stigma associated with its use. They also suggested that counselling courses were now more widely available and affordable to those wanting to undertake the training.

5.4   Conclusion and Lessons Learnt

In the urology field there is prevalence of patients diagnosed with carcinomas. Some of these patients die soon after they are admitted, while others receive treatment, but are then readmitted to the ward at various stages throughout their illness. Ultimately attachments are formed, and subsequent deaths are the cause of increased emotional upsets for the relatives, as well as the healthcare professionals involved in their care. Before I commenced the course, I can remember feeling quite uncomfortable at the prospect of approaching these patients, because I did not have the necessary experience or skill to offer them emotional support. However, I have found that by doing this course, and having acquired necessary knowledge and experience, I have been helped to become more holistic in my approach to patient care. Most pertinent to this approach was the knowledge gained of object relations, because it had given me insight into how individual patients coped with problems. My understanding of object relations and their relevance to patient care is that patients have needs (objects). These needs may be physical, psychological, sociological or religious, and their aim is in satisfaction of the impending need. Whether it is to relieve their pain, to listen to their worries or provide them with emotional support, the relations (e.g. the nurse) should respond with the appropriate gratification to satisfy that need. I also believe that time had been expedited, because I became more adept in my assessment of patients, in my communications with and listening to them, and was therefore more capable of providing them with emotional support.

I would recommend that all trained nurses working for any length of time in the urology ward consider undertaking some form of counselling. Not only would this be of benefit to them on a personal level, in terms of coping with stress-related factors within the clinical environment, but it would also provide ongoing support to patients, their relatives and work colleagues. Having knowledge and experience of counselling would also increase efficiency and efficacy in the care provided.

Since undertaking this course in 1997, the knowledge, understanding and experience gained have been utilised throughout my practice, and will continue to be utilised long after my nursing career has ended. Since becoming the Macmillan Uro-Oncology CNS, 14 years ago, a key requirement to performing this role was that I access regular emotional support, in this case clinical supervision. This activity is designed to enable nurses to talk about their practice and to put into context their thoughts in terms of their patients and colleagues, evaluating painful and difficult experiences and coming to terms with ensuing feelings. The belief is that regular clinical supervision enables nurses to be better prepared to support their patients. However, while I have found this activity beneficial, the psychodynamic course has been instrumental in increasing my ability to confidently, and competently, interact with my patients when dealing with their pain, both physical and emotional, to better understand the inherent dilemma of having to cope with a suspicious or actual diagnosis of cancer, and accordingly provide them with the necessary support, one that aspires to meeting their individual needs.

5.4.1 Second AP(E)L Assignment

The second assignment, 'A reflective view on a current practice and issues relating to this practice', was prepared as an AP(E)L claim that was also awarded 30 credits at level 2 status and the outcomes were used for educational purposes by students and colleagues within the clinical area. At the time of undertaking this AP(E)L project I had been a staff nurse in the urology ward for 5 years.

The following is an edited version of the assignment for this project that reported on the previous change project in the development of the AUR Pathway. It also provides an insight into past practice, and how issues such as staff and bed shortages, and other changes, have impacted care delivery and continue to do so today. The full unedited version included a full definition of urinary retention and the various causes, specifically benign prostatic hyperplasia (BPH), benign enlargement of the prostate gland and clot/haematuria. Focus was placed on AUR in the male patient and on BPH and clot/haematuria, as two of the main causes of AUR (Scholtes 2002; Nichani et al. 2017; Anon 2021).

5.5   A Reflective View on a Current Practice, and Issues Relating to this Practice

In urology nursing, bladder dysfunctions are common problems. One of the most common is acute urinary retention (AUR), a state in which the individual is unable to effectively pass urine from the bladder (Scholtes 2002). An effective management of care is required, of which catheterisation is paramount. Catheterisation is a highly invasive procedure and one that is associated with increased risks and implications, especially urinary tract infections (UTIs), estimated to account for approximately 30–40% of hospital-acquired infections, in which the presence of an indwelling urethral catheter is a major factor in their development (Nichani et al. 2017).

Before the decision is taken to catheterise a patient, researchers have strongly recommended that a comprehensive assessment be undertaken to establish patient's suitability for the procedure, and also to plan management of care with them. There is great emphasis on the selection of catheters and choice of drainage systems in the catheterisation process, and this includes the catheter valve. The catheter valve provides an option of drainage, which facilitates intermittent instead of continuous bladder drainage when appropriate. Healthcare professionals, both doctors and nurses, are recognised as having a central role in this process. Most pertinent in that role is their responsibility to utilise evidence-based practice and research, so that they can make decisions and allocate care from an informed basis. Any decision should be made in participation with the patient and the carer, if there is one, and with support from the healthcare professional. Healthcare professionals have a further responsibility to ensure that patients are fully informed of all the issues relating to their catheters and drainage systems, before gaining their consent to undertake the procedure. Any decision should promote the patient's comfort, dignity and an improved quality of life, so patient education is fundamental to the provision of care.

Intermittent catheterisation (IC) provides a practical alternative to an indwelling catheter. It can be a short- or longer term intervention, and can play a part in the management of post-operative urinary retention. Changes in practice meant that there has been an increasing demand for its use, and all appropriate patients who are willing and able should be offered IC. However, there is a need for much more training with junior doctors and nurses prior to its implementation. Intermittent catheterisation and catheter valve are believed to significantly reduce infection (Nichani et al. 2017; Anon 2021) and are more conducive to maintaining bladder health. Bladder health is maintained through the action of intermittently catheterising and removing the urine from the bladder, and the clamping action of the catheter valve that mimics normal voiding, i.e. allowing the bladder to intermittently fill and empty (Anon 2021). However, their use would be heavily subject to the patient's compliance, and their suitability for use (Nichani et al. 2017).

Clinical governance aims to improve the quality and effectiveness in the NHS (Department of Health 1998a). One of these aims is to identify and reduce risks, and catheter management is one area where this can be achieved. Healthcare professionals therefore have a responsibility to be more proactive in their clinical practice, so that potential risks and complications, i.e. urinary tract infections, cross-contamination and allergies, can be prevented or reduced wherever possible. If establishments are to maintain clinical effectiveness, then they must continuously monitor and improve the services they provide. Auditing and benchmarking help them to achieve this goal. Clinical governance and benchmarking are both frameworks through which NHS organisations are accountable for continually improving the quality of and maintaining high standards of care (Department of Health 1998a).

I have been a nurse for many years and throughout this time I have observed and experienced many changes to the nursing profession. When I reflect on the nursing profession today, and compare it to past practice, I realise that the nature of nursing today in hospital environment has become very acute. Over the years there has been an increase in the demand for shorter length of stay in hospital, but with an even greater number of elderly patients being admitted to hospital, and inevitably with more social problems, there is also a greater demand for beds. This situation had been further exacerbated because there are fewer junior doctors being recruited. In addition, there has also been a reduction in the number of hours that junior doctors are able to work to cover shifts, and most are not trained at an appropriate level to meet demands and maintain high standards. I have observed a steady decline in staffing levels and that wards are smaller, but there remains a demand from the government and the public for high standards of care. Consequently, staff are overstretched, stress levels are increased and morale is lower. Nevertheless, patients deserve optimum care, and although this can be an uphill struggle at times, nurses have a responsibility to provide care, at a level which meets their patients' expectations.

I find the urology field of nursing interesting and rewarding. I regularly undertake mentoring of students and teaching of colleagues in the clinical area, and I am highly aware of the way current protocols, policies and procedures are implemented and try to ensure that correct practice is followed. I have always felt that I should increase my knowledge and skills in this area of practice and have undertaken studies to achieve this. In 2001, I completed the ENB 978 Course. The chosen topics for my assignments increased both my knowledge and awareness of the issues relating to managing patients with indwelling catheters, especially the increased risk of urinary tract infections (UTIs) from an indwelling catheter and subsequent urinary drainage systems. I have also developed a better understanding of the catheter valve and of the significant benefits of its use. Having completed the course, I subsequently implemented, with support from my colleagues, the findings and recommendations in the clinical area. I am pleased to report that these implemented changes had been maintained, and overall have substantially improved catheterisation and catheter management, which includes urinary drainage systems. Associated practices, such as handwashing and catheter rounds, have also improved.

I wanted to undertake further studies relating to my field of practice and to monitor the services we provide, and with this in mind I was asked by the urology nurse specialist to carry out an audit on patients who were admitted to the accident and emergency department (A&E) with acute urinary retention (AUR). The aim of the audit was to determine whether AUR patients were provided with the appropriate urinary drainage system. To monitor these patients, I devised an audit tool, with the appropriate criteria for audit, and these forms were completed on the patient's admission to the ward. A prospective audit was undertaken between August 2002 and January 2003. A total of 20 patients were included in the audit. The first analysis of audit results indicated that many of the criteria listed on audit forms had not been recorded, so medical notes were retrieved as appropriate. However, retrieved notes highlighted areas of inadequate documentation, necessary for the completion of audit forms. Most noticeable was incomplete information pertaining to the catheterisation process. Assessment notes were not always legible to provide clear guidelines for implementing care, and were often not timed or dated. The final analysis showed that of these 20 patients, only 4 (20%) passed their trial without catheter (TWOC), compared to 8 (40%) who failed their TWOC. The overall conclusion suggested that a majority of patients who presented to A&E in AUR met the criteria for discharge home, but were instead admitted to hospital.

These results suggested that A&E and junior urology doctors would benefit from updated information on the management of patients requiring catheterisation, and particularly patients in AUR. The ever-increasing shortages of beds and the constant struggle to meet NHS targets meant that establishments need to identify areas that are in need of improvements and take steps to increase efficiency. To help me get my information across I formulated a poster entitled 'Proposed Management Pathway for Patients Who Present to A&E in Acute Urinary Retention' (AUR) (Fig. 5.2). The pathway was designed with the specific intention of providing guidance to HCPs especially junior doctors in the A&E department, to become more focused when planning care for patients who present to them in AUR. The main emphasis was placed on assessment, by stating its vital importance prior to the implementation of subsequent care. The pathway was also meant to re-enforce the way protocol for care was implemented, and from which optimum results could be achieved. This pathway is meant to provide guidance only; a protocol still needs to be written.

The following reflective account illustrates how I examined issues related to the causes of AUR, catheterisation and management of patients in AUR. I also examine the necessity for a comprehensive assessment, highlighting the risks of infection, selection of catheters and urinary drainage systems that are available, and advantages and disadvantages of their use, and also the nurses' and doctors' involvement in that selection.

In my experience of nursing urology patients with bladder dysfunctions, I have noticed that the patients who develop AUR usually present to the A&E department, either by their general practitioner's referral or on their own initiative. Patients are then assessed, and if appropriate admitted to the ward. The cause of retention is more often than not due to clot/haematuria, which is a condition indicating bleeding from the urinary tract and where clots are formed as bleeding occurs, or due to an enlarged prostate, which is usually the result of a history of benign prostatic hyperplasia (BPH).

The writing of this essay has been educational. This was my first audit, and the first time I had formulated a care pathway, and I found the experience enlightening. I have come to appreciate clinical auditing, and have been made more aware of its importance to the monitoring and improvement of services. Formulating the care pathway was both rewarding and challenging, and it had given me the opportunity to work closely with other team members. The drafted pathway was shown to consultants, members of the medical team, ward colleagues and significant others to obtain feedback. This exercise was very time consuming. The changes took much longer than anticipated, as it was difficult to track down colleagues and nursing staff. Even so, I believed that it was important and necessary to obtain all relevant perspectives. There was overall agreement with the design and input for the pathway, but many changes were suggested. These subsequently improved the poster format, and contributed to the formulation of a constructive teaching tool. However, this project has taught me a valuable lesson, which is when undertaking new projects to manage change, I must never overlook or underestimate those individuals whose views and opinions may become relevant to the project. As pointed out by Broome (Broome 1990), the first step in any change project is to be certain that there is agreement on the core purpose among the most significant people.

Once the final draft of the pathway was completed, I contacted A&E and advised them of my intention to undertake a teaching session with them. This however was met with some dissatisfaction, because I had not involved the staff in A&E in the formulation of the pathway from the onset. This was not intentional, but had nevertheless generated some dissatisfaction. According to Haffer (Haffer 1986), when initiating change, the approach taken should allow the person(s) undergoing the change to participate in identifying the problem, choosing the solutions and implementing the change. This is a wise statement, because I soon came to realise that people get very offended, if they are of the opinion that their views were deliberately excluded in the proposal of a project, for which their help would subsequently be required to implement. Andrews (Andrews 1993) stated, 'openness is a prerequisite to any change, and every individual involved in the change should have access to all available information so that informed decisions can be made. This strategy may be time consuming but as the objective is to change beliefs or attitudes, it may be the most effective and therefore worth the time invested'. The original idea to draft this pathway was meant to provide A&E staff with updated information and guidance for practice, and attempt to increase the efficacy in the way current care was provided to AUR patients. However, in hindsight, doctors agreed that perhaps it would be advantageous if A&E staff were able to undertake, in its entirety, the assessment and implementation of care to these patients when appropriate. I subsequently met with a consultant from A&E and showed him the proposed draft of the pathway, and after discussions a few changes were made. At first, I was disappointed with this setback, but ultimately, wiser to the rules of bureaucracy, regarded it as a valuable learning curve. These changes were incorporated, and on my second meeting with the consultant, the pathway received full approval and, as it would seem, admiration. I then met with the matron who also demonstrated an eagerness to get things moving, as she felt that updated information would be vital.

The teaching session on the pathway was undertaken on eighth August 2003. This went extremely well, and the members of staff who were present seemed very eager to have the pathway implemented. Its subsequent implementation was done on first September 2003. I have since received feedback suggesting that junior doctors have found the pathway very helpful in their assessment and treatment of patients in AUR. It is my intention to monitor the results for 6 months and then re-audit. I presented the results of the audit and the implemented pathway at the audit presentation seminar on 19th September 2003. This was my first attempt at doing this, and while I found it to be 'nerve racking', the experience was enjoyable. Undertaking this project has increased my communication skills, elevated my self-esteem and morale, broadened my knowledge and extended my practice. I have been able to re-evaluate my practice and identify areas where changes are required. I am now more aware of the vital importance of assessment prior to the implementation of care, and realise that current assessment strategy within the clinical area could do with some updating.

Acute urinary retention (AUR) will continue to be the cause of increased distress for the patient and nursing intervention needs to be expedient to achieve the desired outcome. Catheterisation is an essential procedure in the treatment of AUR; however, because of the invasiveness of the procedure, there is a significant risk from infection and the potential for further problems to the patient's health. It is therefore imperative for researchers to implement strategies whereby the onset of bacteria can be effectively prevented or controlled. The role of the nurse is persistently championed, and while this is admirable, caring for patients with catheters and their chosen urinary drainage systems is most definitely a multidisciplinary role. Therefore, in the management of care for patients in AUR, the role of doctors, especially junior doctors, is highly significant. Clinical practice is not a 'static' exercise. The process is changeable; therefore, protocols need to be constantly updated (usually through audit), in particular issues of infection control and managing catheters and urinary drainage systems to promote patient's dignity, self-care and independence, and ultimately an improved quality of life.

Issues surrounding catheterisation are ongoing. Where possible the procedure should be for the short-term duration to minimise complications (Getliffe 1993; Winn 1998). In view of these complications, and to increase the efficacy of care provided for patients when using catheters, intermittent catheterisation as an alternative option of care has recently gained increased support for its use (Winn and Thompson 1998). However, if long-term use of catheters is indicated, then comprehensive assessment (with time frame for reassessment), fully supported by effective education, must be strictly incorporated to ensure highest standards of care for those patients. In practice, every attempt to achieve clinical excellence is expected, but establishments' recruitment and retention of the workforce that is competent, efficient and appropriately skilled are needed to achieve objectives (Addison 2001). Education and training come high on the agenda, with a further assurance that ongoing practice will be regularly monitored and audited, and improvements instigated accordingly to maintain standards (Royle and Walsh 1992).

5.5.1   Summary

There were several updates of the AUR Pathway, the last of which is illustrated in Fig. 5.2. Following implementation of the pathway in 2003, protocol was written and its use incorporated into practice. Responsibility for the AUR Pathway and the information leaflet (monitoring of its use in the A&E department and subsequent updates) was handed over to the urology CNS in 2005. The AUR project was the topic of choice for the dissertation module, in the undertaking of the BSc nursing degree. This project provided an in-depth understanding of issues such as assessment, infection, choice of catheters and appropriate usage, catheter valve, risk management, admission and discharges of patients in a timely manner, consent and other issues, including the healthcare professional (nurses and doctors) role, in the overall process.

5.5.2   First Research Experience

I commenced the level II research module … *'An Introduction to and Understanding of Research Methods in Health Care'* on 21st January 2004. Admittedly, my understanding of research principles and methodology was lacking and I found the course quite difficult. My difficulty was lack of understanding of qualitative and quantitative research, interpreting the findings/results and applying these to practice. This lack of understanding was very evident in my completion of the written assignment for this module. This was a literature review for which I had to evaluate various studies (quantitative and qualitative); compare, contrast and critique informational content; and highlight strengths and weaknesses for each one. On reflection, not my best work! I remember the research lecturer (SM-L) recounting her experiences in Uganda and I found this quite moving. This recount highlighted the many difficulties faced by those living in countries where the most basic resources (such as analgesia) are often difficult to source. It also emphasised the importance of research and its role in advancing care delivery worldwide.

I also remember the module leader expressing his passion for the subject area. On this occasion, after the group returned from lunch, we were discussing the course and the difficulty of grasping certain elements of the research methodology. I was reassured to discover that I was not the only one struggling. As the module leader entered the room, one member of the group stated that he was only interested in passing, not in getting a good grade. The module leader's response to this comment, 'That is no way to think … you should aim high guys … always aim high', had made clear his annoyance. We were all surprised by the module leader's words, although, thinking back on my own academic undertakings, I realise that I have always aimed high.

Despite the initial lack of understanding, I believe that this course was beneficial, in that the learning gained enabled me to make sense of various studies, in terms of interpreting the findings and results and applying these to patient and practice outcomes. I further believe that this research experience was useful in my second research undertaking in 2012.

Unacceptable Behaviour Admittedly, my interactions with patients during my stay in the urology ward and experiences thereof were mostly positive, but as illustrated in the following scenario, some were less positive. I felt that it was important to include this scenario as it highlights the negative impact of antisocial behaviour and why staff should not have to tolerate such behaviour.

It was 23.12.2004, and I was verbally abused by a 17-year-old teenager, who seemed not to have any respect for those around him especially nurses, who had been allocated to his care. More frustratingly, his mother, who was sitting by his bedside, had tried to justify her son's behaviour, by placing the blame on the doctors and nurses. I was very angry, and a part of me had wished that I could have 'slapped' him. Yes, not a very professional thought, but I would not have tolerated such behaviour from my own children. Abuse of any sort is demoralising, especially for the individual to whom the abuse is targeted. It is a behaviour that cuts to the very core. My colleagues had been supportive and advised me to complete an incident form, but it had done little to assuage my frustration. The incident had re-enforced the concern as to why health professionals should *NOT* have to tolerate bad behaviour, which, despite the earlier instigation of the zero-tolerance rule in 1999, was still a cause for concern.

5.6   Dealing with Stressful Situations

It would have been unrealistic for me to think that as a nurse, I could have gone through my career without encountering some stressful situations, as illustrated in two reflective accounts: (1) managing a critical incident, i.e. issues of death, cultural and religious beliefs, and (2) coping with the death of a colleague. I thought that it would be useful to illustrate how such situations could impact the healthcare professional, myself included.

5.6.1   Managing a Critical Incident

Over the years, I have found that nursing and efforts to deliver optimal care to patients could be a hugely stressful affair, for the patient, family and health professional. It was fifth March 2005, and at work, I had my first experience of dealing with a critical incident involving death and cultural and religious issues. This was quite a profound experience, one that I was advised by my nursing colleague to provide an account on what this meant for me and the learning gained. The following is a version of the events, adapted for the reflective component of the competency assessment—in the completion of the level 3, BSc Hons degree course. Reflective account is guided by Gibbs (Laker 1994) reflective model.

5.6.2   Description

Mr. X is 78. He is an Asian gentleman of Muslim religion with end-stage renal disease. In view of his declining health and predicted poor prognosis, following discussion with his family, a 'Do Not Resuscitate' (DNR) order was instigated on 16th February 2005. Family consisted of his wife (who did not speak English) and three sons (two of whom were in attendance when the incident occurred). For simplicity, sons are referred to as number 1 and 2 in this account. Palliative intervention was requested as Mr. X was experiencing difficulty with his breathing. Medication as prescribed was commenced subcutaneously via a syringe driver. Mr. X was nursed in a single-bedded cubicle.

It was Saturday morning, fifth March 2005, and the time was 08.00. The ward was busy, and staffing levels were less than adequate to meet demands. Son No. 1 voiced concerns regarding his father's increasing drowsiness, and requested that I stop the syringe driver. I assured him that I would inform the doctor of his concerns but sadly Mr. X died before I could do so. The family was distraught and insisted that I revive him. I explained that I could not intervene as Mr. X was a DNR, an announcement which was refuted by son No. 2. Mr. X's wife began pulling at me, urging me to revive her husband. Son No. 1 told me to get out as I had not tried to save his father. He then disconnected the syringe driver from Mr. X's arm and left it lying on the bed, which I then picked up. Son No. 2 demanded the syringe. He believed that the contents were responsible for his father's death, and wished to conduct further investigations.

Contacting the medical house officer (HO) took over two hours as they were attending a critical alert call. I informed him of the current situation and requested his immediate attention, but on his arrival to the ward the relatives refused him access to examine Mr. X. HO contacted the on-call registrar, who agreed to intervene. Before this intervention, I explained about the syringe incident, which needed to be retrieved. The family allowed the registrar to certify Mr. X's death. He also explained that if they wished to conduct investigations on the syringe content, then an autopsy would have to be undertaken. As this proposal was unacceptable, the syringe was duly returned.

5.6.3 Feelings

The atmosphere following Mr. X's death was extremely tense, so tense, in fact, that it felt uncomfortable, almost painful. The room was hot and stuffy. I wanted to open the windows, but did not feel confident to do so. Subsequent actions such as son No. 1 telling me to get out, his accusation that I had somehow failed him by not undertaking DNR on his father, son No. 2's behaviour with the syringe and the wife pulling at me were altogether overwhelming. Throughout this time, however, I was very much aware of their sense of loss and hopelessness (Gibbs 1998). I was annoyed that despite numerous attempts to contact the doctor, it took him so long to respond, and I had wondered if a more expedient response would have helped to appease the family's grief. In hindsight, my use of humour (albeit ironic humour) helped me to put occurrence into perspective (Harrison 1995).

5.6.4 Evaluation

This critical incident was insightful. I had learnt that burial within the Muslim culture should take place within 24 h of the patient's death (Smith 1996); consequently, the death of Mr. X on the weekend complicated last office proceedings. While I regard my management of this incident effective, my lack of experience regarding cultural and religious issues was also evident. Nevertheless, subsequent incident management had greatly enhanced my knowledge and experience. Caring for the dying patient is an important part of the care provided by healthcare professionals; hence, doctors should examine their role in this process to improve service outcomes.

5.6.5 Analysis

Mr. X's family was in denial of his imminent death. However, I have since learnt that cultural and religious background affects the way individuals respond to illness and issues relating to death and dying (Nyatanga 1997). If the family accepted that Mr. X was dying, they would have lost hope, and subsequently their ability to cope with ensuing emotions (Karim 2002). Also, feeling that they were isolated in an environment which they perceived as an insensitive feeling of their cultural and spiritual needs (Nyatanga 1997), as well as a poor understanding of the information received (Nyatanga 1997), affected the family's reaction to Mr. X's death. However, working in collaboration with members of the multidisciplinary teams was highly constructive in achieving desired outcomes.

5.6.6 Conclusion

This was a difficult situation, and I now realise that I must consistently update my knowledge and awareness of cultural and religious issues, to ensure that I always adequately address the individual's needs (Nyatanga 1997).

5.6.7 Action Plan

If this situation arose again, I would conduct further discussions with the family to ensure that they fully understood the implications of DNR, and advise them to seek spiritual guidance, if appropriate.

5.6.8 Summary

It has been 14 years since this incidence, and while I have not encountered another, it is one I have never forgotten. This experience was a learning curve, in that it increased my awareness of why, in our attempts to deliver holistic care, it is important to address all salient issues, including cultural and religious issues, and ensure that these are incorporated into the individual's plan of care.

5.6.9   Coping with the Death of a Colleague

Aileen, aged 36 years, was married with two young children, and pregnant with her third child. As the birth of her baby got closer, Aileen was excited at the prospect of meeting him/her. I still see her making plans and looking forward to the birth, and her last days in the ward, before commencing maternity leave. The next thing I remember is the call. I was at home, the time was approximately 7.50 p.m., the phone rang and it was (JC) calling to inform me of Aileen's untimely death. 'What!', I heard myself saying, 'How is that possible?', I asked. JC went on to explain what happened, and it was surreal. Aileen's death had had a huge impact on the team. 3 weeks following her sudden demise (29.04.06), we were finally able to say our goodbyes. The service was lovely, a very fitting tribute, that had accurately captured Aileen's personality and her zest for life. A life tragically cut short at 36 years old, and which would be sorely missed by her husband, children and extended family, all of whom she loved with a passion.

It was now 08.05.2006, nearly 2 months since Aileen's passing, and her absence from the team was still painfully evident.

It was 09.06.2006, and to remember Aileen, the team members had organised a tribute that included her work colleagues, family and friends. The ceremony was extremely emotional, but a fitting tribute nevertheless. While I had only known Aileen for a short while, working with her was never dull. She had a mischievous way about her that often manifested in her saying the most outrageous things that would leave you shaking with laughter. A good feeling that often helped to alleviate any lingering feelings of stress, after a hard day at work. I was flattered to be asked to read the poem *'Phenomenal Woman'* by Maya Angelou at Aileen's ceremony; it accurately captured her tenacity and her love of life. The eulogy, read by the ward manager, was also quite profound. It depicted Aileen's nursing career, her time in the urology ward and, most importantly, the lovely person she was.

Understandably, Aileen's death raised questions. It was after all the twenty-first century, an era in which, thanks to advancements in prenatal nursing care, a woman dying in childbirth was rare. The question therefore was how was it possible that a young woman, who was otherwise fit and healthy, could have died in childbirth. Was negligence a factor? Since her death, analysis of these tragic events has revealed that BAME women are five times more likely to die in childbirth. I guess, we will never know. To this day, Aileen's death is a bitter sweet memory, and remembering how she was can still put a smile on my face.

2006—On my Lonesome   Six months into my post I found myself working on my 'lonesome', while my two colleagues went on maternity leave. While I was not happy with this situation, I burrowed down and got on with it. The first colleague went on leave in February 2006; her leave was scheduled for 6 months, but this was extended. The second colleague went on leave in October 2006, and because her leave was also extended, I was left working on my own for 6 months, and doing so across sites. This was a challenging task, but ultimately, when you are the sole practitioner, you quickly learn to multitask, and more importantly to prioritise your workload. I successfully maintained interactions with my patients, from diagnosis onward, as well as arranging the necessary follow-up referrals. In terms of the joint consultation clinic, I did receive some support to run the clinic from my colleague (JC), for a short while. Obviously, I could not secure face-to-face interactions with all patients at the time of diagnosis, but I was able to arrange telephone interactions for those I was unable to see. I went into an auto-working mode. I was able to meet most of my responsibilities, although this meant that I often worked overtime to keep on top of the workload. Having acknowledged the increased workload and the potential for increased stress on my part, the urology consultants were supportive. In fact, encouragement from one consultant (who suggested that working solo would be good grounding for my career) was reassuring. He may have been right, since I survived to tell the tale and kept my sanity.

5.7   Supportive Study: Honours Degree in Nursing

Having completed studies towards the diploma, I thought that I could now rest for a while before embarking on further study. However, this was a thought with which my colleague, and new mentor, the urology nurse consultant (UNC-WN), did not agree. WN felt that if I were to have a break, I would not undertake the degree. I guess she was convincing, since I commenced the Honours Degree in nursing (BSc Hons. Nursing) on 14th September 2004. The modules completed for this degree course comprised:

- Care of the Adult with Urological Problems.
- Tissue Viability.
- Therapeutics and Challenges for Cancer Care.
- Dissertation: Acute Urinary Retention: Developing a Management Pathway for an Emergency Care Setting.

5.7.1   Care of the Adult with Urological Problems

This module was the first in the degree package, an informative, well-organised and well-executed module. The knowledge and learning gained enhanced my understanding of urological problems (benign and cancerous pathology) and its management, as well as implications for an individual's health.

5.7.2   Therapeutics and Challenges for Cancer Care

This 30-credits module was a mandatory requirement of the MUCNS role that provided me with an in-depth understanding of the principles of cancer practice and its management. I commenced this module in May 2005, 2 months prior to applying for the MUCNS post.

5.7.3   Tissue Viability Module

The following assignment entitled *'Factors most likely to influence the role of nutrition in the wound healing process'* has been edited to provide a rationale for choice of topic area, implications for practice, conclusion and lessons learnt, an update on the wound-healing process and reflection on a possible case of bias. The reader is directed to the published article 'Nutrition and wound healing: the necessity of assessment' (Anderson 2005) for a more in-depth insight into nutrition and wound-healing process and the importance of assessment in this. As a urology nurse, caring for patients with wounds was rare. However, the merger with the surgical ward had presented the opportunity to care for one particular patient whose management had highlighted some interesting notations, most especially poor preoperative nutritional status and its impact on wound healing (Collins 2002). The patient in question was Mrs. Ward, a lady in her 80s, who following her initial discharge home after major surgery had suffered a rapid decline in her general health, and consequently the development of a large, highly exuding, sacral pressure sore for which she was readmitted to hospital for debridement. Suffice to say, the management of Mrs. Ward's situation resulted in a full recovery. A review of the literature examined the evidence to establish how various factors may have impacted Mrs. Ward's health and her subsequent recovery (Reynolds 2001; Todorovic 2002). Since nutrition and wound healing are integral parts of delivering holistic care to patients, I felt that it was important to explore the issues presented.

The role of nutrition in wound healing is well established (Reynolds 2001; Todorovic 2002). It has also been established that nurses need to understand the role of specific nutrients in wound healing, if they are to provide patients with optimal care (Shepherd 2003). Nurses also need to understand the importance of assessment and the use of rigorous assessment tools in its undertaking (Shepherd 2003; Russell 2000; Guigoz et al. 2002), as well as being able to interpret results appropriately, a requirement that had signified a need for education in this area (Cartwright 2002), as well as accurate documentation (Rollins 1997; Haydock and Hill 1986). Nutrition is vital to health and well-being (Reynolds 2001; Todorovic 2002), and crucial in a holistic approach to wound healing as said by Todorovic (Reynolds 2001). Many factors are presumed to influence nutrition during wound healing, but a detailed discussion is beyond the scope of this review. Focus is therefore placed on the most relevant factors, identified as assessment (Shepherd 2003; Russell 2000; Guigoz et al. 2002), and highlighting the role of the nurse and members of the multidisciplinary team (MDT) in the overall management of care (Shepherd 2003; Russell 2000; Guigoz et al. 2002). The role of vital nutrients, specifically proteins, in their relation to malnutrition and the manifestation of protein-energy malnutrition (PEM), is also discussed (Russell 2000).

Implications for Future Practice   A review of the literature has indicated that poor preoperative nutritional status adversely affects wound healing (Collins 2002). Conversely, dietary intervention could significantly improve or accelerate the process (Reynolds 2001), provided that strategies are implemented early enough to prevent a catabolic-induced decline in lean muscle mass (Himes 1999). Certainly, given the speed of deterioration observed in the patient's general condition, and the subsequent development of her wound, it could be argued that preoperatively she was in a malnourished state and that further deterioration occurred post-operatively. Review had further shown that nurses must acknowledge the implications of malnutrition on health and wound healing, and in so doing ensure that a holistic nutritional assessment is undertaken in the early preoperative period to identify presenting problems and instigate measures to prevent or delay further complications (Shepherd 2003; Russell 2000; Guigoz et al. 2002). Regular yearly educational updates to increase practitioners' awareness of nutrition and its impact on the wound-healing process would be highly beneficial (Cartwright 2002).

5.8   Conclusion and Lessons Learnt

This literature review has demonstrated that protein-energy malnutrition remains prevalent among hospitalised and long-term care facility patients, particularly the elderly. It is further demonstrated that this condition may begin before admission, and fuels concerns that frequently a stay in hospital may result in significant worsening of the problem (Himes 1999). The subject of nutrition and wound healing is an area where the nurse is clearly recognised as having a central role in the overall management of care, but equally specific members of the multidisciplinary teams also have significant roles to play. According to Thomas (Thomas 1996), 'the consistent relationship between nutritional status and complications forms the cornerstone of nutritional support, yet there is controversy about the ability of nutritional support to reduce complications or to increase wound healing'. Undoubtedly, nutrients play a vital role in the wound-healing process, but how much is unclear. What is clear, however, is that malnutrition has a significant impact on the wound-healing outcome, and accurate patient assessments are essential to the identification of problems and the devising of suitable interventions to achieve desirable patient outcomes. Continued research is vital to enable practitioners to deliver high-quality evidence-based care to their patients.

An Update on the Wound-Healing Process The evidence verifies a clear progression in research and technology, as well as some striking improvements in caring for wounds and the wound-healing process (Ovington 2007; Swezey 2011; Harding 2015). Between the 1900s and the twenty-first century, advances in dressing technology have led to a new proliferation of topical products that do more than just cover and conceal, but facilitate the healing process as well as address specific issues in nonhealing wounds. The advent of growth factors and other biosynthetics, such as collagen, began the movement to an interactive dressing (Ovington 2007; Swezey 2011; Harding 2015). Emphasis has remained on the importance of an assessment, one that includes a full patient examination and patient history (Swezey 2011), as well as the individual's nutritional status, and considering their role in securing effective patient outcomes (Anderson 2010; Quain and Khardori 2015). From this reflection, I was acutely reminded of my past involvement with wound management. This memory pertains to several patients with wounds, but specifically working as a bank nurse and my involvement in nursing a lady, also in her 80s, with an extremely large sacral pressure sore. However, because she was nutritionally compromised, all efforts to treat her wound had been futile, and sadly, unlike Mrs. Ward, she died. The use of egg whites and oxygen on open wounds, the paraffin gauze for the treatment of a leg ulcer and, much later, the use of maggots in the debridement of wounds remain vivid in my memory, and highlight just how far we have progressed. Ultimately, the evidence has emphasised the role of good nutrition in the wound-healing process and its continued importance in securing effective health outcomes.

Reflection on a Possible Case of Bias/Racism To undertake the Tissue Viability Module, I needed an appropriate mentor, so I contacted the tissue viability consultant (TVC), who was happy to perform the mentorship role. After I had completed the written assignment and submitted it to the university, my mentor contacted me. She thought that my assignment was very good, and suggested that I publish my work. She also asked me to email the assignment to her so that she could place it in the correct format for publishing. As I had never published anything prior to her suggestion, I was sceptical, so much so that I did not immediately respond to her request. During this time, I had received the final mark for my assignment, a 'C' grade. Considering how much work I had put into this assignment I was disappointed, and to be honest puzzled by what I considered to be a significant under-marking of my work. I relayed my disappointment to my mentor, and questioned the decision to publish. I was under the impression that only A- and B-graded assignments were suitable for publication. My mentor was surprised, and quickly dismissed the grade awarded, since she believed that it was not representative of my work. She reiterated her request for me to email the assignment to her, and advised me to challenge the grade with the university module leader.

On contacting the module leader, and voicing my concerns regarding the 'C' grade, she maintained that the assignment was correctly graded. I felt that her explanation was contradictory, as the comments she made did not align with the stated criteria for awarding me this grade. I was disappointed with this mark, and I felt that my work had been under-marked. I wondered if this low grade was due to bias or even racism on the part of the module leader. Nonetheless, I was reassured by my mentor's belief in the quality of the assignment produced. True to her word, she edited the assignment, placed it in the correct format and, after advising me of what changes to make, submitted it to the BJN. Following submission, and subsequent completion of minor additional changes requested by the BJN, the article entitled *'Nutrition and Wound Healing: A Need for Assessment'* resulted in my first ever publication (Anderson 2005)—a great feeling! The lessons learned from this are the following: do not be afraid to challenge decisions, stand your ground and believe in yourself. In this instance, my confidence had taken a knock, and initially had led to some self-doubts. Even so, my mentor's belief in me encouraged me to continue writing, and I went on to write and publish a further 19 articles over the past 14 years.

5.8.1   The Dissertation Project—Acute Urinary Retention: Developing a Management Pathway for an Emergency Care Setting

This was a 10,000-words project that had brought together the outcomes from three audits, the first undertaken in 2002, with subsequent re-audits occurring in 2004 and 2006. Focus was placed on change and its implementation into practice.

Following discussions with the urology clinical nurse specialist (UCNS), it was decided to investigate whether admission to hospital was the best management strategy for these patients. An audit of these patients was subsequently undertaken with the results indicating a need to initiate a change in the current management of AUR patients in A&E. The audit results also demonstrated that nursing staff and medical staff, specifically junior doctors, were in need of updated information in the treatment of AUR patients. Observations noted that over a period of 18 months, a number of patients with AUR (on average, 3–5 per month) were admitted to the urology ward, when arguably most should have been discharged home. In view of the ever-increasing shortage of hospital beds and the constant struggle to meet NHS targets, establishments need to identify areas that are in need of improvements and take steps to increase efficiency. This project reported on the development of the AUR Pathway in an A&E in the UK through the process of change with the nurse assuming the role of change agent.

5.9   Conclusion and Lessons Learnt

This project enabled me to focus on change and its impact on developing innovative strategies to instigate improvements into practice. I have learnt that the status of the person who proposes the change has great bearing on the manner in which it is accepted (Haynes 1992). Ideally, change in nursing practice should be instigated by someone who possesses appropriate knowledge and ability, and who is also a leader. Chaucer once said, *'time and tide wait for no man'. In other words, 'time stops for no one'* (Lemon 2005*)*. In the same way that we cannot stop time, neither can we stop the onset of change, or indeed the pace in which it occurs. I was forced to acknowledge the wisdom of Chaucer's words, as time was a significant drawback in the undertaking of these projects.

I fully appreciate that ongoing examination of clinical practice is essential to identify problem areas and devise strategies to achieve successful practice outcomes. Ultimately, the key to achieving this objective is a management strategy that seeks to forge team participation, by acknowledging and respecting team participants' contribution to the change project. Essentially, nurses require time to reflect on their practice. However, with increasing work pressures, applying valuable time to reflection, when it could be better applied to caring for patients, is perhaps a little unrealistic (Williams and Lowes 2001). My reflection on this project has been painful, especially in light of the uncertainties created by current changes within the

NHS. Conversely, the experience is educational, as it enhanced my learning and developed my expertise in clinical practice (Scanlan and Chernomas 1997).

The completion of this project led to the invitation by SM-L to give a talk to students on the current BSc degree course on what it was like, to suggest ways in which their approach to its completion could be improved and to present the AUR Pathway to the university lecturers and students. I was also asked to supervise one of the students on this current BSc degree course, who, interestingly, was the same student who had gone on to complete the master's degree with me in 2010–2012, and accordingly presented our work to the university.

5.9.1 2019—Summary

Hopefully, this chapter has provided the reader with an insight into urology nursing and the principles of practice in terms of the urology ward, types of patients and procedures, and background on healthcare professionals, typically how knowledge, experience, competency levels and working as a team, combined with relevant teaching support, contributed to improving their learning and accordingly patient and practice outcomes. It also shows how my undertaking of various studies, including audit and experiences gained, helped me to initiate change in practice. Working in this field of nursing provided me with many positive experiences, ones that were made possible by the support of colleagues who encouraged me to become the very best that I could be. Admittedly, my experiences from nursing patients with urological cancers were especially beneficial, since I believe that they played a part in obtaining the MUCNS role.

Chapter 6 provides an overview of the management of urological cancers. This includes the role of the multidisciplinary teams, specifically the MUCNS, and highlights key elements of the role in this management.

References

Addison R (2001) Catheterisation: a guide to the role of the nurse, teaching supplement
Anderson B (2005) Nutrition and wound healing: the necessity of assessment. Br J Nurs [Internet] 14(Sup5):S30–S38. https://doi.org/10.12968/bjon.2005.14.Sup5.19955
Anderson B (2010) A perspective on changing dynamics in nursing over the past 20 years. Br J Nurs 19(18):1190–1191. [Internet]. http://tinyurl
Anderson B, Khadra A (2006) Acute urinary retention: developing an A&E management pathway. Br J Nurs 15(8):434–438. [Internet]. http://www.ncbi.nlm.nih.gov/pubmed/16723949
Andrews M (1993) Importance of nursing leadership in implementing change. Br J Nurs 2(8):437–439. [Internet]. https://doi.org/10.12968/bjon.1993.2.8.437
Anon (2021) Urinary catheterisation—Better Health Channel [[Internet] Cited: 2021 Feb 17]. www.betterhealth.vic.gov.au/health/conditionsandtreatments/urinary-catheteris…
Blackwell (1994) Blackwell's dictionary of nursing. Blackwell Scientific, Oxford
Broome A (1990) Managing change. In: Managing change. Macmillan, Basingstoke
Cartwright A (2002) Nutritional assessment as part of wound management. Nurs Times 98(44):62–63. [Internet]. http://www.ncbi.nlm.nih.gov/pubmed/12451754

Collins N (2002) Which tube-feeding formulas help wounds heal best? Nursing (Lond) 32(2):4–5

Cube (1997) The Croydon college company: booklet of introduction on foundation and diploma in psychodynamic counselling. The Croydon College Company, Croydon

Department of Health (1998a) A first-class service: quality in the new NHS. London NHS Executive. https://www.betterhealth.vic.gov.au/health/conditionsandtreatments/urinary-cathet erisation?viewAsPdf=true

Erickson E (1985) The eight ages of man, childhood and society, Pelican

Getliffe K (1993) Informed choices for long-term benefits. The management of catheters in continence care. Prof Nurse 9(2):122–126. [Internet]. http://www.ncbi.nlm.nih.gov/pubmed/8234379

Gibbs G (1998) Learning by doing, a guide to teaching and learning methods. Oxford Brookes University, Oxford. [Internet] [cited 2020 Oct 25]. http://www.glos.ac.uk/gdn/gibbs/index.htm

Guigoz Y, Lauque S, Vellas BJ (2002) Identifying the elderly at risk for malnutrition. The mini nutritional assessment. Clin Geriatr Med 18(4):737–757. [Internet]. http://www.ncbi.nlm.nih.gov/pubmed/12608501

Haffer A (1986) Facilitating change: choosing the appropriate strategy. J Nurs Adm 16(4):18–22

Harding K (2015) Innovation and wound healing. J Wound Care 24(Supplement 4):7–13. [Internet]. https://doi.org/10.12968/jowc.2015.24.Sup4b.7

Harrison N (1995) Using humour as an educational technique. Prof Nurse 11(3):198–199. [Internet]. http://www.ncbi.nlm.nih.gov/pubmed/8552694

Haydock DA, Hill GL (1986) Impaired wound healing in surgical patients with varying degrees of malnutrition. J Parenter Enter Nutr 10(6):550–554. [Internet]. https://doi.org/10.1177/0148607186010006550

Haynes S (1992) Let the change come from within the process of change in nursing. Prof Nurse 7(19):635–638

Hildebrand P (1995) Beyond mid-life crisis: a psychodynamic approach to ageing. Sheldon Press

Himes D (1999) Protein-calorie malnutrition and involuntary weight loss: the role of aggressive nutritional intervention in wound healing. Ostomy Wound Manag [Internet] 45(3):46–51. 54–5. http://www.ncbi.nlm.nih.gov/pubmed/10347519

Karim K (2002) Informing cancer patients: truth telling and culture. Cancer Nurs Pract 2:3

Klein J (1987) Our need for others and its roots in infancy. Routledge, London

Laker C (ed) (1994) Urological nursing. Scutari Press, Harrow, pp 194–195

Lemon J (2005) Opening convocation remarks. Susquehanna, University, Office of the President. [Internet]. [cited 2019 Feb 10]. http://www.susqu.edu/president/convocation05.htm

National Cancer Action Team, Taylor C, Ramirez A (2009) Multidisciplinary team members' views about MDT working: Results from a survey commissioned by the National Cancer Action Team [Internet]. [cited 2020 Jan 20]. http://www.ncin.org.uk/view?rid=137

Nichani S, Fitterman N, Lukela M, Crocker J (2017) Urinary tract infection. 2017 hospital medicine revised core competencies. J Hosp Med 12:4. S40-S41l10.12788/jhm.3030. [Internet]. https://www.journalofhospitalmedicine.com/jhospmed/article/165937/hospital-medicine/urinary-tract-infection-2017-hospital-medicine-revised

Noonan E (1983) Counselling young people, London, UK

Nursing Explorer (2019) What is urology nursing? [Internet]. nursingexplorer.com. [cited 2020 Oct 13]. https://www.nursingexplorer.com/careers/urology-nursing

Nyatanga B (1997) Cultural issues in palliative care. Int J Palliat Nurs 3(4):203–208. [Internet]. http://www.ncbi.nlm.nih.gov/pubmed/29328849

Ovington LG (2007) Advances in wound dressings. Clin Dermatol 25(1):33–38. [Internet]. http://www.ncbi.nlm.nih.gov/pubmed/17276199

Persad R (2021) Kidney stones: causes, symptoms and treatments, Bupa UK [Internet]. [cited 2021 Oct 13]. https://www.bupa.co.uk/health-information/urinary-bladder-problems/kidney-stones

Quain AM, Khardori NM (2015) Nutrition in wound care management: a comprehensive overview. Wounds 27(12):327–335. a Compend Clin Res Pract [Internet]. http://www.ncbi.nlm.nih.gov/pubmed/27447105

Reber AS (1995) The Penguin dictionary of psychology, 2nd edn. Penguin Books, London, UK

Reynolds TM (2001) The future of nutrition and wound healing. J Tissue Viability 11(1):5–13. [Internet]. http://www.ncbi.nlm.nih.gov/pubmed/11949310

Rollins H (1997) Nutrition and wound healing. Nurs Stand 11(51):49–51. [Internet]. http://www. ncbi.nlm.nih.gov/pubmed/14618895

Royle JR, Walsh M (eds) (1992) Watson's medical-surgical nursing and related physiology. Bailliere, London

Russell L (2000) Malnutrition and pressure ulcers: nutritional assessment tools. Br J Nurs 9(4):44–49. -undefined

Salzberger-Wittenberg I (1970) Psycho-analytic insight and relationships [Internet]. London; [cited 2020 Oct 13]. https://www.amazon.co.uk/Psycho-Analytic-Insight-Relationships-Salzberger-Wittenberg-Paperback/dp/B00IJ0TVVW/ref=sr_1_1?dchild=1&keywords=psych oanalytic+insight+and+relationships+1970&qid=1602596002&s=books&sr=1-1

Scanlan JM, Chernomas WM (1997) Developing the reflective teacher. J Adv Nurs [Internet] 25(6):1138–1143. https://doi.org/10.1046/j.1365-2648.1997.19970251138.x

Scholtes S (2002) Management of clot retention following urological surgery. Nurs Times 98(28):48–50

Segal J (1992) Introduction on the work of Melanie Klein, chapter 2, Klein's major theoretical contributions. Sage Publications

Shepherd AA (2003) Nutrition for optimum wound healing. Nurs Stand 18(6):55–58. [Internet]. http://www.ncbi.nlm.nih.gov/pubmed/14618895

Smith JW (1996) Cultural and spiritual issues in palliative care. J Cancer Care 5(4):173–178

Swezey L (2011) Wound dressing and wound healing—changing philosophy. woundeducators.com

Thomas DR (1996) Nutritional factors affecting wound healing. Ostomy Wound Manage 42(5):40–42, 44–6, 48–9. [Internet] http://www.ncbi.nlm.nih.gov/pubmed/8717012

Todorovic V (2002) Food and wounds: nutritional factors in wound formation and healing. Br J Community Nurs 43(4):46–48

Waterlow M (2001) Treating depression, mental health matters

Williams G, Lowes L (2001) Reflection: possible strategies to improve its use by qualified staff. Br J Nurs 10(22):1482–1489

Winn C (1998) Complications with urinary catheters. Prof Nurse 13(5 Suppl):S7-10. [Internet]. http://www.ncbi.nlm.nih.gov/pubmed/9526422

Winn C, Thompson J (1998) Urinary catheters for intermittent use. Prof Nurse 13(8):541–548. [Internet]. http://www.ncbi.nlm.nih.gov/pubmed/9653298

Winnicott DW (1991) The child, the family, and the outside world. Penguin Psychology, London

A Perspective on Uro-Oncology Management and the Macmillan Uro-Oncology CNS (MUCNS) Role in this Management

6

6.1 Urological Cancers: Types, Diagnosis, Management, Treatments

Urological cancers encompass five types of tumours: bladder, prostate, kidney, testicular and penile (Cancer Research UK 2019). For all types, management and treatments are determined by the relevant risk category (i.e. whether the disease is low, intermediate or high risk, with management assigned according to the relevant risk category), patient's age, fitness status, grade and stage of the disease (Cancer Research UK 2019; National Institute for Health and Care Excellence [NICE] 2015), and most importantly patient's choice, preferably one that is made only after receiving all the relevant information and having the level of risks explained (National Collaborating Centre for Cancer 2014). Emphasis is placed on early diagnosis and treatment in facilitating more favourable patient and practice outcomes (World Health Organization [WHO] 2021).

For a more detailed explanation on current statistical evaluations for urological cancers, including diagnosis, management and treatments, the reader is referred to the Cancer Research UK website (Cancer Research UK 2019).

Bladder cancer is the tenth most common cancer in the UK, accounting for 3% of all new cancer cases. Bladder cancer is associated with a number of risk factors. The main risk is increasing age but smoking and exposure to some industrial chemicals also increase risk (Babjuk et al. 2015; Witjes et al. 2015). Bladder cancer tumours are graded (G1–3) and staged (T1–4) (Babjuk et al. 2015; Witjes et al. 2015). Disease is categorised as non-muscle-invasive bladder cancer (NMIBC), high-risk non-muscle-invasive bladder cancer (HRNMIBC), muscle-invasive bladder cancer (MIBC) and metastatic bladder cancer (MBC) (Babjuk et al. 2015; Witjes et al. 2015).

Treatments include intravesical (directly into the bladder) therapies (Vahr et al. 2015), chemotherapy, mitomycin C (MMC), immunotherapy, Bacillus Calmette-Guérin (BCG) (Babjuk et al. 2015), chemo-hyperthermia (CHT) and electromotive drug administration (EMDA) (Di Stasi et al. 2011; Kwong et al. 2013). Surgery

© Springer Nature Switzerland AG 2022
B. Anderson, *A Uro-Oncology Nurse Specialist's Reflection on her Practice Journey*, https://doi.org/10.1007/978-3-030-94199-4_6

includes cystectomy and transurethral resection of bladder tumour (TURBT), systemic chemotherapy and radiotherapy (Witjes et al. 2015). (Please refer to Anderson (Anderson 2018a) Part 1 and (Anderson 2018b) Part 2 for a detailed explanation on the management and treatment of bladder cancer, including the role of smoking in its development.)

Prostate cancer is the most common cancer in males in the UK, accounting for 26% of all new cancer cases (Cancer Research UK 2019). This disease is more common in Black males than White males, and least common in Asian males (Cancer Research UK 2019).

Treatment of prostate cancer includes active surveillance (AS), surgery, radiotherapy, hormone therapy and chemotherapy (Cancer Research UK 2019).

Kidney cancer is the seventh most common cancer in the UK, accounting for 4% of all new cancer cases (Cancer Research UK 2019). It is estimated that 56% of patients diagnosed with kidney cancer will have surgery to remove the tumour as part of their primary cancer treatment followed by 8% who will have radiotherapy and 13% who will have chemotherapy (Cancer Research UK 2019). Patients diagnosed with advanced disease generally have immunotherapy as the current recommended treatment of choice as it has proven beneficial in extending survival and improving quality-of-life outcomes.

Testicular cancer is the 17th most common cancer in males in the UK, accounting for 1% of all new cancer cases in males (Cancer Research UK 2019). Testicular cancer usually occurs in young and middle-aged men with ages ranging between 15 and 65 years plus. Overall survival has increased in the last 40 years in the UK probably due to the use of combination surgery and chemotherapy (Cancer Research UK 2019).

Penile cancer is a cancer of the penis and is relatively rare in the UK. It can develop anywhere on the penis, but is most common under the foreskin in men who have not been circumcised or on the head of the penis (the glans) (Cancer Research UK 2019). The most common types of treatments for penile cancer include surgery, radiation therapy and chemotherapy (Cancer Research UK 2019).

Central to the management of urological cancers is the urology multidisciplinary team (*Box 6.1*), in which the Macmillan Uro-Oncology Clinical Nurse Specialist (MUCNS) role is pivotal.

Box 6.1 Members of the Urology Multidisciplinary Team
- MDT coordinator.
- Consultant urologists.
- Consultant clinical oncologists.
- Urology specialist registrars.
- Macmillan Uro-Oncology Clinical Nurse Specialists (MUCNS).
- Consultant radiologists.
- Consultant histopathologists.
- Specialist multidisciplinary team (SMDT).

Changes to Urology Cancer Management in Local Practice Between 1997 and 2005, all of these cancers were managed within the urology ward, but with subsequent reconfiguration of services were later separated out from the benign pathology. Bladder, prostate, kidney and testicular cancers continued to be managed locally within the Trust, but with referrals being made as appropriate to other secondary or tertiary care sectors. Penile cancer management had passed to another Secondary Care Trust within the specialist urology field, where it has been managed by the same specialist consultant, who previously managed these patients in the local Trust, where he worked as part of the urology team, and still does today, albeit on a lesser level.

Between 2005 and 2019, a further reconfiguration of urology cancer management took place. This included working in closer unison with clinicians from the tertiary and secondary care sectors to secure a joint decision-making venture that aimed to ensure that management and treatment decisions are made in the best interest of patients and that care is actioned within the government's targeted specifications.

Diagnostic Imaging In the UK, in the diagnosis and treatment of urological cancers, the '2-week wait' is the most expedient route to securing a diagnosis (National Institute for Health and Care Excellence [NICE] 2015), while the confirmation of a diagnosis and the selection of the most appropriate treatment are reliant on specific diagnostic imaging, as illustrated in Table 6.1 (Witjes et al. 2015). Position emission tomography (PET) scans are an invaluable addition to practice and can predict more

Table 6.1 Diagnostic imaging

Computed tomography (CT)	A CT scan is a cross-sectional, three-dimensional image of an internal body part produced by computed tomography chiefly for diagnostic purposes
Magnetic resonance imaging (MRI)	An MRI scan produces detailed images of the body using powerful magnets, radio waves and a computer
Nuclear medicine bone scan (BS)	A bone scan is a nuclear medicine imaging technique of the bone. It can help diagnose a number of bone conditions, including cancer of the bone or metastasis
Choline C-11 PET (positron emission tomography) scan	This is an imaging test used to help detect sites of prostate cancer that has returned despite treatment (recurrent prostate cancer). It may be used when other imaging has not been helpful. Choline C-11 PET scan is a scan that uses a special chemical tracer called choline C-11 injection
PSMA (prostate-specific membrane antigen) PET-CT scan	The PSMA scan is used to stage prostate cancer in patients who have had a positive prostate biopsy and in patients who have had their prostate removed but now present with increasing levels of PSA (a prostate activity marker) in their blood indicating that their cancer may have recurred. For the identification of more advanced localised disease, i.e. disease that has spread outside the margins, specifically within the prostate
FDG-PET/CT scan (fluorine-18-fluorodeoxyglucose position emission tomography scan)	This scan is a pivotal imaging modality for cancer imaging, assisting diagnosis, staging of patients with newly diagnosed malignancy and restaging following therapy and surveillance. It is particularly useful in diagnosing bladder cancer that has spread outside the margins

Source: (Witjes et al. 2015)

accurately treatment outcomes (Witjes et al. 2015). Appropriateness for choice of staging is dependent on age, grade and stage of disease, and on choice of treatment, i.e. surgery, chemotherapy or radiotherapy. Recent evidence has shown that PET scans are more effective in detecting more advanced localised disease than the usual nuclear medicine bone scan (Witjes et al. 2015). In local practice, the choline PET scan was often the imaging of choice; however, to avoid occlusion of the imaging, it must be performed prior to starting the patient on hormone therapy, a necessity that has often delayed the commencement of treatment. The PSMA PET scan on the other hand can be performed after the patient has begun treatment with hormone therapy, and as such can expedite management. However, as observed in local practice, increases in the demand for the choline PET scans, combined with the intermittent lack of availability of choline, had significantly raised the pressures on the relevant establishment to honour requests, a situation that was further compounded by targets (National Institute for Health and Care Excellence [NICE] 2015), which placed the emphasis not only on honouring the request for these scans, but that these were performed in line with meeting the target specification and avoiding an eminent fine. Admittedly, it was a difficult and equally stressful task.

6.2   An Overview of the MUCNS Role

The MUCNS role is integral to the provision of direct patient care at an advanced level. This is based on knowledge and experience, and indirectly as an educator, consultant, researcher, change agent and staff advocate (Thompson and Watson 2003; Hamric 2005) (Fig. 6.1).

The following recounting of the events provides an overview of the MUCNS (Me) role and how the role was developed and highlights various elements of the role in the management of patients diagnosed with urological cancer. My intent is to provide the reader with greater understanding of how various activities contributed to increasing my knowledge, experience and competency to perform the role, and accordingly improving both patient and practice outcomes. The recounting of the events utilises case study accounts, with reference made to various publications and their relevance to the topic area being discussed. In terms of academia, the various modules explain my interactions with patients and accordingly my ability to support them.

In 2005, the decision to separate the cancer pathology (uro-oncology) from the benign pathology resulted in the MUCNS role. I believe that the knowledge and experience gained over the previous 8 years were beneficial in securing me the role, which I commenced on first August 2005 and held until my retirement on 22nd October 2019. The role comprised working with the existing MUCNS and members of the urology multidisciplinary team (UMDT) to provide holistic care to patients who were newly diagnosed with urological cancers or had been told that this was a possibility. Other elements of the role included visiting and providing support to patients in the wards, in the outpatients' department and over the telephone; attending and supporting the weekly UMDT meetings and the Joint

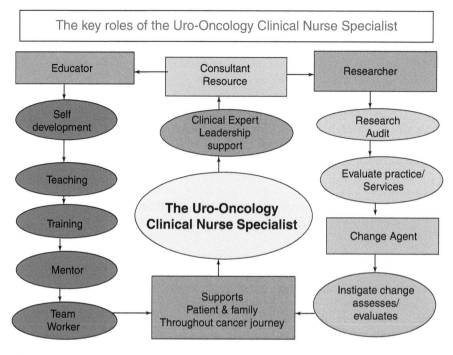

Fig. 6.1   Source: Devised by Beverley Anderson (2005)

Consultation Cancer Clinic (JCC); and importantly working in conjunction with members of relevant multidisciplinary teams to ensure that care was delivered in line with meeting government targets and the standards within the Manual for Cancer Services.

Key Worker Role   This was pivotal in supporting patients during and following the receipt of a cancer diagnosis ('the breaking of bad news') from the urology consultant, and it was also important in subsequent discussions regarding the patient's choice of treatment and management plans (McGuigan 2009), prior to making their final decision. The MUCNS knowledge of diagnosis, treatment modalities and associated risks is central in supporting a patient's final decision (Macmillan Cancer Support 2014). Providing appropriate support and guidance includes effective communication and supporting this with relevant information booklets and leaflets, the majority of which is provided by Macmillan Cancer Support (for all urological cancers) and Prostate Cancer UK (PCUK) for prostate cancer.

The MUCNS is crucial to coordinating care pathways, particularly where patients are treated between different Trusts (as is the case in local practice). Following the receipt of the diagnosis, I would then arrange an appointment in the JCC to see either the consultant urological surgeon or the consultant clinical oncologist to discuss recommended management and treatment options pending the specialist MDT decision (surgery, active surveillance, radiotherapy and chemotherapy). Following a decision, the patient is referred to the appropriate secondary or tertiary care sector to expedite their care. I would then liaise with my counterpart at these sites to ensure that they were fully apprised of all relevant information pertaining to the patient and their specified management/care.

Unfortunately, my interaction with these patients is discontinued at this point (they would now have access to a CNS at the secondary and tertiary care sector), but was usually re-established upon their referral back to the local Trust. The MUCNS group then takes up the responsibility for future monitoring and follow-up, until such time that the patient is referred back to their GP in the community.

6.3   Caring for Patients Diagnosed with Bladder, Prostate, Kidney and Testicular Cancers in Local Practice

Bladder Cancer In local practice, my role as MUCNS involves interacting and caring for patients (male and female), who are diagnosed with NMIBC, MIBC and metastatic bladder (Babjuk et al. 2015; Witjes et al. 2015) cancer, but mostly my interactions are with patients diagnosed with NMIBC, specifically in the delivery of nurse-led services for the aforementioned intravesical therapies (Vahr et al. 2015). For those patients diagnosed with MIBC and metastatic cancer, my interactions usually include meeting patients at the receipt of their diagnosis, where I provided the necessary support that included reassurance, relevant information, my contact details and arranging an appointment in the JCC where I maintained this support.

The following case studies provide an insight into my interactions with and the experiences gained from caring for two patients diagnosed with bladder cancer.

6.3.1   Case Study

I first met Mr. Lawson, a gentleman in his early 70s, in the JCC while receiving his diagnosis from the consultant. He was diagnosed with an aggressive form of bladder cancer, at the muscle-invasive stage, for which surgery (radical cystectomy) was the initial choice of management. Unfortunately, unforeseen delays in commencing treatment resulted in a progression of the disease and accordingly manifested symptoms of increased pain and worsened haematuria, which meant that surgery was no longer a viable option. Mr. Lawson was subsequently admitted to hospital. At this point, the only feasible option of treatment was palliative radiotherapy, where the objective was to effectively manage his symptoms of increased pain and worsened haematuria. On visiting Mr. Lawson, in the ward, I was quite surprised at how quickly his general health had deteriorated. He was clearly in a lot of pain and as he was moderately disorientated, it was difficult to communicate with him. Sadly, Mr. Lawson did not benefit from radiotherapy treatment as he died soon after this admission. Here, the importance of early diagnosis and expedient treatment is clearly highlighted in achieving more favourable outcomes (World Health Organization [WHO] 2021).

6.3.2 Case Study

As I reflect back to my time in the urology ward (1997–2005) and as a senior registered nurse (RN), I clearly remember quite a few patients who were diagnosed with MIBC and malignant bladder cancer, of which one particular patient remains vivid in my mind. Mr. Roberts, a gentleman of Caucasian background, who was in his mid-60s, was diagnosed with bladder cancer that had advanced; as all curative and control options of treatments were exhausted, his remaining option had been a palliative approach to care, which included effective pain control and continuous bladder irrigation to manage the persistent haematuria. Mr. Roberts had accepted his diagnosis and prognosis and had come to terms with the reality of his imminent death (the doctors had given him a few weeks to live); however, he had other ideas. He, apparently, had a lot to sort out and was not ready to give up the fight. My memory of Mr. Robert's time with us in the urology ward is of him mobilising up and down the ward, pushing the drip stand with the irrigation fluid and bag attached and still smiling. The bleeding eventually subsided and his request to be discharged home was granted. He extended his predicted prognosis by nearly 4 months, but sadly succumbed to his illness a few weeks after his discharge. He was an inspiration to the members of the urology team who contributed to his care.

Publications Over the past 14 years, there have been several publications on bladder cancer (Anderson 2018a; Anderson 2018b; Anderson and Naish 2008a; Anderson and Naish 2008b; Anderson and Naish 2008c; Anderson and Naish 2008d; Anderson 2009; Anderson 2013), aimed at providing an in-depth insight and understanding on this subject area.

Prostate Cancer Caring for patients diagnosed with prostate cancer was a large part of my MUCNS role. Overall, my interactions and experiences, especially with the newly diagnosed patient, were enjoyable and extremely enlightening.

As previously noted, early diagnosis and treatment are crucial to achieving more favourable patient and practice outcomes (World Health Organization [WHO] 2021), a notation that is very true for prostate cancer and especially for men of African descents (Cancer Research UK 2019). However, when I reflect back on practice, I am surprised that my only experience of actually caring for a patient of African descent with prostate cancer on a practical level had been while working as an agency nurse, in a secondary care hospital. This gentleman, who was in his late 40s and of African-Caribbean background, had been in the end stages of the disease and its impact on his overall health was sobering. At that time, I must admit that I had not fully acknowledged the role played by screening and its importance to establishing an early diagnosis and initiating subsequent treatment. I did, however, acknowledge that securing improvements in this area necessitated increased awareness of this importance among men of African descents. A necessity that received closer scrutiny in my role as the MUCNS.

Publications There are several publications on prostate cancer (Anderson 2010a; Anderson 2015; Anderson 2017; Anderson et al. 2013; Anderson and Marshall-Lucette 2016), to which the reader is directed for a wider understanding of the disease and its management.

Kidney Cancer Caring for patients diagnosed with kidney was also a large part of my MUCNS role. As observed in local practice, for most patients, a CT scan was usually an accurate determination of a clinical diagnosis of kidney cancer. Also observed was that not all surgeries were for a cancerous pathology. Sometimes surgery was performed to remove non-cancerous growths (such as large cysts) that had the potential to obstruct kidney function (National Cancer Institute 2018) and accordingly impact the patient's renal health and quality of life.

Over the past 14 years, I was involved in the care of many kidney cancer patients, most of whom were newly diagnosed with low-risk, localised disease. Here, surgery was the recommended treatment of choice, the intent of which was to secure a cure and more favourable quality-of-life outcomes. For patients diagnosed with aggressive disease, as in advanced metastases, chemotherapy and radiotherapy were the usual treatments of choice; although the outcomes were less favourable. For patients whose disease had progressed following treatment with surgery, or at subsequent follow-up, additional treatment with immunotherapy was the recommended treatment of choice (National Cancer Institute 2018). Here, liaison between secondary care and tertiary care sectors (as in referrals to the consultant oncologist to seek an opinion on the most appropriate management) was the usual approach to care.

In determining care, a routine referral to the specialist renal MDT was important in ratifying any management decisions for this patient group.

In the case of advanced metastatic kidney cancer, as illustrated in the following case study, sometimes a diagnosis could be emotionally devastating, for both patients and health professionals alike. This account was used for the undertaking of master's degree in 2011.

6.3.3   Case Study—Issue: The Breaking of Bad News (BBN)

It was a Tuesday afternoon in January 2006. At approx. 14.10, I received a phone call from the nurse in outpatients' clinic, and the consultant requested that I see a patient. This was an unscheduled appointment, urgent referral from GP, for suspected kidney cancer. I met Leanne, a 39-year-old mother of four children, with the eldest 21 and the youngest 2 years old.

A CT scan had diagnosed an incidental finding of advanced metastatic kidney cancer—a particularly traumatic diagnosis that was further compounded by the fact that Leanne's presentation was completely unplanned. Leanne had been with her long-term partner for 25 years, and while they had discussed marriage and got engaged in the early stages of their relationship they had never married. The resulting effect for Leanne and her family was extreme emotional distress, especially for her mother who had accompanied her to the outpatients' appointment, and a high level of concern for the consultant and me. Having explained the diagnosis, the available treatment options (chemotherapy) and the potential risks and implications, Leanne had then asked the consultant what the benefits of surgery would be. The consultant explained that because her disease was so advanced, surgery may do little to improve her outcomes, and if she did have surgery, she would still require chemotherapy after.

Leanne was so scared at this time. It was evident that she was clutching at anything that would extend her life, and as such had convinced the consultant to perform surgery (despite the predicted outcome). She was referred to the tertiary care centre to discuss additional treatment intervention with chemotherapy, post-surgery, and was promised a prognosis of between 18 months and 3 years. Leanne proceeded to have surgery but sadly, due to a significant decline in her general health, she was unable to have the planned chemotherapy. The promised prognosis of between 18 months and 3 years reduced to 4 months—she died in May 2006.

6.4 Reflection and Learning Gained

Following surgery Leanne visualised an extended time, to celebrate her 40th birthday, to get married and to have more time with her children. Sadly, it was a visualisation that was not meant to be. On reflection the inherent risks to Leanne's decision about her management related to whether the decision made was in her best interest. In choosing to have surgery Leanne opted for the procedure that she believed would extend her life, but sadly this was not the case. However, in hindsight, I believe that it would have been impossible to deter her from going down this route, and realising this, the consultant had no choice but to agree to her request to have surgery.

This situation was made even more difficult since the outpatient's department was not conducive to breaking bad news. It is well documented that the delivery of bad news should be done in a private location, but in my experience, the outpatient department was not the most ideally suited environment for this undertaking and dealing with the implications thereof (McGuigan 2009).

This was particularly evident on this occasion. This was a very busy clinic, and since space was limited, the only room available for me to see Leanne after the receipt of bad news from the consultant was a room in the ENT section within the outpatient's department. I was very conscious that this was an inappropriate space for dealing with bad news and providing the necessary support, even so I believe I handled the situation well.

After introducing myself again to Leanne and her mother and apologising for having to give her such bad news, I proceeded to ask her how she felt. With the pain and distress blatantly obvious, she looked at me and said, 'Am I going to die?' 'I can't die, what will happen to my children?' At this moment, feeling unsure of how honest I should be, I looked her in the eye and asked just how honest did she want me to be, to which her response was, 'Very!' This was an extremely emotional time. Having re-explained the diagnosis and the actual potential implications to this, Leanne had expressed her wish to celebrate her 40th birthday and to get married. Her mother had tried to support her, but in voicing the telling words, 'this is not right; this should not be happening', her own emotional turmoil was laid bare.

Leanne had gone on to have surgery. I supported her as best as I could, by visiting her in the hospital ward and on her subsequent discharge home with telephone conversations to see how she was getting on. It was obvious that she was struggling. While I believed that I had provided Leanne with the best support, I was also unsure of just how effective this support had been—an uncertainty that was assuaged by Leanne's subsequent feedback stating that my being there had made a difference.

It is understandable that Leanne's subsequent death had had a huge emotional impact on me, in particular visions of my own mortality. I desperately wanted her to have the extra time she needed to 'get her house in order'. As such, I did question whether not having the surgery would have given her more time.

6.5   Conclusion and Lessons Learnt

Admittedly, in January 2006, one year into my role as MUCNS, my knowledge of kidney cancer was still being developed, and my experience of how I should interact with these patients, following this type of diagnosis, was still in its infancy. Nevertheless, I believe that my knowledge of kidney cancer and my understanding of the disease impact, combined with the knowledge and experience gained from the psychodynamic counselling course, were beneficial in providing the necessary physical and emotional support. Without a doubt, Leanne's diagnosis had impacted me emotionally, and I am aware that this impact was compounded by the fact that she was relatively young and that she had children. As a nurse and a mother, the duality of those roles coincided to speak to my own discomforts in trying to comprehend what Leanne had gone through. Going forward, I have been involved in similar cases of breaking bad news, although, admittedly, I had been better placed emotionally to deal with the ensuing fallout.

This experience of kidney cancer had been one of several. The second case study relates to a 48-year-old lady, also diagnosed with advanced metastatic renal cell carcinoma in 2013, and the fallout from this diagnosis. Readers are directed to the Anderson (Anderson 2019a) article for a detailed explanation and understanding of the events.

Testicular Cancer   In local practice, a patient with suspected testicular cancer is usually referred via the 2-week rule (TWR) referral pathway. Since speed is of essence in the diagnosis and treatment of this cancer, patients will, following assessment and an ultrasound scan, be fast-tracked for surgery, inguinal orchidectomy, within 24 hours, plus/minus a referral to the tertiary care centre (TCC) for further assessment and consideration of additional treatment with chemotherapy. Subsequent histology from this orchidectomy is routinely discussed at the local UMDT, where histology results will normally confirm if referral to the TCC was still necessitated. However, while a referral for chemotherapy may not be indicated, some patients are referred anyway for trial purposes. I have observed that while diagnosis was still more prevalent among the younger male, diagnosis in the older male (65 years plus group) had increased.

Due to the speed in diagnosis and subsequent treatment, the opportunity for the MUCNS to routinely interact upfront with these patients was often lacking. Usually, interaction would only occur if the MUCNS team was informed of the patient's appointment and a MUCNS had then met the patient in clinic where he/she provided the appropriate emotional and informational support, including contact details to initiate future contact. This support might also include (pending the patient's consent and appropriateness) a referral for sperm harvesting and banking. During my 14 years as MUCNS I have been made aware of a small majority of patients who have been referred with a suspicious testicular diagnosis (usually via the UMDT), but had only interacted with three patients, the youngest of whom was 12 years old. The lack of MUCNS interaction with these patients was recently highlighted in local practice by my line manager who was eager for this to become more accessible to this group of patients.

There has been no actual publication for testicular cancer; however, through a case study discussion, I did address issues pertaining to diagnosis and management in the realms of survivorship and the various stages of survival in my undertaking of the Surviving Cancer Course in 2009.

Penile Cancer Identification of penile cancer cases is rare in local practice, but as previously explained, if and when a diagnosis was made, these are routinely transferred to the specialist team at another secondary care hospital within the local cancer network group of hospitals. There has been no publication for penile cancer; however, as outlined in the following case studies, my experiences with two patients (1998–2001) left a lasting impression on me.

6.5.1 Case Study

Mr. Gerrard, a 57-year-old gentleman, was an author and a divorcee with two teenage sons. He was diagnosed with penile cancer, a diagnosis for which he was intermittently readmitted to the urology ward for over 3 years (the true definition of a returnee). Mr. Gerrard was the first patient I had known with penile cancer, a part of the body which before then I had not consciously associated with cancer. He was an extremely pleasant gentleman who was always friendly to the nurses. I remember that he would always ask me how I was and during our interactions had often spoken to me about his writing exploits. He suggested that I should consider writing since he believed that there was a book in everyone. Thinking back on Mr. Gerrard's final admission I clearly remember thinking that he was a shadow of the man he once was, with the incredible weight loss, general malaise, unshaven face and evident lack of enthusiasm for life. He had lost not only the fight, but sadly also the battle. Often, while caring for Mr. Gerard, his frame and build subsequently reminded me of Mr. Young, my first cancer diagnosis and subsequent death in 1974. Different cancer diagnosis, but the same degree of decline in health. Mr. Gerrard had returned home to his second family who gave him a fitting send off on his final journey.

6.5.2 Case Study

My only other experience of penile cancer had been with a gentleman in his late 70s, whom I visited in his home in the community with the district nurse (DN) during the Enrolled Nurse Conversion Course in the 1990s. This gentleman had had a total penectomy and was being followed up by the DN for change of dressings and relevant support. As I observed the resulting wound from the loss of the penis, I was eager to learn if this change in body image affected his self-perceived notions of masculinity. Bearing in mind the sensitivity of the situation I asked the question and was surprised by his honesty. For him, being alive was the overriding importance. Unfortunately, like so many others, I did not get to witness the outcome of this cancer diagnosis.

6.6   Audit and the Delivery of Nurse-Led Services

The Prostate-Specific Antigen (PSA) Telephone Follow-Up Clinic Since coming into post in 2005, one of my initial responsibilities was to look at ways to improve the structure of the urology joint consultation clinic (JCC), in an attempt to improve the service provided to patients and increase overall efficiency within this clinic. Anecdotal evidence of patients' feedback highlighted significant dissatisfaction with the current method of service provision. Dissatisfaction was mostly related to the long waits in the outpatients' clinic to see the doctor. Not only was this situation frustrating, but it was also expensive, due to the high cost of hospital parking if they drove to site. Admittedly, a few patients refused telephone follow-up as they preferred face-to-face consultations with the doctor in the outpatients' clinic, and others had 'hinted' that despite the evident problems, it was a day out, and they enjoyed coming to the clinic to see the doctor. Nevertheless, ongoing observations of service provision had indicated that too many patients were attending the clinic for their PSA follow-up appointment and that many of these patients were inappropriate 'attenders', since their PSA history signified levels that were clinically stable and had been for some time. As such, they could be easily followed up in another way, i.e. over the telephone. This conclusion had led to the creation of the *prostate-specific antigen (PSA) telephone follow-up clinic*, to which I recruited suitable patients. Recruitment involved devising a simple leaflet that explained the clinic protocol and the types of patients who were suitable for this type of follow-up. Patients were selected at their appointment, after the consultant had determined their suitability for telephone follow-up and had explained the potential benefits of this service. If a patient was happy to be followed up in this way, I then introduced myself and asked them to complete the leaflet which signified their agreement to being enrolled into the clinic. In support of this clinic, I also devised the PSA telephone follow-up leaflet (*Appendix II*) to provide patients with more information about the service.

The PSA Telephone Follow-Up Audit   The PSA telephone follow-up clinic commenced in January 2006 and I conducted my first audit 5 months later. Results revealed that even though this service was still in its infancy, patients were happy with the care received. Following encouragement from my line manager, I presented this audit at the Pan London Conference in 2006. As a new beginner to presenting my work in front of a large audience, I was anxious. In fact, I was so nervous that I nearly 'bolted'. My presentation did not meet my expectations on that day, but with practice, I was able to find my comfort zone within public speaking; however, to this day, the nerves while less severe still persist.

A second audit of this clinic was undertaken in 2009, the results of which were used in the second stand-alone project for the master's degree in 2010. This PSA telephone follow-up clinic ran for 11 years. Over this time, a total of 93 patients were recruited of which a number had returned to follow-up in the urology outpatients' clinic and sadly some had died. The number of patients still being followed up in this clinic by the end of November 2017 reduced to 41, and as per guidance regarding the long-term follow-up of stable prostate cancer patients, all were discharged back to their respective GPs to be followed up in the community, with the appropriate instructions in place to ensure safe and timely referrals back to secondary care if so indicated.

The Bladder Cancer Nurse-Led Clinic   The second nurse-led service is the weekly chemotherapy clinic, which delivers the aforementioned intravesical treatments of BCG and MMC (Vahr et al. 2015) to patients who have been previously diagnosed or have been newly diagnosed with non-muscle-invasive bladder cancer (NMIBC). Diagnosis of NMIBC has increased significantly over the years, and consequently the number of patients being referred for these treatments has also increased. I took over the running of this nurse-led service in 2005, initially on my own (between 2005 and 2006), and later working in conjunction with another MUCNS until my retirement in October 2019.

Practitioner Competency   Integral to the running of this clinic is the practitioner's competence. This requires knowledge of the disease, diagnosis, treatment modalities and associated risks of these, to enable them to provide patients with clear and concise information about their care (Macmillan Cancer Support 2014). All practitioners must be appropriately trained to administer treatments to patients (Lamm et al. 2000). Training includes an initial full-day induction on the aforementioned treatments and subsequent practice sessions, followed by yearly half-day updates. Practitioners must also consider the cost of treatments. Because of the lifetime need for surveillance, treatment of recurrent tumours and costs associated with maintenance therapies, bladder cancer poses a significant economic burden (Jacobs et al. 2010). In demonstrating competency, the practitioner must ensure that they obtain the patient's consent (an ethical and a legal requirement) to this undertaking (Department of Health [DH] 2009) and that in delivering this treatment the patient's privacy and dignity are maintained (Doult 2009).

Patient Information   Integral to the delivery of this service is the provision of Trust-specific patient information leaflets about the treatment regime, side effects and role of smoking in the development of bladder cancer (*refer to Appendix II*). The overall consensus from patients' feedback is that these leaflets are extremely useful.

The evidence suggests that bladder cancer is more prevalent in people of Caucasian background and less prevalent in people from Black, Asian and Minority Ethnic (BAME) backgrounds (Cancer Research UK 2021). In regard to the chemotherapy clinic, I can affirm that over the past 14 years, the majority of patients referred for these treatments were of Caucasian backgrounds, from the UK and Europe. Referrals included males and females, but with males outnumbering females by at least 3:1. Referrals from BAME backgrounds were at a lesser level, which supports the lower prevalence in diagnosis of bladder cancer in this group. For patients from Black Minority Ethnic (BME) backgrounds, referrals were less than those of Asian backgrounds, although in comparison to women referrals for men were higher. This notation was apparent up until 2019, when a total of two BME women had been referred for this treatment.

The Bladder Cancer Audit   The inspiration for this audit was aroused during my interactions with patients in the chemotherapy clinic, when the realisation that most of these patients were either current smokers or ex-smokers piqued my curiosity. Since the evidence suggests that smoking is the predominant cause in the development of bladder cancer (Vahr et al. 2015), it seemed prudent to conduct further exploration. Accordingly, discussions with my colleague, the urology nurse consultant (WN), resulted in an extremely beneficial brainstorming session from which we accrued a significant amount of credible evidence pertaining to smoking and its link to bladder cancer. This then led to an audit of patients who presented to this nurse-led clinic having received or were receiving treatment with either MMC or BCG therapies. The audit aims were to establish if the findings in the literature supported the theory that smoking was indeed the predominant risk factor in the development of bladder cancer. Not only did the results support this theory, but it also underlined the importance of health promotion and education in increasing patients' awareness of this risk and in enabling them to take responsibility for their health (Morris 2019;

National Institute for Health and Care Excellence [NICE] 2017). This audit resulted in the bladder series publications (Anderson and Naish 2008a; Anderson and Naish 2008b; Anderson and Naish 2008c; Anderson and Naish 2008d).

6.6.1   2019—Summary

Nurse-led services remain an integral part of clinical practice. In regard to the bladder cancer clinic, I have noted that unforeseen problems with follow-up care, as in the performance of cystoscopies (under local and general anaesthetics) after BCG and MMC treatments within the 6–8-weekly interval, did impact the delivery of service despite efforts to minimise this. Nevertheless, the overall consensus from various 'friends and family' feedbacks is that this nurse-led activity delivers a robust service and that patients were satisfied with the care received.

Thinking back on my endeavour to deliver education and health promotion, I have come to the conclusion that while I had a responsibility to highlight the relevant risks of continued smoking and the benefits of stopping, expecting patients who have smoked for most of their lives to stop the habit in their 70s, 80s or 90s was somewhat unrealistic. Nonetheless, it was an important undertaking, the aim of which was to provide the necessary support to enable patients to take responsibility for their health, and accordingly make an informed decision on whether they should stop smoking.

In my continued attempts to improve efficiency within this clinic, I devised a spreadsheet that has proven useful for tracking patients' progress during the 1-year regime and in ensuring that maintenance treatments are delivered in a timely manner.

6.7   Reassuring Distractions

In this context, reassuring distractions relate to catheterising patients prior to delivering intravesical treatments in the nurse-led chemotherapy clinic. Over the years, I have come to appreciate that the insertion of a *urinary* catheter is an invasive procedure that can incite fear, anxiety and embarrassment, especially in the predominantly male patients I have had to perform this upon. Trauma experienced during a previous catheterisation only serves to add to the vulnerability that these men feel in such instances. Integral to deflecting these emotions is the practitioner's competency to skilfully perform catheterisation and the beneficial effects of humour and breathing techniques in this.

Utilising Humour   The insertion of a urinary catheter is an integral part of delivering intravesical treatments (BCG and MMC) to patients. Over the past 14 years, in my attempts to support patients emotionally during incredibly vulnerable moments in their lives, I have found humour essential (Harrison 1995) in building the rapport needed to deflect fear, anxiety and remove any embarrassment. However, as experience has shown, humour must be used appropriately, as it could easily be misinterpreted in its use as an insult or a sign of disrespect (Harrison 1995). For this reason, it is important to assess each situation individually as it goes hand in hand with the needs of each patient. Continuity of care is crucial to positive medical outcomes, and it afforded me the chance to hone my instincts when dealing with patients and understanding how they would respond to my careful applications of humour. An interesting observation was that some patients (men and women) had often taken the initiative to inject humour into the equation, particularly if they were feeling fearful or embarrassed.

However, the use of humour was not always successful. There were patients (mostly men) who were so nervous that I could do nothing to reassure them. My memories of such moments take me back to patients with their eyes tightly closed and bodies extremely tense with no sense of relief in sight. In the performance of catheterisation, my competence and skill were crucial to securing a successful outcome. I may not have been able to reassure the patient, but talking to them enabled me to insert the catheter, instil the treatment and often remove the catheter before they had even realised that it was all over. In this moment, the astonished look of surprise and subsequent retort of 'Is it all done … wow, that wasn't as bad as I thought' was incredibly gratifying. Often, positive experiences such as these meant that future treatments were less stressful.

I should point out that while my use of humour did attain a degree of success, I understand that some practitioners may not feel comfortable utilising such a technique in their practice. However, in creating safer and less stress-induced experiences for patients, I do believe that it is fundamental for practitioners to find methods to connect with patients in order to support their physical and emotional well-being.

Beneficial Breathing Having made reference to compromised breathing in Chap. 2, I felt that it would be useful to highlight the reassuring effect of this technique in enabling patients to relax during catheterisation and their receipt of intravesical treatments. Often, I had been able to quell the fears and anxieties of patients in regard to the procedure and for the most part I was able to bring them some form of comfort just by talking to them. However, during the last 2 years of delivering this nurse-led service, I had noticed that the younger men who were being referred presented with greater levels of anxiety prior to being catheterised for treatments. In my attempts to calm their fears and encourage them to relax, I began using breathing techniques for support. In this instance, I encouraged the patient to focus on their breathing (breathing in deeply and slowly exhaling) and not on the task at hand. For me, the usefulness of this exercise was verified by subsequent patient remarks, such as 'Is it done', and the evident relief on their face, when I said, 'Yes, it is'. In some cases, the expression of relief was often followed by tears and an enthusiastic thank you. Unlike my previous notations of compromised breathing (where the individual struggled to breathe, and for which the appropriate gratification had been inhalers, oxygen and nebulisers), in this context, breathing is the appropriate gratification. Breathing is a key technique in the act of meditation, shifting consciousness to benefit psychological well-being. Breathing techniques are known to reduce stress levels and help regulate the bodies' reaction to stress which is why I believe that it is so effective as it provides patients with the tools they need to overcome their fears and anxieties during the right moments.

2005–2017—Extended Elements of the MUCNS Role   In my role as MUCNS, my responsibility for providing support to my patients often extended to their spouses, in particular wives, many of whom were NHS employees (secretaries, ward clerks and nursing colleagues). The majority of these patients were men, who had been diagnosed with prostate cancer, some of whom had survived the disease following treatment, and some who, sadly, had died soon after diagnosis and subsequent treatment. As I personally observed in practice, when a diagnosis of prostate cancer is given to a patient, usually wives are affected just as much (if not more, in certain cases) by the news as their husbands are, and hence were equally deserving of the MUCNS support.

Often, I would run into these wives in the hospital corridor, on the stairs or just in common places where our paths happen to cross. After the usual question of how they were doing, I would find myself listening to an update on the husbands' progress, following which I would offer the appropriate advice, information, explanation and reassurance. In some cases, this interaction was a little uncomfortable, but knowing that they valued my support was also rewarding. From a personal perspective, my interactions and experiences with these wives forced me to think about my own husband and how I would cope if he were to be diagnosed with prostate cancer. Just thinking about it evoked a sense of fear and anxiety within me, feelings that were perhaps not that dissimilar to those of these wives I conversated with.

6.8   Personal Insights from the Patient's Perspective (2)

For this second personal insight, I have elected to reflect on my experience of enduring the magnetic resonance imaging (MRI) scan. I felt that it was important to illustrate how this experience informed my knowledge and accordingly my interactions with patients.

An MRI or magnetic resonance imaging is a radiology technique scan that uses magnetism, radio waves and a computer to produce images of body structures. The MRI scanner is basically a tube surrounded by a giant circular magnet. The procedure involves the patient being placed on a moveable bed that is inserted into the magnet (Shiel 2019).

From listening to patients and comparing their experiences to my own, an apt description of the MRI scanner is of a coffin-like equipment, in which the individual's claustrophobic fears are heightened. This is a situation that is further compounded by the loud banging noise that resonates from the MRI while it is scanning. It is further compounded by a very bright light that hangs from the ceiling directly over the patient's head which is close to the individual's face and can be quite unnerving. Working as the MUCNS, I often supported newly diagnosed men with prostate cancer for whom an MRI scan was often necessitated to determine any underlying abnormality or pathology. For most patients, having this scan is quite straightforward, but for some it is quite a difficult task, especially if they suffer with a fear of enclosed spaces (claustrophobia). On reflection, I must confess to my sometimes flippant retorts to patients, 'oh, it's not that bad, you'll be fine', in regard to their concerns regarding undergoing the procedure. The following account highlights my own experience of having an MRI and my subsequent acknowledgement of my patient's fears.

In July 2007, I had an accident that resulted in me sustaining a tear in the rotator cuff in my right shoulder for which, unfortunately, surgery was necessary. An MRI was required to enhance internal visualisation during the surgery. Having had no prior experience of an MRI, I eagerly agreed to have the procedure. On the day of my appointment, the MRI technician was very informative. She had explained the procedure to me, including what to expect, everything except, perhaps most importantly, to keep my eyes closed as I entered into the scanner. Since music was considered beneficial to helping the patient to relax, the technician had asked me to select a musical piece—I selected Ella Fitzgerald. I am sitting outside the scanner on the moveable bed, with gown and headphones on. The technician asked me if I was ready, and I said, 'Yes, I was'. At this point, I had not a hint of nerves evident. I laid down on the moveable bed and it slowly proceeded into the scanner, my head getting closer to the opening as I was slowly edged into the tunnel. With my head and most of my body inserted, I am directly beneath this bright light that is literally inches from my nose. My eyes are fixated; this is much too close! 'Oh, my lord', the coffin-like experience! I could feel the fear rising, a fear and a feeling of being buried alive is all encompassing—I began to panic. I remember hearing the technician's voice, and even though her words seemed far away, she was asking me if I was ok? The light, so bright. I tried to close my eyes, but the brightness persisted. It is hard to breathe. I heard myself saying, 'Nooooh, I'm not …, please, please pull me out!'. I am aware of the moveable bed being slowly recalled, and I am eventually outside the tunnel. I can now breathe more easily, but still the dreaded feeling of being buried alive remains in the pit of my stomach.

The technician said that I did not have to do test if I felt uncomfortable. 'Yes, I do', I said … 'the consultant requires the scan to assess the tear in my shoulder and the extent of the damage prior to surgery …, so I do have to have the MRI'. 'Ok', she said …, 'if you are sure'. Second attempt. Headphones on again, Ella's voice mellowing in the background. The conveyor bed advances towards the tunnel, and this time, I kept my eyes tightly closed—the problem is you cannot unsee what has been seen. The noise is extremely loud; I can hardly hear Ella—her voice is drowned out by the persistent clunking. Even though my eyes remained tightly shut, the bright light seems to have penetrated beyond the lids. 'You can do this', I quietly voiced to myself. In an attempt to allay my fears, I focused on my breathing, counted back from a hundred and thought of something soothing—a memory from my childhood, cornfields swaying in the breeze. The light is so intense, and in my attempt to thwart its intensity, I slowly moved my right hand to pull the blanket up over my face at which point the technician's voice staunchly intervenes: 'Please do not move … you will distort the images'. She attempted to reassure me, 'Not long to go'. 20 minutes had felt like 20 hours. I am finally at the other end of the scanner; my head slowly emerges, and it is such a relief. The technician asked me if I was ok? 'Yes', I said, but I was not. I felt sick, and with tears running down my cheeks, I realised just how scared I was.

Never again I thought, not unless I am anaesthetised. In fact, I had said exactly that to the consultant when I met with him later. He had smiled and thanked me for having the MRI. He stated that he appreciated that it was a difficult procedure but it was essential to determine his approach to performing my surgery. I returned to work in the afternoon and had felt sick, fearful and very strange, for the rest of the day. However, in light of this experience, I now understood how my patients felt in terms of their concerns regarding the MRI procedure, specifically their fears of enclosed spaces. I went on to have my surgery in March 2008, and as a result of my personal MRI experience, in the provision of care going forward, I endeavoured to see things from my patients' perspective, and as such stopped being flippant about their fears and concerns.

6.9   2019—In-Team Relationships

A team is defined as a group of individuals working together to achieve their goal (Thompson 2008). As I have observed in practice, when various personalities are thrown together in a team, if the communication between team members and across the team was poor, this often resulted in in-team bickering, conflict, power struggles and 'bully-boy' tactics, as each member of the team seeks to find their niche within the group and establish their position within the team's hierarchy. A case of 'too many cooks …', combined with demeaning and condescending communication, and the outcome is likely to be a reduction in the individual's self-esteem, morale and confidence (Thompson 2008; Ali 2017; Doyle 2020). It is not a situation that is conducive to establishing an effective working environment, or a space in which learning can flourish, but more importantly an atmosphere like this often inhibits an individual's ability to grow and excel, where their efforts are acknowledged and appreciated and their opinions valued and respected. Considering that most nurses spend a significant amount of their life working, I believe that it is reasonable to expect that the environment in which they work is conducive to motivating a high level of performance, boosting confidence and overall job satisfaction (Doyle 2020; Anderson 2010b).

Ultimately, the key to team cohesiveness is leadership and the ability to communicate effectively (Thompson 2008). Essentially, as health professionals, we have a responsibility to work in unison, and to communicate effectively, with the people (in this case team members) we interact with (Ali 2017; Doyle 2020). I am not naïve; I am aware that not all members of a team will get on with each other. As my mum used to say, 'Your spirit won't take to everyone'. Nonetheless, in terms of nursing and working as a team, there is the unspoken requirement for professionalism, which necessitates all team members working together. However, experience has shown that such an objective can be difficult to accomplish. As explained in Chap. 1, change, regardless of whether it is planned or unplanned, will cause ensuing resistance and stress (Oguejiofo 2018); hence, an effective leadership and management strategy is key to securing successful outcomes for everyone (Lancaster and Lancaster 1982). The following account addresses the implementation of change into practice. Admittedly, prior to this, there had been some rumbling of disquiet within the MUCNS team, one that had been heightened by the enlarging of the team. Following the implemented change, the receipt of a complaint and the resulting impact of poor communication and poor leadership had significantly increased the disquiet in the MUCNS and within current practice (Anderson 2019b).

The Change Strategy The implemented change was a new strategy, for which the objective was to increase overall efficiency in the management of two cancer pathways (prostate and bladder), and consequently improve the patient's health, ensuing experiences as well as practice outcomes. It was also a way to expedite care, in line with meeting the government's target specifications (*Table 1.1, Chap. 1*) (National Institute for Health and Care Excellence [NICE] 2015). This innovative strategy entitled telephone assessment consultation (TAC) provided an efficient service to those patients who had been referred by their GPs via the two-week rule (TWR) waiting times standard on the rapid prostate and bladder pathways. Pending an assessment, these patients are then fast-tracked to receive the necessary diagnostic tests to exclude or confirm a diagnosis, and determine subsequent management. This is a nurse-led service, for which the chief drivers of its delivery are the MUCNS team, in conjunction with doctors and other members of the MDT.

The initial TAC clinic for prostate cancer patients was commenced in 2016, followed by bladder patients in 2018. Subsequent reviews of this service showed that TAC was beneficial in terms of improving referral pathways and patient throughput, and overall efficiency in patient and practice outcomes, although these had been at a cost. The implemented change and its subsequent management had a noticeable impact on the MUCNS team. As stated by Burns (Burns 1993), if a change is introduced too quickly and changes again, before recipients of the change have had a chance to adapt, will incite tension and stress. Unfortunately, following the implementation of this change, management did not allow the necessary time for it to be embedded into practice before proposing an addition to the initial change, a decision that led to increased workloads, pressure and friction within the MUCNS team.

There were also changes to working patterns, namely time management (MUCNS regularly worked unpaid overtime to manage the workload), resulting in less time to honour other responsibilities, such as attending and running various clinics, in line with meeting the patient's needs. As previously explained in Chap. 1, a crucial part of the MUCNS role is their presence in clinic when a patient receives their diagnosis, and spending time with the patient after diagnosis to provide the appropriate support and reassurance (Stringer 2008; McClain 2012). However, due to the increased pressures of work, meeting this expectation was difficult to fulfil—a difficulty that was clearly highlighted on one particular occasion.

The JCC clinic was extremely busy; with 4 consultants in attendance and only 2 MUCNS to manage the overall workload, it was impossible to provide MUCNS support to all patients. In this instance, both my colleague and I felt that patients were being short-changed—an upsetting acknowledgement, since providing patient support was a key part of our role. Added to this situation had been the issue of poor communication. As highlighted in Anderson (Anderson 2019a) for some senior nursing professionals, there is an assumed hierarchy of entitlement, in the way these individuals communicated with their peers. A patronising and disrespectful attitude had impacted negatively the MUCNS team, in that having implied doubts with regard to the individual's professional standing, and their competency to perform their role, incited in them a lack of confidence and reduction in self-esteem, and accordingly discomfort and disharmony within the clinical environment.

This situation was further compounded by the receipt of a complaint against the MUCNS team, for which the lack of effective management had left certain team members feeling let down, unsupported or, for want of a better word, betrayed by the very individuals who were meant to support them. There is ample evidence to show that within the healthcare system, complaints are par for the course, but with effective management, in which effective communication is crucial, it is possible to secure positive outcomes for all concerned (Ali 2017; Doyle 2020). Some may argue that the MUCNS team was perhaps too sensitive, or had taken the complaint too personally, but to this my response would be, 'Those who feels it, knows it'. Based on my personal experience, if you are the unfortunate recipient of that complaint, its receipt is very personal, and the ensuing feelings are very justified (Anderson 2019b).

Reflection Reflection on this undertaking has highlighted the same issues (team-working, power, control, poor communication, leadership) as previously addressed in the power risk and leadership modules. In my reflection on recent in-team issues, there were definitely elements of competitiveness, and a craving for control and power, which combined with strong evidence of poor communication had led to the conflict within the MUCNS group.

It could be argued that this is a subjective view, but when I reflect back to the early years (1974–1976), my time in the urology ward (1997–2005) and my experiences of teamworking then, compared to that of the current MUCNS team, the true meaning of effective teamworking becomes apparent. My memory of that sense of belonging, support and respect for each other's skills still burns bright, something which I am sad to say was never truly evident, at least not on the same level, within my current team. If I am honest, I have found cancer nursing more competitive, and in some ways less supportive, and while I cannot generalise across all cancer groups, there is an evident lack of warmth and compassion when compared with my early nursing experiences. In terms of fun, while elements of this had been apparent in the earlier years in the urology ward, and in some ways still are, the feeling of belonging is less marked, while elements of stress are more pronounced. Sadly, these issues came to the fore, even more so in the last months of my nursing journey.

Arguably, the relentless culture that is change had intervened once more, and for me had played a final role in what I can only describe as a disorganised chaos within my team. It resulted in an extremely uncomfortable working environment. Admittedly, at this stage of my journey, I would have preferred not to have encountered change, or to have experienced the subsequent feelings of pain and discomfort that emanated from its implementation.

6.9.1   Conclusion and Lessons Learnt

In summary, it would be fair to say that working in teams can be stressful, and is especially so if the relationships within those teams are strained to begin with. There are a number of factors that can impact teamworking, of which the implementation of change into practice can be particularly damaging. As observed in local practice, while the implementation of change can be beneficial in terms of improving both patient and practice outcomes, a failure to effectively manage the implemented change can result in increased stress, anxiety and difficult teamworking. The evidence has shown that within the healthcare establishment, health professionals are often overworked and overstressed; hence, while the instigation of change may be perceived by some as a welcomed strategy, others will invariably view its instigation as a burden, adding to an already arduous workload (UKEssays 2018), a conclusion with which I fully concur. However, the evidence has also shown that if the change is managed effectively, it is possible to achieve the desired outcomes for patients, health practitioners and the organisation. Central to achieving this outcome is effective communication and leadership. Reflecting on my past experiences of poor communications, and remembering their ensuing effect, I remain steadfast in my belief that those responsible (including myself) for delivering this basic but very important activity must remain vigilant of the inherent risks, and always strive to minimise the potential for a negative impact, arising from poor communications, on the recipients.

Chapter 7 provides a summary on the completion of the MSc in advanced practice project, highlighting the modules undertaken and their relevance in the completion of the project. My interactions with PCUK are highlighted, including a current update on the Charity's activities.

References

Ali M (2017) Communication skills 1: benefits of effective communication for patients. Nurs Times 113(12):18–19

Anderson B (2009) Understanding the role of smoking in the aetiology of bladder cancer. Br J Community Nurs 14(9):385–392

Anderson B (2010a) The benefits to nurse-led telephone follow-up for prostate cancer. Br J Nurs 19(17):1085–1090. [Internet]. http://www.ncbi.nlm.nih.gov/pubmed/20871511

Anderson B (2010b) A perspective on changing dynamics in nursing over the past 20 years. Br J Nurs 19(18):1190–1191. [Internet] http://tinyurl

Anderson B (2013) Detecting and treating bladder cancer. Br J Nurs 22(11):628–628. [Internet]. http://www.ncbi.nlm.nih.gov/pubmed/23899731

Anderson B (2015) Cancer treatment: at what cost? Nurs Resid Care 17(3):173–174. https://doi.org/10.12968/nrec.2015.17.3.173. [Internet]

Anderson B (2017) An insight into the patient's response to a diagnosis of urological cancer. Br J Nurs [Internet]. 26(18):S4–12. http://www.ncbi.nlm.nih.gov/pubmed/29034698

Anderson B (2018a) Bladder cancer: overview and disease management. Part 1: non-muscle-invasive bladder cancer. Br J Nurs 27(9):S27–S37. [Internet]. http://www.magonlinelibrary.com/doi/10.12968/bjon.2018.27.9.S27

Anderson B (2018b) Bladder cancer: overview and management. Part 2: muscle-invasive and metastatic bladder cancer. Br J Nurs 27(18):S8–20. [Internet]. http://www.magonlinelibrary.com/doi/10.12968/bjon.2018.27.18.S8

Anderson B (2019a) Reflecting on the communication process in health care. Part 1: clinical practice-breaking bad news. Br J Nurs 28(13):858. [Internet]. http://www.ncbi.nlm.nih.gov/pubmed/31303035

Anderson B (2019b) Reflecting on the communication process in health care. Part 2: the management of complaints. Br J Nurs 28(14):927–929. [Internet]. http://www.ncbi.nlm.nih.gov/pubmed/3130303517

Anderson B, Marshall L, Webb P (2013) African and afro-Caribbean men's experiences of prostate cancer. Br J Nurs 22(22):1296–1307

Anderson B, Marshall-Lucette S (2016) Prostate cancer among Jamaican men: exploring the evidence for higher risk. Br J Nurs 25(19):2–7

Anderson B, Naish W (2008a) Bladder cancer and smoking. Part 1: addressing the associated risk factors. Br J Nurs 17(18):1182–1186. [Internet]. http://www.ncbi.nlm.nih.gov/pubmed/18946399

Anderson B, Naish W (2008b) Bladder cancer and smoking. Part 2: diagnosis and management. Br J Nurs 17(19):1240–1245. [Internet] http://www.ncbi.nlm.nih.gov/pubmed/18974695

Anderson B, Naish W (2008c) Bladder cancer and smoking. Part 3: influence of perceptions and beliefs. Br J Nurs 17(20):1292–1297. [Internet] http://www.ncbi.nlm.nih.gov/pubmed/19043336

Anderson B, Naish W (2008d) Bladder cancer and smoking. Part 4: efficacy of health promotion. Br J Nurs 17(21):1340–1344. [Internet] http://www.ncbi.nlm.nih.gov/pubmed/19060816

Babjuk M, Böhle A, Burger M, Compérat E, Kaasinen E, Palou J, et al. (2015) Guidelines on Non-muscle-invasive Bladder Cancer (Ta, T1 and CIS) [Internet]. [cited 2019 Oct 19]. https://uroweb.org/wp-content/uploads/EAU-Guidelines-Non-muscle-invasive-Bladder-Cancer-2015-v1.pdf

Burns R (1993) Managing people in changing times : coping with change in the workplace : 9 practical guide. Allen & Unwin, St. Leonards, NSW

Cancer Research UK (2019) Statistics by cancer type [Internet]. cancerresearchuk.org. [cited 2020 Sep 22]. https://www.cancerresearchuk.org/health-professional/cancer-statistics/statistics-by-cancer-type

Cancer Research UK (2021) Cancer incidence by ethnicity [Internet]. cancerresearchuk.org. [cited 2021 Sept, 9]. https://www.cancerresearchuk.org/health-professional/cancer-statistics/incidence/ethnicity

Department of Health [DH] (2009) Reference guide to consent for examination or treatment, Second edition. [Internet]. [cited 2021 Sept 5]. https://assets.publishing.service.gov.uk/government/uploads/system/uploads/attachment_data/file/138296/dh_103653__1_.pdf

Di Stasi SM, Liberati E, Micali F, Valenti M, Masedu F, Di Stasi SM et al (2011) Electromotive instillation of mitomycin immediately before transurethral resection for patients with primary urothelial non-muscle invasive bladder cancer: a randomised controlled trial. Lancet Oncol 12:871–879. [Internet] www.thelancet.com/oncology

Doult B (2009) Cautious welcome for pledge to eliminate mixed-sex wards. Nurs Stand 23(22):11

Doyle A (2020) Communication skills for workplace success [Internet]. thebalancereers.com. [cited 2020 Oct 13]. https://www.thebalance.com/communication-skills-list-2063779

Hamric AB (2005) Advanced practice nursing: an integrative approach [internet], 3rd edn. Elsevier Health Sciences. [cited 2020 Oct 7]. https://www.amazon.co.uk/Advanced-Practice-Nursing-Integrative-Approach/dp/0721603300/ref=sr_1_6?dchild=1&keywords=Advanced+Practice+Nursing%3A+An+integrative+approach&qid=1602073620&s=books&sr=1-6

Harrison N (1995) Using humour as an educational technique. Prof Nurse [Internet] 11(3):198–199. http://www.ncbi.nlm.nih.gov/pubmed/8552694

Jacobs BL, Lee CT, Montie JE (2010) Bladder Cancer in 2010: how far have we come? CA Cancer J Clin 60(4):244–272. [Internet]. https://acsjournals.onlinelibrary.wiley.com/doi/full/10.3322/caac.20077

Kwong T, Tana A, Ayres B, Perry M, Bailey M, Issa R (2013) Hyperthermic mitomycin C in the treatment of high risk non-muscle invasive bladder cancer—is it effective and safe? A regional centre's experience. Int J Surg 11(8):731. [Internet]. https://linkinghub.elsevier.com/retrieve/pii/S1743919113009321

Lamm DL, Blumenstein BA, Crissman JD, Montie JE, Gottesman JE, Lowe BA et al (2000) Maintenance bacillus Calmette-Guerin immunotherapy for recurrent TA, T1 and carcinoma in situ transitional cell carcinoma of the bladder: a randomized Southwest Oncology Group Study. J Urol 163(4):1124–1129. [Internet]. http://www.ncbi.nlm.nih.gov/pubmed/10737480

Lancaster J, Lancaster W (1982) The nurse as a change agent: concepts for advanced nursing practice. St Louis, MO

Macmillan Cancer Support (2014) Cancer clinical nurse specialists. Impact brief series. [Internet]. [cited 2021 Sept 6] https://www.macmillan.org.uk/documents/aboutus/research/impactbriefs/clinicalnursespecialists2015new.pdf

McClain G (2012) Healthcare professionals: acknowledging emotional reactions in newly-diagnosed patients [Internet]. Just Got Diagnosed. [cited 2016 Jul 18]. http://www.justgotdiagnosed.com

McGuigan D (2009) Communicating bad news to patients: a reflective approach. Nurs Stand [Internet] 23(31):51–56. http://www.ncbi.nlm.nih.gov/pubmed/19413074

Morris K (2019) Health promotion and health education for professional nurse. Prof Nurse. [Internet]. [cited 2021 Sept 5]. https://www.myassignmentservices.com/blog/health-promotion-and-health-education-for-professional-nurse

National Cancer Institute (2018) FDA approves Nivolumab and Ipilimumab combination for advanced kidney cancer [Internet]. cancer.gov. [cited 2020 Jul 13]. https://www.cancer.gov/news-events/cancer-currents-blog/2018/kidney-cancer-fda-nivolumab-ipilimumab-first-line

National Collaborating Centre for Cancer (2014) Bladder cancer: diagnosis and management. Clinical guideline methods, evidence and recommendations [Internet]. [cited 2018 Jan 21]. https://www.nice.org.uk/guidance/ng2/documents/bladder-cancer-clinical-guideline-draft-for-consultation2

National Institute for Health and Care Excellence [NICE] (2015) Suspected cancer: recognition and referral NICE guideline [NG12] [Internet]. [cited 2020 Oct 5]. www.nice.org.uk/guidance/ng12

National Institute for Health and Care Excellence [NICE] (2017). Smoking: supporting people to stop. Published August 2013, updated 2017. [NG92] [Internet]. [cited 2021 Sept 5]. https://www.nice.org.uk/guidance/ng92/

Oguejiofo N (2018) Change theories in nursing [Internet]. bizfluent.com. [cited 2020 Oct 13]. https://bizfluent.com/about-5544426-change-theories-nursing.html

Shiel WC (2019) Magnetic resonance imaging (MRI) scan definition and facts [Internet]. medicinenet.com. [cited 2019 Nov 12]. https://www.medicinenet.com/mri_scan/article.htm

Stringer S (2008) Psychosocial impact of cancer. Cancer Nurs Pract 7(7):32–37

Thompson DR, Watson R (2003) Advanced nursing practice: what is it? Int J Nurs Pract 9(3):129–130. https://doi.org/10.1046/j.1440-172X.2003.00424.x. [Internet]

Thompson LL (2008) Making the team: a guide for managers [internet], 3rd edn. Pearson, Upper Saddle River, NJ. https://www.amazon.co.uk/MakingTeam-Managers-Leigh-Thompson/dp/0134484207/ref=sr_1_fkmr0_1?dchild=1&keywords=Making+the+team+%3A+a+guide

+for+managers+%283rd+ed.%29.+Pearson%2FPrentice+Hall&qid=1602583451&s=books
&sr=1-1-fkmr0

UKEssays. (2018) Changes in roles and responsibilities of nurses in the modernisation of the NHS [Internet]. ukessays.com. [cited 2019 Oct 19]. https://www.ukessays.com/essays/nursing/changes-in-roles-and-responsibilities-of-nurses-in-the-modernisation-of-nhs-nursing-essay.php?vref=1

Vahr S, De Blok W, Love-Retinger N, Thoft B, Turner JB, Villa G, et al. (2015) Evidence-based Guidelines for Best Practice in Urological Health Care Intravesical instillation with mitomycin C or bacillus Calmette-Guérin in non-muscle invasive bladder cancer [Internet]. [cited 2020 Oct 25]. https://nurses.uroweb.org/wp-content/uploads/EAUN15-Guideline-Intravesical-instillation.pdf

Witjes JA, Compérat E, Cowan NC, De Santis M, Gakis G, James N, et al. (2015) Guidelines on muscle-invasive and metastatic bladder cancer [Internet]. [cited 2019 Oct 19]. https://uroweb.org/wp-content/uploads/EAU-Guidelines-Muscle-invasive-and-Metastatic-Bladder-Cancer-2015-v1.pdf

World Health Organization [WHO] (2021) Promoting cancer early diagnosis [Internet]. [cited: 2021 March 25]. https://www.who.int/activities/promoting-cancer-early-diagnosis

Educational and Practical Aids to Enhancing Practice

7

7.1 Reflection on the Completion of the Master's Degree in Advanced Practice Project

Having completed the BSc study and receiving the subsequent award in 2007, I thought this was it, as far as studies was concerned, but my mentor (WN) had other ideas. Her familiar words of encouragement were convincing … 'Bev, I know you did not want to do anymore studying, but how about doing the Master's degree to complete your academic journey?'. I looked her keenly in the eye, and with a smile framing my lips said, 'If I decide to do this study, will you leave me alone?' 'Yes', she said, also with a sly smile. Having agreed to do this study, I thought carefully about the possible topic areas, but had not managed to identify a suitable one—not until a few weeks later, when I received an email from my supervisor for the previous BSc course (SM-L), inviting me to enrol on the master's degree in advanced practice course, which she would be running. She felt that the course would be hugely beneficial to my current role and practice. Seemingly, I was destined to do the master's degree, so I proceeded to apply for the 2009 intake. However, as this course was full, I was advised by the university to apply for enrolment on the 2010 course, and to avoid wasting the year that I should look into undertaking stand-alone modules at level 7, to obtain credits towards the course in 2010. Subsequent conversations with my line manager and my mentor (WN) confirmed that they were happy for me to undertake this study, which comprised the following modules:

Stand-Alone modules prior to commencing MSc project included:
- The surviving cancer module.
- An overview of prostate cancer and highlighting the role of nurse-led services in long-term management.
- Defining the role of the clinical nurse specialist in cancer (oncology) care.

© Springer Nature Switzerland AG 2022
B. Anderson, *A Uro-Oncology Nurse Specialist's Reflection on her Practice Journey*, https://doi.org/10.1007/978-3-030-94199-4_7

Set group of modules on commencing the MSc project included:
- The Research Proposal.
- Research Project Planning and Management.
- Power, Risk and Decision-Making in Contemporary Partnership Contexts.
- Leadership in Advanced Practice.
- Personal and Professional Development in Advanced Practice.
- The Research Project.

7.1.1   The Surviving Cancer Module

Until well into the twentieth century, most cancer diagnoses were universally fatal. However, increasing advancement in diagnostics and treatment modalities has resulted in some phenomenal achievements and significant increases in the number of people who were now living with cancer rather than dying from the disease (survivorship) (National Cancer Institute 2008).

The survival process is divided into three stages: acute survival (diagnosis and treatment), extended survival (re-entry) and permanent survival (living life). No specific time frames exist for the stages, nor do all patients experience all stages (Self 2005; Decker et al. 2007; Morgan 2009).

For the surviving cancer module, I illustrated the various stages of survival through the case study of two patients, Jack and Nicholas, both referred by their GPs as a 2-week rule to the urology team. Jack, a 55-year-old self-employed solicitor, was diagnosed with locally advanced prostate cancer. He was married to Emily, a self-employed gardener, and together they had three daughters, aged 21, 19 and 16.

Nicholas was a 16-year-old young man, diagnosed with early localised testicular cancer who had recently completed his GCSE. He lived with his parents and was the eldest of four children comprising a sister who was 15, a brother who was 14 and a sister who was 11.

Working through the stages of survival allowed me to appreciate the impact of a cancer diagnosis on both Jack and Nicholas' lives and some of the challenges faced as a result. These include making decisions about their care (Self 2005; Morgan 2009); dealing with sexual problems (Fan 2002; Brandenburg et al. 2005; Fergus et al. 2002; Postovsky et al. 2003); psychosocial concerns—employment, financial and insurance problems (Waring and Wallace 2000; Itano and Taoka 2005); education (Hewitt and Ganz 2007); psychological concerns—uncertainty and fears of recurrence (Fan 2002; Itano and Taoka 2005; Rosella 1994); coping with the cessation/side effects of treatments (Skaali et al. 2009); and dealing with quality-of-life issues (Morgan 2009; Pemberger et al. 2005).

In this context, I was able to understand my role as well as the consultant urologist role in their management, in which the provision of emotional, and especially informational, support is imperative (Fergus et al. 2002; Tarrant et al. 2008). It has been shown that providing patients with the appropriate support gives them a degree of personal control over decision-making and they generally have higher quality-of-life outcomes (Hoffman and Stovall 2006).

Before undertaking the surviving cancer course, I was aware of some of the potential problems that were likely to be encountered by my patients following the receipt of a diagnosis (i.e. psychological and psychosocial concerns and the impact of treatments on quality of life) but perhaps I did not fully appreciate the true extent of this impact. Undertaking the course afforded me a true insight into the effects on my patients' lives, and accordingly I was better able to support them.

It is 10 years since I completed this course, and Jack had sadly succumbed to his illness. Both prostate and testicular cancer management has progressed to include more sophisticated approaches to care. There has been no publication on testicular cancer; however, Nicholas' case study had increased my insight into this cancer as well as my knowledge and experience in this field and my ability to support relevant patients.

7.1.2 An Overview of Prostate Cancer and Highlighting the Role of Nurse-Led Services in Long-Term Management

This was the second stand-alone module to be undertaken as part of the MSc advanced practice project. It highlighted the important role that audit plays in the monitoring of practice to identify areas that are in need of improvements, and in devising innovations that will either improve or change practice. In this instance focus was placed on the MUCNS role in the delivery of this nurse-led service. This activity resulted in the publication of 'The Benefits of Nurse-Led Telephone Follow-Up', Anderson (Anderson 2010), to which the reader is directed for a more in-depth account on this topic area.

7.1.3 Defining the Role of the Clinical Nurse Specialist in Cancer (Oncology) Care

This project provided an overview of the specialist nurse in cancer care, with focus placed on the MUCNS, demonstrating how the role sits within the remit of the multidisciplinary team (MDT), highlighting the role's importance in the management of those patients diagnosed with urological cancers (Frank-Stomberg and Johnson 2008; Leary et al. 2008a; Macmillan Cancer Support 2014) and providing the necessary reassurance and support (Bishop 2006) to counter the ensuing psychological and psychosocial impact of the diagnosis (Driscoll 2007; Anderson 2014). The psychological impact of cancer care on healthcare professionals (specifically nurses), and the availability of support (Driscoll 2007; Anderson 2014), is discussed as well as dealing with the problems encountered in the delivery of this service.

This module resulted in the subsequent publication of Anderson (Anderson 2014), to which the reader is directed for an in-depth understanding of the issues discussed.

7.1.4   Power, Risk and Decision-Making in Contemporary Partnership Contexts (Power Risk) Module

This module comprised two parts. Part 1 critically explored the ethical issue of consent in an incident involving Mr. AB, a gentleman in his late 70s, who was diagnosed with non-muscle-invasive bladder cancer (NMIBC) and referred for intravesical treatment, initially with chemotherapy followed by immunotherapy as chemotherapy had failed. The role of the urology consultant, the Macmillan Uro-Oncology CNS (MUCNS) (me) and the son-in-law was explained in Mr. AB's care.

Part 2 critically explored the group activities undertaken for the course. Unfortunately, due to the length of assignments, I am unable to illustrate the full recounting of the events. I have therefore provided a summarised version of the events for both parts, illustrating how elements of power (Box 7.1) (French and Raven 1959; Lukes 2005) are demonstrated in clinical practice and in groups/teams, and highlighting the inherent risks.

Autonomy refers to the regard for the right of individuals to hold view, to make choices and to make decisions based on their personal values and beliefs (Beauchamp and Childress 2007). Integral to this is **consent** (Royal College of Nursing 2005), which to be valid must be given voluntarily by a mentally competent patient and without pressure from other parties (The Mental Capacity Act) (Department for Constitutional Affairs 2007). Informed consent and risk communication (Royal College of Nursing 2005; Edwards et al. 1998; Bowling and Ebrahim 2001) are closely related concepts of the decision-making process (Elwyn et al. 1999); as such, the provision of clear and concise information (Leydon et al. 2000) about the diagnosis, treatments and incurred risks and benefits is imperative (Edwards et al. 1998; Bowling and Ebrahim 2001). The principle of autonomy is closely related to empowerment (helping people gain greater control over their lives) (Thompson

---

Box 7.1 Types of Power
- **'Expert power':** power that derives from subordinates' assumptions that the power holder possesses superior skills and abilities
- **'Informational power':** power based on the potential use of informational resources, including rational argument, persuasion or factual data
- **'Legitimate power':** power based on an individual's socially sanctioned claim to a position or role that gives the occupant the right to require and demand compliance with his/her directives
- **'Lukes, One-dimensional power':** refers to the power involved in decision-making ... and the power of one person or group to achieve their ends, possibly contrary to the interests of others.

Source: (French and Raven 1959; Lukes 2005).

2007) and as such is closely linked to the notion of power (French and Raven 1959; Lukes 2005). Here, power is often demonstrated by hierarchical status, knowledge and expertise, and use of language (Braye and Preston-Shoot 1995).

7.2   Part 1: Consent—An Issue of Concern

At his first outpatient's appointment to receive his diagnosis, Mr. AB was accompanied by his son-in-law, who had previously asked the consultant not to tell Mr. AB that he had cancer, or that the treatment of choice was chemotherapy. He believed that the news would be too distressing for Mr. AB. The consultant agreed to this request and because I (the MUCNS) was not present at this consultation, he inadvertently placed me in the difficult position of being compliant in a decision that I believed was ethically and morally wrong. Under English law, a relative does not have the right to make a decision on behalf of a patient (Evans and Over 1997). By neglecting to provide Mr. AB with a full disclosure of all information (Leydon et al. 2000), including the relevant risks and benefits (Edwards et al. 1998; Bowling and Ebrahim 2001), it could be argued that the combined actions of the consultant and the son-in-law demonstrated a lack of respect for his autonomy and thus his right to make informed decisions about his care (Royal College of Nursing 2005). Consequently, risks of unforeseen complications from treatments could result in Mr. AB seeking legal advice, and accordingly placing the consultant, the MUCNS and the healthcare organisation at risk of litigation (Dimond 2008).

Unfortunately, this is not an isolated incidence. Experience has taught me that in the delivery of healthcare, the rules that govern decision-making are not always clearly defined. While the clinician's obligation is first and foremost, to respect the patient's autonomy, an obligation in which consent and being truthful are imperative (Royal College of Nursing 2005; Department for Constitutional Affairs 2007), sometimes it is necessary to extend the rules to incorporate the relatives' needs (Evans and Over 1997), despite the evident risks (Edwards et al. 1998; Bowling and Ebrahim 2001). As the MUCNS, my role was to ensure that Mr. AB received a full disclosure of his diagnosis (including the inherent risks and complications) before obtaining his consent to receive subsequent treatments. In making decisions about his care, I also had a responsibility to ensure that this was supported with the relevant information (Leydon et al. 2000) and that proposed care was in his best interest (Leathard and Goodinson-McLaren 2007). Fortunately, at Mr. AB's second appointment to discuss immunotherapy treatment, I was able to honour this responsibility.

7.3   Part 2: Reflection on Group Activity

The evidence has shown that in group activities, respect for individual's autonomy is crucial to ensuring empowerment, developing confidence, boosting self-esteem, enhancing skills, enabling group cohesiveness and working in partnership (Forsyth 2010; Miller 2001). As previously stated, the principle of autonomy is closely related to empowerment and is closely linked to the notion of power (French and Raven 1959; Lukes 2005); thus in group/team activities, making decisions can lead to the emergence of risks, and accordingly conflict and animosity within the group (Miller 2001; Thompson and Nadler 2000). In terms of working in partnership, it is acknowledged that the 'differences in power, status and experience can sabotage working together … the challenge is to share power in a way that empowers each person to contribute equally to the task' (Miller 2001; Thompson and Nadler 2000).

My group comprised of myself, from a nursing background, and three additional members, all from a social work background. The group was tasked with identifying a role-play scenario for a group presentation to be executed at the final session. I suggested a scenario around consent, which was initially accepted and then rejected in favour of a mental health scenario.

While I was initially disappointed with this outcome (mostly because I was concerned that my lack of knowledge and experience would likely limit my contribution to group discussions), I was willing to work towards achieving the objective. However, I was aware that selecting a mental health scenario shifted discussions to the social work team members' areas of expertise (Smith 2008), and that there was an unequal distribution of power (French and Raven 1959; Lukes 2005), albeit one that could have reversed if the consent scenario was selected.

There was a distinct interplay of power associated with the need to retain the locus of control (French and Raven 1959; Lukes 2005), which was demonstrated in their use of knowledge and prior experience of the task, withholding information and use of language in controlling discourses (French and Raven 1959; Lukes 2005). I also believe that team members were extremely reluctant to move outside their area of expertise (comfort zone), while I was forced to move outside mine.

On the day of the groups' presentations, our presentation went well, although more theoretical input would have been useful. While all presentations met the required criteria, group three's presentation was well researched, organised and executed, and clearly demonstrated their ability to work in a contemporary partnership context. Reflection on the events revealed that the issues that emerged from the group's dynamics were classic in the way they exactly mirrored group behaviour as detailed by Forsyth (Forsyth 2010), Miller et al. (Miller 2001) and Thompson (Thompson and Nadler 2000). Nonetheless, I acknowledge that the power-play tactics that ensue during the group normalisation process and the manoeuvring for positions of power within the group were an inherent part of the process (Miller 2001; Thompson and Nadler 2000).

7.4   Conclusion and Lessons Learnt

I must admit that while I did not initially acknowledge the relevance of this module to my practice, in hindsight, it was extremely relevant. The course highlighted the inherent problems arising as a result of the demonstration of power within individual workforce and the subsequent impact on those concerned, namely, clients/patients, service users, employers and employees. Issues around consent are clearly highlighted in terms of empowering patients (through information) to take control when making decisions about their health/care. Regarding group/teamworking, power is explicitly underlined in terms of how it could be used to disempower/undermine others and accordingly impact their confidence and self-esteem.

Admittedly, in completing this module, I did feel empowered to address future problems at work. With regard to my healthcare role, I was able to recognise how power could be used in the decision-making process, especially its potential to disempower and alienate others. As such, I was mindful to ensure that when interacting with patients, colleagues and students, I always respected their autonomy, specifically their right to make decisions, which in essence are formulated from an informed basis.

This module complemented the later undertaken leadership in advanced practice module, in that it also addressed salient issues, such as consent, power and poor communication, and the ensuing impact on in-team relationships (Anderson 2019) (as previously illustrated in Chap. 6, 'In-Team Relationships').

7.4.1 Leadership in Advanced Practice Module

Leadership and Management The literature highlights three styles of leadership: transactional (authoritarian), transformational (democratic) and non-transactional (laissez-faire) (Marquis and Huston 2009; Brady Germain and Cummings 2010). In healthcare, Burns (Burns 1978) identifies two types of leaders in management: the transactional leader (the traditional manager, concerned with the day-to-day operations) and the transformational leader (the manager, who is committed, has a vision and is able to empower others with this vision) (Marquis and Huston 2009; Brady Germain and Cummings 2010). The belief is that if leadership is to be effective, some measure of power (defined as the capacity to influence others) must support it (Dwamena et al. 2008). Here, power includes elements of empowerment and authority (French and Raven 1959; Lukes 2005).

This module critically analysed leadership in the context of advanced practice. Content included an exploration of leadership theories (Marquis and Huston 2009; Brady Germain and Cummings 2010) and highlighting how key components of the process, such as power differentials (French and Raven 1959; Lukes 2005), were demonstrated in clinical practice in terms of the patient and healthcare professional. My role as the Macmillan Uro-Oncology Clinical Nurse Specialist (MUCNS) was explained in leadership issue 1, the management of patients following the receipt of a diagnosis of urological cancer ('the breaking of bad news') (Finlay 2005) from the urology consultant in the outpatient department and how I demonstrated leadership in this instance. In terms of my MUCNS role, leadership issue 2 illustrated how my experience of poor leadership and poor communication impacted my confidence and my self-esteem. The following accounts are summarised versions of the events.

Leadership Issue (1)—'Breaking Bad News' In my role as MUCNS, one of my responsibilities is to ensure that patients are represented during and following the receipt of bad news (Finlay 2005) from the consultant, and accordingly provide them with the appropriate support (emotional, communicational and informational) in an attempt to counter the impact of this news (Leydon et al. 2000). Reflecting on my interactions with these patients in local practice and using a transformational leadership approach to evaluate and analyse my provision of this support, I concluded that my approach to managing difficult situations, such as breaking bad news (Finlay 2005), was appropriate. In terms of demonstrating leadership, I believe that providing patients with emotional, communicational and informational support following the receipt of bad news helped to empower them to take control of their situation and accordingly make decisions that were in their best interest (Leydon et al. 2000).

Reflection had also highlighted my interactions with patients with learning disabilities and how I demonstrated leadership in this instance. One such patient was Peter, who was diagnosed with advanced prostate cancer. His situation was particularly poignant as it highlighted issues around autonomy, i.e. his ability to communicate effectively, his understanding of information received and his ability to make decisions about his care or indeed give his consent to these. Having to explain to Peter that he had prostate cancer, and that we needed to start him on treatment, was quite challenging. I found that I was explaining things to the carer and not to Peter as he seemed not to understand what was going on. In fact, he was more interested in having a cup of tea and a biscuit. I did voice my concerns to the consultant, but the consensus was that Peter needed treatment—a decision he felt that had been made in his best interest.

I was later contacted by the matron from Peter's care home. She was eager to confirm that Peter's treatment had indeed been selected on the basis that it was in his best interest, i.e. was the treatment selected because it was the most appropriate to treat Peter's cancer, or was it considered suitable because of his learning disability. I assured her that in Peter's case this was the most appropriate treatment for his type of cancer. However, in these situations, I have learnt that decisions are not always clear-cut. As clinicians, sometimes the individual may wonder if the decisions they make are indeed in the best interests of the patient. At this point, a referral to the Mental Capacity Act (Department for Constitutional Affairs 2007) had proven beneficial. In Peter's case, my liaison with the Trust's learning disability nurse was also beneficial in providing him with additional support.

Leadership Issue (2)—Poor Communication For this activity I had elected to examine my line manager's management of the proposed move from my office of 5 years (which I had developed with the assistance of the general manager), from a dark and dingy cupboard to a bright airy space overlooking the car park, to presumably accommodate three other people. Needless to say, I was unhappy with this proposal, as I would be moving to a much smaller office. Also, because the Trust had just employed a new urology nurse consultant (with whom I would be sharing this office), the smaller space would be inadequate to meeting both our working needs, an observation which seemed unimportant to my line manager. Unhappy about the move, I asked my line manager if I had a choice in the decision, to which she strongly affirmed that I did not and went on to remind me that the office belonged to the Trust.

Unfortunately, subsequent efforts to expedite the move encountered a number of delays and some unpleasantness. Facilitating this move was not as straightforward as my line manager envisaged. Attempts to get **WORKS** to fit the new office (using current office resources, including shelving) had proven difficult. It had taken several identified dates and several cancellations, as well as subsequent attempts to arrange for them to take measurements, provide start date and undertake the work. Nevertheless, a final date was ascertained. In the final week prior to this move, with the promise that the work would be completed on the Friday evening and subsequent agreement with my line manager, the move was scheduled for the following Monday. I was still unhappy to be moving, but had come to terms with it.

However, a stressful situation was about to become more so. As previously explained, part of my role as the MUCNS is the provision of the nurse-led service that delivered intravesical chemotherapy and immunotherapy agents to patients diagnosed with non-muscle-invasive bladder cancer, on a Friday, between 09:00 and 13:00 h from one of the Trust's hospitals. On this particular Friday, I completed the clinic and had made the usual return to my base hospital. As I pulled into the car park, I looked up to my office window where I observed the evident movements in my office. With a sinking feeling in my stomach, I alighted the stairs, entered the corridor to my office, knocked on the door and, on opening, observed a meeting between my line manager and several other persons. The look on my face must have reflected my surprise, a surprise that seemingly did not register with my line manager who proceeded to close the door, an action that had left me temporarily dumbfounded. While this observation was surprising, even more so was the notation of various contents from my office (computer, answerphone and other items) outside my door in the corridor.

Feeling hurt and upset, I called my colleague on the other site and, as tears stung my eyes, reiterated what had occurred. Unfortunately, her attempt to comfort me had little effect. With no office, no computer and no answerphone, I was unable to complete my duties (mainly documentation and returning patients' calls) for the day. I waited until my line manager completed the meeting and returned to her office, at which point I had asked her why she had taken over my office before the agreed move date on Monday. Her response was even more hurtful. She stated that she needed the room to conduct the meeting and that she had more important things to think about than my office moves. To add insult to injury, she further suggested that I should not be such a baby, and as the new office was not yet ready that I should go home, and once again closed the door in my face. At this moment, I remember feeling a strong sense of powerlessness and of being bullied by my line manager, simply because she had the authority and the power to do so. Her actions had led to an increase in my stress levels and a reduction in self-esteem and morale. In fact, I had never felt more demoralised.

Leadership/Management Approach Transformational leadership is an approach that motivates followers to perform to their full potential over time by influencing a change in perceptions and providing a sense of direction (Marquis and Huston 2009). A transformational approach to managing the situation would have influenced me in accepting the proposed changes, maintained my self-esteem and morale, which is in contrast to the line manager's approach (transactional) which led to anger, frustration, disillusionment and disempowerment.

Action Taken to Regain Control In an attempt to take back power and to restore my confidence and self-esteem, I confronted the problem by requesting a one-to-one with my line manager, which she surprisingly agreed to. On the day itself, and even before I sat down, she attempted to justify her behaviour by stating that she was very disappointed with how I reacted to this situation, and went on to explain why. Initially, her explanation was quite dismissive of my feelings, but motivated by a sense of being disrespected and my need to be listened to, I kept calm. Once I was allowed to speak, I was mindful not to be angry. Instead, I exercised tact and diplomacy to highlight my concerns, and to ensure that they would be taken seriously. I pointed out to my line manager that while she may be disappointed with my reaction to the situation, I was equally disappointed with her management of said situation. I went on to explain that had she taken the time to listen to my concerns, and had taken my feelings into account, I may have been more amenable to the move. I went on to say that as my manager, she had a responsibility to support me in doing a job that was extremely stressful and to ensure that I had the required resources to do so effectively. I pointed out that she had moved me out of an office space that had been adequate for my work, and into a much smaller workspace that was totally inadequate. This was further compounded by the fact that she had given me assurances regarding the move, but had subsequently reneged on them. We are, after all, professionals and deserve to be treated as such. I felt I had to take this step to regain my self-respect. Had I not done so, I believe that my self-confidence and self-worth in terms of how I felt about my role could have been affected.

7.5   Conclusion and Lessons Learnt

This module highlighted similarities with the power risk module in terms of poor communication and power. It had also reminded me of my first experience of poor communication in 1974 and of the ensuing tears and feelings of being disheartened. This feeling had underlined the importance of why we should communicate effectively with the people we interact with in life. Reflecting on my own approach to communicating with others, while I realise that I have made mistakes, and that the younger me was perhaps a little 'bullish' over the years, I believe that the mature me has excelled in this area. The line manager in this leadership 2 issue was a modern matron, and when I reflect back on the matrons in the 1970s and on my interactions with them, I must admit that the way I was treated in this instance has tainted my perception of the modern matron, although in fairness, it would be wrong to tarnish all modern matrons with the same brush. According to Snoddon (Snoddon 2010) change is an inherent part of professional life; thus, leadership is a prerequisite for the development of practice and central to our expectations for tomorrow's healthcare professionals. However, based on my experiences over the years, I acknowledge that not everyone is a leader, nor wishes to be at the forefront. Some people are content to remain in the 'shadows' while directing operations.

7.6   Personal and Professional Development in Advanced Practice

This penultimate module for the master's project illustrated my personal and professional journey from a senior urology staff nurse to an advanced Macmillan Uro-Oncology Clinical Nurse Specialist (MUCNS).

The module comprised two parts: the reflective component, which aimed to take the reader on a journey through the MUCNS experiences and present the learning outcomes realised, and the portfolio component, which was designed to provide the reader with an understanding of the activities undertaken and how they contributed to my personal and professional development. Reflection is guided by Driscoll (Driscoll 2000) model of reflection, which is inspired by Borton's (Borton 1970) 'What–So What–Now What?' model which provided an operational framework from which the reflection was discussed. All information is anonymised to respect confidentiality (Nursing and Midwifery Council 2008). Reflection included evaluation, linking with the Royal College of Nursing's (RCN) seven domains and competencies for advanced nurse practitioner (ANP) which were indicated within the text by a bracketed number(s) for cross-referencing, with further linkage to the portfolio. A relationship between the evidence and the RCN's advanced practice competencies (Royal College of Nursing 2010) was represented by an evidence matrix connecting the specified evidence to the relevant domain. Additional information was presented in relevant appendices.

The following version of the events (recounted in real time) provides the reader with an insight into my journey thus far, and how various study undertakings complemented my role, my practice and the wider uro-oncology community. Content also includes acknowledgements of my performance within practice.

7.7   Background to Topic Area

The term 'advanced nurse practitioner' (ANP) is increasingly being used in the UK to acknowledge practice and its associated competences (Royal College of Nursing 2010). Specialist nurses are required to demonstrate that they have knowledge and expertise befitting their role (Nursing and Midwifery Council (NMC) 2005; Department of Health 2010), illustrating that they are safe to practice (Royal College of Nursing 2010). The CNS role was the first ANP role to be implemented (Department of Health 2010). However, studies have shown disparities both in expectations and performance of individuals (Doherty 2009; Thompson and Watson 2003; Leary et al. 2008b). There is agreement that standardised levels of practice, identified by healthcare professionals, employers, commissioners and the public, would provide greater clarity and help to resolve continued controversy (Handley 2010; National Cancer Action Team et al. 2010). Consequently, the RCN's seven core domains of competency for advanced practitioners (Box 7.2) were devised (Royal College of Nursing 2010).

The CNS Role in Cancer Care—Current Status In cancer care, the prerequisite is that CNSs are at graduate level, with the expectation of having a master's degree (National Cancer Action Team) (National Cancer Action Team et al. 2010); arguably, reality does not reflect this. Nevertheless, cancer CNSs are clinical experts in evidence-based nursing practice in their specialty and practice autonomously in diagnosis and treatment while working to promote patient health and well-being (Hewett and Ross 2012). As the MUCNS, I work within secondary care in a urology department of a district general hospital. While I work autonomously, this involves working across boundaries within a multidisciplinary context involving the primary, secondary and tertiary care sectors. The role encompasses several components including effective communicator (Hamric et al. 2005), responsibility for particular aspects of care and managing the cli-

---

Box 7.2 RCN's Seven Core Domains of Competency
1. Management of client health status.
2. The nurse-client relationship.
3. The teaching-coaching function.
4. Professional role.
5. Managing and negotiating the healthcare delivery system.
6. Monitoring and ensuring the quality of healthcare practice.
7. Cultural competences.

Source: RCN (Royal College of Nursing 2010).

ents' care pathway while delivering nurse-led services (Lewis et al. 2009). In this context, the primary focus is helping patients understand their disease and treatment options once a diagnosis has been confirmed and offering emotional and psychosocial support while acting as the patient's key worker in line with national guidance (National Institute for Health and Care Excellence [NICE] 2004; Department of Health 2007).

What? Description In 2005 my role as senior staff nurse, working in a urology ward, had reached an impasse. I was at this time likely to be performing at advanced beginner stage (Benner 1984). I developed my practice in urology nursing and its management through skill acquisition partly by undertaking traditional medical roles (i.e. cannulation, venepuncture, male catheterisation) (Benner 2004).

During this journey, I had undertaken audits with the aim of improving care, devised and implemented into practice through several patient information leaflets. In my experience of dealing with sensitive issues (namely cultural and religious issues around death and dying), I utilised reflection in making sense of and learning from the situation, while a previously undertaken counselling course highlighted my capability in dealing with complex emotional issues. Acknowledgement of these increasing capabilities emphasised my readiness to progress in my career and apply for the MUCNS post.

On appointment I was required to undertake a BSc, which included a cancer module that helped me to develop my skills in breaking bad news. Here, clinical supervision has proved beneficial in managing complex emotional issues. Delivering nurse-led services is integral to the role and improved practice outcomes (Lewis et al. 2009). Regular examinations of these services have resulted in publications, which are used to support learning, in-house and within the wider context.

In undertaking of the MSc, I completed several modules (three work-based learning modules, research methods, surviving cancer, power risk and leadership in advanced practice, research project planning and management). These have been instrumental in enhancing my practice. Personal experience of 'bad' leadership highlighted the importance and benefits of transformational leadership (Marquis and Huston 2009), specifically in motivating teams and individuals. Knowledge of teaching and learning theory enhanced my clinical care with individual patients. My role as key worker is highlighted in providing information and support following BBN and empowering individuals to make decisions about their health.

So What? Analysis Reflection on my professional journey has highlighted some apprehension in the initial and interim stages, regarding my ability for this new challenge. The first 2 weeks in post highlighted a degree of discomfort and a lack of confidence in my ability to provide a patient with the level of support required following BBN. The memory is almost tangible, but in hindsight, the experience was vital in shaping my future management of BBN. Three years later, I again encountered another BBN experience, this time I was given the opportunity to re-enact and explore my feelings on a 3-day advanced communications course (National Institute for Health and Care Excellence [NICE] 2004). Completion of the surviving cancer course gave greater understanding of patients' problems following a diagnosis of cancer, while work-based learning projects enabled evaluation of the role in context. Reflection highlighted issues in regard to the cost-effectiveness of the MUCNS (Handley 2010). Notably, costs are key to delivering quality patient-centred care, and to a greater extent my survival as a CNS (Handley 2010). There may be difficulty in associating the CNS role with tangible benefits (Tarrant et al. 2008); thus, in times of austerity, the role is often the first to be reviewed if resources are constrained (Handley 2010). In response to this, chargeable activities were recorded, both quantifying actions and generating income, and a greater emphasis was placed on the role of the CNS in the quality of care (Benner 2001).

A variety of initiatives established my commitment to leadership, quality assurance and practice development. These include regular evaluations of practice through audit, being involved in clinical trials, developing patient information and publications, undertaking study to enhance my role conducting patient assessments and actioning care accordingly. I have found that through the MSc in advanced practice, I have developed confidence in my ability to question issues relating to patient care (Department of Health 2005). The combined modules have increased my knowledge and extended my practice as an advanced practitioner and although this view is subjective, I have become more critical and assertive in challenging decisions in my patients' best interest. The previously undertaken counselling course combined with the surviving cancer course and experience of emotional intelligence has improved my ability to provide emotional support to my patients (Department of Health 2010). On reflection, the way I dealt with BBN at the start of my journey is very different to my approach today. Admittedly, this is in part attributable to enriched experiential learning based on increased insight into my patients' problems (Department of Health 2010) combined with the added benefits of life's learning.

The course has highlighted the importance of research, audit, teaching and mentoring, in accordance with the RCN's seven domains of competencies as an ANP. Having completed this intensive study, I believe that I am more informed about my practice, and have become a more effective practitioner, from an emotional and practical perspective (Department of Health 2010). However, in regard to the leadership module, while I did not see myself as a leader at the outset, completing the transformational leadership exercise and modules towards the

MSc advanced practice, I now visualise myself as a leader and I am able to identify the leadership components of my role as well as others' perception of me as such.

Now What? Proposed Actions Following the Event This reflection has highlighted continued development needs outlined in the SWOT (strengths, weaknesses, opportunities and threats) analysis in year 2 that had created a progression action plan for future practice. Overall, this has been a valuable learning curve, one that enhances my role as an advanced practitioner and the care I deliver to patients. While I cannot quantify this development, I have found a renewed confidence to challenge, question and critique clinical decisions and will continue to do so. In regard to my practice and me, critical reflection reinforces the fact that cancer is an intensely demanding field; thus, having the appropriate knowledge and expertise combined with working in a multidisciplinary context is crucial to ensuring a management strategy that is tailored to meeting the needs of those affected by the disease (Department of Health 2010). I will endeavour to utilise knowledge gained from the course in promoting and sharing practice within the organisation through continuous professional development, teaching, mentoring and coaching activities (Lewis et al. 2009).

In these times of austerity, the ANP role remains at risk; thus, I realise the importance of avoiding complacency in my approach to practice. Even at this stage, I cannot claim to know everything about my area of expertise. Treatments and management modalities are continually changing; the challenge on my part is in keeping apprised of current and future developments to enable me to provide optimum care to my patients. In regard to my area of expertise and experiential leaning, I realise that some of the richest sources of learning are achieved from my attendance at consultant-led clinics, multidisciplinary team and audit meetings. As the advanced practitioner, I will continue to utilise this facility while promoting my role and determining its effectiveness within the hierarchy (Lewis et al. 2009), ultimately ensuring that the patient remains at the forefront.

7.8 Embracing Acknowledgements of my Performance

A key requirement of this module was that I garnered information about my personal practice, specifically how others perceived my competency in the performance of the MUCNS role and my mentoring ability in terms of their academic undertakings/achievements. If I am honest, I was a little uncomfortable with this exercise, but receiving acknowledgement for my achievements was a significant boost to my confidence, morale and self-esteem.

The following Service User Comments are a testament to my performance:

---

(1) I wanted to write formally to say how impressed I was by RN Beverley Anderson when talking to her about a patient whilst I was on-call. She was very professional in her attitude, but still clearly cared very much for the patient, and was able to give me a very clear picture of his situation in the last period of his life. Her communication skills were excellent. I hope that my appreciation can be conveyed to her.

MM, Consultant in Palliative Medicine

10/2003

(2) Beverley Anderson the Uro-Oncology nurse is known not only for her valued expertise in Uro-oncology but also for her knowledge and expertise in critically analysing research and formatting assignments. I am recently undertaking modules to complete my nursing degree and rely on Beverley for support and help with assignments. Fortunately, Beverley is a person who is always willing, enthusiastic and allows for time in her hectic schedule to help and give advice with essay writing, which she also does in her private time due to work commitments.

If Beverley was not available to provide her input I would struggle to achieve and complete a nursing degree. Her knowledge on formatting and structure of essay writing is invaluable.

JC, urology CNS

03/2012

(3) Beverley Anderson has been a referee for peer-reviewed clinical articles for the *British Journal of Nursing* since 2010. She responds to our invitations promptly and provides constructive feedback for our authors to help them bring their work up to a publishable standard for the *BJN*, while also keeping in mind our readership and current guidelines.

AP, Editor

British Journal of Nursing

03/2012

(4) I have worked with Beverley for the past 4 years both as a colleague and as a 'mentee' whilst working at … Day Surgery Unit.

I have observed Beverley performing variant roles to a number of individuals, some staff, students and service users, and I have also had the privilege of attending two of her study days workshops; the first one being how to administer Mitomycin and BCG, the benefits of the drugs, the safe way to administer and the protocol for using the drugs.

During the times I have worked with, and alongside Beverley, I found her to be very knowledgeable and informative, hardworking, and supportive not only to myself but to her patients and to students whom we have on placement on the unit from time to time. Many of her patients who are more often patients in the day surgery unit at some time or another have always commented on how supportive Beverley has been to them helping them to cope through the difficult journey of their illness, sometimes it is apparent that they think she is always working at this unit site as her name is first one, they called or inquire of when they come in for their check-ups.

As a mentor Beverley is very encouraging, she also challenges her students to progress in their studies and to find other avenues to improve their knowledge base, she is also very eager to teach and support students as she always seems to have an article for them to look into and gain more insight.

I have much appreciation for Beverley as she has helped me and guided me through my own personal development as a nurse.

TW, Ward Sister

04/2012

---

(5) Beverley Anderson has mentored me during my diploma course which I completed in 2006. I am currently undertaking a distant learning degree course and Beverley has agreed to mentor me again. Beverley has helped me develop critical thinking and improve my writing style. She has supported me, giving me encouragement and constructive feedback on my assignments.

She has an immense understanding of what constitutes a great essay. She shows limitless patience and has the ability to translate the incomprehensible to the understandable. She does this through facilitating reflection and this then leads to improvement. She is able to motivate me to maintain my momentum through her enthusiasm for teaching, learning and preceptorship. I would not have managed to complete this degree module without her support and guidance.

YM, CNS Urology
04/2012

(6) This report relates to Beverley's role in helping medical students undertake a research project as part of their undergraduate degree. The projects lasted 6 weeks at the end of which each student has to produce a poster describing their project. The students choose a broad subject in which to devise their project and their progress is supported by a supervisor.

In the past 3 years I have supervised students whose projects meet the description 'the Patient Experience in Bladder Cancer'. Four of these students have worked with Beverley studying patients attending for intra-vesical BCG treatment.

Beverley's help has been invaluable. The students have a very short period of time in which to devise a project, set it up, conduct it satisfactorily, analyse the results and draw conclusions. One of the main challenges is to involve enough patients to make the study meaningful. By involving the BCG patients this has been possible.

For many students this is their first encounter with a patient. Beverley has put the students at their ease, introduced them to the patients, and gently coached them in managing the patients appropriately. As a result, the patients have been very willing participants and there have been no complaints. This degree of co-operation is not always found as the patients are often interviewed several times and are asked to complete questionnaires. Without Beverley's contribution there is absolutely no doubt that the projects would not have been so successful. The students and I owe Beverley a considerable debt of gratitude.

JB, Honorary Consultant Urologist and Senior Lecturer.
05/2012

7.9 Summary

The undertaking of this module was extremely enlightening in terms of my practice, knowledge, experience and learning gained. I believe that in my performance of the MUCNS role, I achieved the initial goal, in that I advanced from a novice to an intuitive and expert practitioner in my field of practice.

7.9.1 Research Project: 'An Exploration into African and Afro-Caribbean Men's Understanding of Prostate Cancer and its Associated Risks'

The aim of this qualitative phenomenological study was to investigate and provide insight into African and Afro-Caribbean (A&AC) men's understanding of prostate cancer and its associated risks. The purpose was to ascertain whether a focused health promotional strategy, and more specific UK-based research, was necessary in this area to increase these men's awareness of the associated risks and accordingly encourage them to seek help earlier in the process. Not only did the findings support the aim and purpose for this study, but they also highlighted the importance of several key factors and their role in increasing awareness among these men.

This study resulted in the subsequent publication entitled African and Afro-Caribbean men's experiences of prostate cancer (Anderson et al. 2013), to which the reader is directed for a detailed understanding of the study's undertaking and its outcomes.

7.10 Reflection on Project Outcomes, Follow-Up Study and my Interactions with PCUK

Panama Experience The study findings were subsequently presented at the *International Society of Nurses in Cancer Care (ISNCC)* in Panama City in September 2014. This was an interesting and informative conference that provided a worldwide insight into cancer care and its management in low- and middle-income countries, noting similarities between issues such as working long hours, low pay, staff shortages, gaining access to training and specifically funding issues, which seemingly are not that dissimilar to those experienced in Western countries. The session outlining cancer care in Uganda revealed that due to a lack of effective analgesia, such as morphine and morphine-based drugs, clinicians were often forced to offer cancer patients paracetamol as an analgesia. To a cancer nurse this revelation was humbling, and I admit that I did feel that I was fortunate to have access to some of the best cancer care in the world.

This venture was part-funded by PCUK and Macmillan Cancer Support.

Enhanced Skills I can honestly say that the undertaking of this study was hugely beneficial in that I gained an invaluable insight into research and an understanding of its importance in the furtherance of clinical practice and in ensuring the best outcomes for patients. The learning gained extended my knowledge and experience of prostate cancer and accordingly my ability to support *all* men diagnosed with the disease, especially those of African descent.

Continued monitoring on the progress of this research study has shown that it is a worthwhile addition to the evidence base. Since its publication in 2013, it has garnered significant interest from other parties, an observation that is verified by ongoing monitoring, which is being conducted by ResearchGate.

The Poster This study included the formation of a poster that comprised the four main themes identified. It was used to present the study findings to various audiences, which included the university, my local Trust and the PCUK team.

The Follow-Up Study During the undertaking of the interviews for the initial study of Anderson et al. (Anderson et al. 2013), participants had found the conclusion that prostate cancer was more prevalent in men of African descents perplexing, but even more perplexing was the suggestion that, in comparison to other African-Caribbean men, the disease was more prevalent and more aggressive in Jamaican men. To the participants, this was a puzzling phenomenon, one they felt that warranted further exploration. Exploration resulted in the follow-up study and subsequent publication entitled '*Prostate Cancer Among Jamaican Men: Exploring the Evidence for Higher Risk*' in 2015, Anderson and Marshall-Lucette (Anderson and Marshall-Lucette 2016), to which the reader is directed for a more in-depth report on the study's undertaking and its outcomes.

African-Caribbean Cancer Consortium (AC3) Invitation Prior to conducting this study and to enable me to garner a greater understanding of this puzzling phenomenon I contacted Professor Camille Ragin, an Associate Professor from the Cancer Prevention and Control Program, who resides in Philadelphia, for feedback on her thoughts on this topic area. The discussions with Professor Ragin were extremely beneficial in regard to formulating and conducting the study, so in recognition of this fact, I emailed a copy of the published article to her. She thought that the article was outstanding and wondered if I had given any thoughts to doing more research in the area of prostate cancer in Jamaican/Caribbean men, and whether I was interested in joining their collaborative network—the African-Caribbean Cancer Consortium (AC3)—a network that links the team together so that they remain abreast with research highlights and accomplishment and enables members to connect and carry out collaborative studies. Needless to say, I accepted the Professor's offer. However, due to increasing pressures of work, I was unable to fulfil my promise to the Consortium. Feeling guilty, and a little concerned about my membership, I contacted the Professor who reassured me that once a member of the AC3, I was a member for life. She further reassured me that through emails I would be kept updated on the Consortium's many activities—a promise she has honoured to this day.

My Interactions with PCUK I had been interacting with PCUK since I obtained the MUCNS post in 2005 and over this time had come to appreciate the significant role the Charity has played in those men diagnosed with prostate cancer as well as my role in this. Integral to this role was the circulation of key information to patients within local practice (e.g. leaflets and booklets) either at the time of their diagnosis or at other times of interaction throughout their care.

Over this time, I was involved in various PCUK study sessions and volunteering activities that were designed to enhance the healthcare professional's knowledge and expertise in managing prostate cancer and accordingly improving the patient experience and practice outcomes.

Study sessions included meeting various individuals and learning about the service provided by PCUK to men diagnosed with prostate cancer, specifically those of

African descent; participating in a telephone evaluation of the PCUK Educational Programme; and a pilot research activity to evaluate the post-surgery pack and to establish whether these would be beneficial to patients following robotic-assisted laparoscopic prostatectomy (RALP) for the treatment of prostate cancer.

While all study sessions and volunteering activities were hugely beneficial, two were particularly interesting. The Prostate Cancer UK 1 in 4 Roadshow event in 2015 was designed to increase awareness among men from the African-Caribbean community of their risk of developing prostate cancer. This event highlighted how these men responded to educational strategies, specifically how they perceived health messages and how these incited fear and anxiety, and accordingly either encouraging or deterring them to seek help, as in presenting for screening. It was also interesting, but not surprising (I noted same response in local practice), to see how much importance these men placed on religion, in that the power of belief would protect them from being diagnosed with prostate cancer. The session had also affirmed the role of women (wives, mothers and daughters) in encouraging these men to present for vital screening.

The 2016 prostate cancer study day sessions highlighted where we are at in terms of new technology and advancements in prostate cancer management (i.e. robotic-assisted laparoscopic radical prostatectomy (RALRP)) and how this has contributed to enhancing the patient experience and health outcomes. The presentation on the problems faced by the lesbian, gay, bisexual, transgender (LGBT) community, specifically those faced by the gay men diagnosed with prostate cancer, was extremely insightful in terms of breaking down barriers and changing perceptions around sexual orientation and sexuality, and how this could impact the individual's decision in terms of choice of treatment and considering the resulting impact on quality-of-life outcomes. I must admit that while my interaction in local practice with a gay man diagnosed with prostate cancer was fairly infrequent, obtaining an insight into their mindset following the diagnosis was useful in highlighting the potential sensitivities; as such, I believe that I was better equipped to support future patients.

A Current Perspective on Prostate Cancer In February 2020, a recent report (Prostate Cancer UK 2020) affirms that there were 49,029 diagnoses of prostate cancer in 2018, meaning that for the first time ever prostate cancer has overtaken breast cancer as the most commonly diagnosed cancer in England. Nevertheless, PCUK believes that this new data is positive, since the explanation for the higher increase in diagnosis is likely the raised awareness resulting in earlier diagnosis and in more men having a PSA test. However, with a subsequent report from Men United suggesting that for the first time ever the number of men dying from prostate cancer in the UK has exceeded 12,000 in 1 year, the PCUK challenge of continued research in this area is even greater.

I believe that the content of this chapter provides an accurate depiction of my roles in the management of those patients diagnosed with urological cancers and the importance of training, knowledge, insight and understanding into this field of practice in enabling the MUCNS to perform at the highest level while providing patients with care that ultimately improves their experiences and health outcomes.

Chapter 8 provides a personal reflection on coping with bad news relating to various cancers with reference made to how the personal and the professional interrelate in principle.

References

Anderson B (2010) The benefits to nurse-led telephone follow-up for prostate cancer. Br J Nurs 19(17):1085–1090

Anderson B (2014) Challenges for the clinical nurse specialist in uro-oncology care. Br J Nurs 23(Sup10):S18–22. [Internet]. May [cited 2020 Oct 1]. https://doi.org/10.12968/bjon.2014.23.Sup10.S18

Anderson B (2019) Reflecting on the communication process in health care. Part 1: clinical practice-breaking bad news. Br J Nurs 28(13):858–863. [Internet] http://www.ncbi.nlm.nih.gov/pubmed/31303035

Anderson B, Marshall-Lucette S (2016) Prostate cancer among Jamaican men: exploring the evidence for higher risk. Br J Nurs 25(19):1046–1051. [Internet]. https://doi.org/10.12968/bjon.2016.25.19.1046

Anderson B, Marshall-Lucette S, Webb P (2013) African and Afro-Caribbean men's experiences of prostate cancer. Br J Nurs 22(22):1296–1298, 1300–2, 1304–7. [Internet]. http://www.ncbi.nlm.nih.gov/pubmed/24335867

Beauchamp TL, Childress JF (2007) Principles of biomedical ethics, 5th edn. Oxford University Press, New York, NY

Benner P (1984) From novice to expert: excellence and power in clinical nursing practice. Addison-Wesley Pub. Co., Menlo Park, CA

Benner P (2001) From novice to expert: excellence and power in clinical nursing practice. Commemorat. Upper Saddle River, NJ, Prentice Hall Health

Benner P (2004) Using the Dreyfus model of skill acquisition to describe and interpret skill acquisition and clinical judgment in nursing practice and education [internet]. Bull Sci Technol Soc 24:188–199. [cited 2020 Oct 1]. https://doi.org/10.1177/0270467604265061

Bishop V (2006) Clinical supervision in practice: some questions, answers and guidelines for professionals in health and social care, vol 11–26, 2nd edn. Palgrave Macmillan, Basingstoke, pp 46–48

Borton T (1970) Reach, touch, and teach : student concerns and process education. McGraw-Hill, New York, NY

Bowling A, Ebrahim S (2001) Measuring patients' preferences for treatment and perceptions of risk. Qual Health Care 10(suppl1):i2–i8. [Internet]. www.qualityhealthcare.com

Brady Germain P, Cummings GG (2010) The influence of nursing leadership on nurse performance: a systematic literature review. J Nurs Manage 18(4):425–439. [Internet]. https://doi.org/10.1111/j.1365-2834.2010.01100.x

Brandenburg D, Grover L, Quinn B (2005) Intimacy & sexuality for cancer patients and their partners: a booklet of tips & ideas for your journey of recovery [Internet]. [cited 2020 Oct 1]. https://www.newcastle-hospitals.org.uk/downloads/CancerServicesSlides/Intimacy_and_Sexuality__For_Cancer_Patients_and_their_Partners.pdf

Braye S, Preston-Shoot M (1995) Empowering practice in social care. Open University Press, p 216

Burns JM (1978) Leadership. Harper and Row, New York

Decker CL, Haase JE, Bell CJ (2007) Uncertainty in adolescents and young adults with cancer. Oncol Nurs Forum 34(3):681–688. [Internet]. http://onf.ons.org/onf/34/3/uncertainty-adolescents-and-young-adults-cancer

Department for Constitutional Affairs (2007) Mental Capacity Act 2005: Code of Practice. Issued by the Lord Chancellor on 23 April 2007 in accordance with sections 42 and 43 of the Act

[Internet]. [cited 2010 Jun 14]. https://assets.publishing.service.gov.uk/government/uploads/system/uploads/attachment_data/file/921428/Mental-capacity-act-code-of-practice.pdf

Department of Health (2005) Payment by results consultation: preparing for 2005, London

Department of Health (2007) Cancer reform strategy [Internet]. www.nhs.uk. [cited 2020 Oct 1]. https://www.nhs.uk/NHSEngland/NSF/Documents/CancerReformStrategy.pdf

Department of Health (2010) Advanced level nursing: a position statement [Internet]. Gov.uk. https://assets.publishing.service.gov.uk/government/uploads/system/uploads/attachment_data/file/215935/dh_121738.pdf

Dimond B (2008) Legal aspects of nursing, 5th edn. Pearson/Longman, London

Doherty L (2009) NMC and RCN begin talks over regulation of nurse practitioners. Nurs Stand 24(13):5

Driscoll J (2000) Practising clinical supervision: a reflective approach [internet], 2nd edn. Baillière Tindall, Edinburgh. [cited 2020 Oct 7]. https://www.amazon.co.uk/Practising-Clinical-Supervision-Reflective-Approach/dp/0702024198/ref=sr_1_fkmr0_1?dchild=1&keywords=Practising+Clinical+Supervision%3A+A+Reflective+Approach+for+Healthcare+Professionals.&qid=1602081072&sr=8-1-fkmr0

Driscoll J (2007) Practising clinical supervision: a reflective approach for healthcare professionals, vol 3-22, 2nd edn. Balliere Tindall/Elsevier, Oxford, pp 150–151

Dwamena FC, Han C, Smith RC (2008) Breaking bad news: a patient-centred approach to delivering an unexpected cancer diagnosis. Semin Med Pract 11:11–20. [Internet] www.turner-white.com

Edwards A, Matthews E, Pill R, Bloor M (1998) Communication about risk: the responses of primary care professionals to standardizing the "language of risk" and communication tools. Fam Pract 15(4):301–307. [Internet]. https://doi.org/10.1093/fampra/15.4.301

Elwyn G, Edwards A, Kinnersley P (1999) Shared decision-making in primary care: the neglected second half of the consultation. Br J Gen Pract 49(443):477–482. [Internet] http://www.ncbi.nlm.nih.gov/pubmed/10562751

Evans JSBT, Over DE (1997) Are people rational? Yes, no and sometimes. Psychologist 10(9):403–406

Fan A (2002) Psychological and psychosocial effects of prostate cancer. Nurs Stand 17(13):33–37. [Internet] http://www.ncbi.nlm.nih.gov/pubmed/12572219

Fergus KD, Gray RE, Fitch MI (2002) Sexual dysfunction and the preservation of manhood: experiences of men with prostate cancer. J Health Psychol 7(3):303–316. https://doi.org/10.1177/1359105302007003223. [Internet]

Finlay L (2005) Powerful relationships. Nurs Manag 12(2):32–35. [Internet]. https://doi.org/10.7748/nm2005.05.12.2.32.c2024

Forsyth DR (2010) Group dynamics, 5th edn. Wadsworth/Cengage Learning, Belmont, CA

Frank-Stomberg M, Johnson J (2008) Oncology nursing: past, present, and future. Nurs Clin North Am 43(2):ix–xii

French JRP, Raven B (1959) The bases of social power. In: Studies in social power. Institute for Social Research, University of Michigan, Michigan, MI

Hamric AB, Spross JA, Hanson CM (2005) Advanced practice nursing : an integrative approach, 3rd edn. Saunders, St Louis, Mo

Handley A (2010) Specialists face up to more cuts. Nurs Stand 24(20):20–21. https://doi.org/10.7748/ns.24.20.20.s25. [Internet]

Hewett J, Ross E (2012) Views of specialist head and neck nurses about changes in their role. Cancer Nurs Pract 11(2):34–37. [Internet]. www.cancernursingpractice.co.uk

Hewitt M, Ganz PA (2007) Implementing cancer survivorship care planning [internet]. National Academies Press, Washington, D.C.. [cited 2020 Oct 6]. http://www.nap.edu/catalog/11739

Hoffman B, Stovall E (2006) Survivorship perspectives and advocacy. J Clin Oncol 24(32):5154–5159. [Internet]. https://doi.org/10.1200/JCO.2006.06.5300

Itano J, Taoka KN (eds) (2005) Core curriculum for oncology nursing, 4th edn. Elsevier Saunders, St Louis, Mo

Leary A, Crouch H, Lezard A, Rawcliffe C, Boden L, Richardson A (2008a) Dimensions of clinical nurse specialist work in the UK. Nurs Stand 23(15):40–44. https://doi.org/10.7748/ns2008.12.23.15.40.c6737. [Internet]

Leary A, Crouch H, Lezard A, Rawcliffe C, Boden L, Richardson A (2008b) Dimensions of clinical nurse specialist work in the UK. Nurs Stand 23(15):40–44. [Internet]. https://doi.org/10.7748/ns2008.12.23.15.40.c6737

Leathard A, Goodinson-McLaren S (2007) In: Leathard A (ed) Ethics: contemporary challenges in health and social care [internet]. Policy Press, Bristol. [cited 2020 Oct 7]. https://www.amazon.co.uk/Ethics-Contemporary-challenges-health-social/dp/1861347553/ref=sr_1_1?dchild=1&keywords='Ethics%3A+Contemporary+challenges+in+health+and+social+care'%2C&qid=1602064291&s=books&sr=1-1

Lewis R, Neal RD, Williams NH, France B, Wilkinson C, Hendry M et al (2009) Nurse-led vs. conventional physician-led follow-up for patients with cancer: systematic review. J Adv Nurs 65(4):706–723. https://doi.org/10.1111/j.1365-2648.2008.04927.x. [Internet]

Leydon GM, Boulton M, Moynihan C, Jones A, Mossman J, Boudioni M et al (2000) Cancer patients' information needs and information seeking behaviour: in depth interview study. BMJ 320(7239):909–913. [Internet]. https://doi.org/10.1136/bmj.320.7239.909

Lukes S (2005) Power: a radical view, 2nd edn. Palgrave Macmillan Ltd., Basingstoke

Macmillan Cancer Support (2014) Cancer clinical nurse specialists. Impact brief series. [Internet]. [cited 2021 Sept 6]. https://www.macmillan.org.uk/documents/aboutus/research/impactbriefs/clinicalnursespecialists2015new.pdf

Marquis BL, Huston CJ (2009) Leadership roles and management functions in nursing: theory and application, 6th edn. Lippincott Williams & Wilkins, Philadelphia, PA

Miller C (2001) Interprofessional practice in health and social care : challenging the shared learning agenda. Hodder Education, London

Morgan MA (2009) Cancer survivorship: history, quality-of-life issues, and the evolving multidisciplinary approach to implementation of cancer survivorship care plans. Oncol Nurs Forum 36(4):429–436. [Internet] http://onf.ons.org/onf/36/4/cancer-survivorship-history-quality-life-issues-and-evolving-multidisciplinary-approach

National Cancer Action Team, Warwick M, Trevatt P, Leary A (2010) Clinical nurse specialists in cancer care; provision, proportion and performance: a census of the cancer specialist nurse workforce in England. London; 2010

National Cancer Institute (2008) About cancer survivorship research : history [Internet]. cancercontrol.cancer.gov. [cited 2009 Oct 30]. http://cancercontrol.cancer.gov/ocs/history.html

National Institute for Health and Care Excellence [NICE] (2004) Improving supportive and palliative care for adults with cancer. Cancer service guideline [CSG4] [Internet]. National Institute for Clinical Excellence; [cited 2020 Oct 23]. https://www.nice.org.uk/guidance/csg463

Nursing and Midwifery Council (2008) The code: standards of conduct, performance and ethics for nurses and midwives [Internet]. [cited 2020 Oct 23]. https://www.nmc.org.uk/globalassets/sitedocuments/standards/nmc-old-code-

Nursing and Midwifery Council (NMC) (2005) Implementation of a framework for the standard for post registration nursing. Agendum 27.1, December, 2005. London, UK: Royal College of Nursing

Pemberger S, Jagsch R, Frey E, Felder-Puig R, Gadner H, Kryspin-Exner I et al (2005) Quality of life in long-term childhood cancer survivors and the relation of late effects and subjective Well-being. Support Care Cancer 13(1):49–56. https://doi.org/10.1007/s00520-004-0724-0. [Internet]

Postovsky S, Lightman A, Aminpour D, Elhasid R, Peretz M, Ben AMW (2003) Sperm cryopreservation in adolescents with newly diagnosed cancer. Med Pediatr Oncol 40(6):355–359. [Internet] http://www.ncbi.nlm.nih.gov/pubmed/12692802

Prostate Cancer UK (2020) Prostate cancer now most commonly diagnosed cancer in England [Internet]. prostatecanceruk.org. [cited 2020 Oct 13]. https://prostatecanceruk.org/about-us/news-and-views/2020/1/prostate-cancer-now-most-commonly-diagnosed-cancer-in-england

Rosella JD (1994) Testicular cancer health education: an integrative review. J Adv Nurs 20(4):666–671. https://doi.org/10.1046/j.1365-2648.1994.20040666.x. [Internet]

Royal College of Nursing (2005) Informed consent in health and social care research: RCN guidance for nurses. London

Royal College of Nursing (2010) Advanced nurse practitioners: an RCN guide to the advanced nurse practitioner role, competencies and programme accreditation. Royal College of Nursing, London

Self MC (2005) Surviving with scars: the long-term psychosocial consequences of teenage cancer. In: Cancer and the adolescent [internet], 2nd edn. Blackwell Science Ltd, Oxford, pp 183–200. https://doi.org/10.1002/9780470994733.ch17

Skaali T, Fosså SD, Bremnes R, Dahl O, Haaland CF, Hauge ER et al (2009) Fear of recurrence in long-term testicular cancer survivors. Psychooncology 18(6):580–588. https://doi.org/10.1002/pon.1437. [Internet]

Smith R (2008) Social work and power [internet]. Palgrave Macmillan, Basingstoke. [cited 2020 Oct 7] https://www.amazon.co.uk/Social-Work-Power-Reshaping/dp/1403991243/ref=sr_1_1?dchild=1&keywords=Social+Work+and+Power'.&qid=1602065067&s=books&sr=1-1

Snoddon J (2010) Case management of long-term conditions : principles and practice for nurses. Wiley-Blackwell, Chichester, West Sussex

Tarrant C, Sinfield P, Agarwal S, Baker R (2008) Is seeing a specialist nurse associated with positive experiences of care? The role and value of specialist nurses in prostate cancer care. BMC Heal Serv Res (8):65. [Internet] http://www.ncbi.nlm.nih.gov/pubmed/18371192

Thompson DR, Watson R (2003) Advanced nursing practice: what is it? Int J Nurs Pract 9(3):129–130. https://doi.org/10.1046/j.1440-172X.2003.00424.x. [Internet]

Thompson L, Nadler J (2000) Judgemental biases in conflict resolution and how to overcome them. In: Deutsch M, Coleman PT (eds) The handbook of conflict resolution : theory and practice. Jossey-Bass, San Francisco, CA, pp 213–235. 2008.pdf

Thompson N (2007) Power and empowerment (theory into practice) [internet]. Russell House Publishing, Lyme Regis. [cited 2020 Oct 7]. 9781903855997

Waring AB, Wallace WHB (2000) Subfertility following treatment for childhood cancer. Hosp Med 61(8):550–557. https://doi.org/10.12968/hosp.2000.61.8.1398. [Internet]

Coping with 'the Breaking of Bad News': Personal and Professional Perspectives

Types of Cancers There are more than 100 different types of cancer. Each type is classified by the type of cell the cancer originates from (Hull 2017). There are six major types of cancer, including carcinomas, sarcomas, myelomas, leukaemia, lymphomas and mixed types (including blastomas). Carcinomas, the most commonly diagnosed cancers, originate in the skin, lungs, breasts, pancreas and other organs and glands. Sarcoma is a cancer that begins in the connective or supportive tissues such as bone, cartilage, fat, muscle or blood vessels (WebMD 2020).

Osteosarcoma Osteosarcoma is a highly malignant form of bone cancer. Osteosarcomas can be either primary or secondary, and as explained by the Macmillan Cancer Support (Macmillan Cancer Support 2019), these have differing demographics:

1. Primary osteosarcoma: This typically occurs in young patients (10–20 years old) with 75% taking place before the age of 20 because the growth centres of the bone are more active during puberty/adolescence, with slight male predominance.
2. Secondary osteosarcoma: This occurs in the elderly, usually secondary to malignant degeneration of Paget's disease, extensive bone infarcts or post-radiotherapy for other conditions.

Diagnosis The disease is usually diagnosed in several grades and stages: parosteal, low grade, periosteal, intermediate grade, telangiectatic and small-cell osteosarcoma.

Classical symptoms include bone pain, increasing in severity at night, localised swelling, pins and needles, and loss of power/grip.

This chapter provides the reader with an honest account of my personal experience of cancer through case study presentations of several cancers: brain, liver, ovarian, breast, colorectal, prostate, pancreatic, osteosarcoma and ovarian,

© Springer Nature Switzerland AG 2022
B. Anderson, *A Uro-Oncology Nurse Specialist's Reflection on her Practice Journey*, https://doi.org/10.1007/978-3-030-94199-4_8

respectively, and where appropriate, comparisons are made between personal and professional experiences, and how these interrelate in principle is explained. Consent and confidentiality are maintained; hence for all entries, apart from Owen, names have been changed.

Case study accounts are entitled: close—colleagues and acquaintances; close enough—friends; too close—family; and painfully close—Owen's story, depicting his experience of being diagnosed with cancer. In this context, close refers to comfort level: In other words, is the diagnosis and the ensuing feelings too close for comfort?

8.1   Close

In terms of colleagues and acquaintances, reflection has highlighted many individuals with whom I have interacted, both personally and professionally, who had been diagnosed and treated for cancer and had subsequently died. In terms of comfort level, the diagnosis and subsequent death had been close, in that it had incited feelings of sadness for the loss of life, and the ensuing impact on the family. These deaths had also heightened my sense of fear, in terms of my mortality.

8.2   Close Enough

8.2.1   Aaron

Aaron was a boisterous and mischievous 12-year-old boy, who had been diagnosed with an untreatable brain tumour. At 12 years old, he had his whole life ahead of him, and had just begun to give a glimpse of the man he would become. I remember receiving the news about Aaron's situation from his dad and his mum, Eleanor. Apparently, a report from Aaron's school had stated that he had been sleeping in class and not paying attention, although, in speaking to Aaron, it was revealed that he had found it hard to concentrate in class and was sleeping because he felt tired all the time. Sadly, subsequent tests (carried out in the private sector) had revealed a brain tumour, and that this was inoperable. Life is a continuum, with a beginning, middle and an ending. I remember thinking that life is so cruel, sometimes. My son Owen, not quite 1 year old at the time, and Aaron, 12 years old, were at different stages of this continuum, but with their whole lives, and the potential experiences and memories, still to be realised. 'Why is this happening?', I silently asked myself. I remember visiting Aaron, and saying to him, 'You must fight', and his response, 'I'm trying Bev, really, I am', and at that moment, my overwhelming need to hug and protect him somehow. Over the next few months, numerous tests had confirmed that Aaron's tumour was fast growing, and since it was inoperable, the only care available to him was palliative. During the next few months of Aaron's life, he had been intermittently cared for by his family at home. I remember, on one particular occasion, visiting him, only to find that quite a few family friends were also visiting, and we all congregated in Aaron's room. He was in his bed, in the middle of the room, and no longer fully conscious. The nasogastric tube (NGT) that was inserted via his nose into his stomach had become dislodged, and his mum (Eleanor) had asked me if I could reinsert it, so that she could administer his medications. I was feeling nervous; all eyes in the room were focused on me and what I was doing, but I successfully reinserted the tube.

The emotional burden of the situation was apparent, and as a mother, I had felt almost impotent to make a real difference. Here is a young boy, who was being cheated out of his hopes and dreams. His parents, siblings, extended family and friends were also cheated out of knowing the man he would become and sharing in his accomplishments. As Aaron's condition deteriorated, he had slipped into a state of unconsciousness, and accordingly had been admitted to the local hospice, where friends and family had visited him on a regular basis. It was at this moment that I realised that this was the same hospice that I had visited as a pupil nurse, as part of my training in 1973. That something should threaten your child's life is a mother's worst nightmare, and when that threat becomes real, that nightmare is magnified. As I have learnt over the years, grief, and the way it is dealt with, is very personal for each individual, but difficult as it may be, it is better to release the tears, to grieve, to feel and to face the reality of the situation sooner rather than later. However, in my experience, people will only deal with their grief when it is emotionally safe to do so. This is a coping strategy that is designed to stop the individual from being overwhelmed by grief, and as such, for some people coming to terms with their loss could take years, as it did in Eleanor's case.

As we all stood around the graveside, Aaron's dad was crying, uninhibited by the presence of other mourners, also deeply affected by his open expression of grief. Mum, on the other hand, had remained numb-like. The glazed look, and loss of light in her eyes, expressed the emptiness she felt inside. In this instance, the quote 'No parent should have to bury a child ... No mother should have to bury a son or Mothers are not meant to bury sons; it is not in the natural order of things' (Guirgis 2005) is very apt.

On reflection, it would be fair to say that Eleanor had not coped well with her son's death. I remember clearly the telephone call that had been surprising, since we were not that close, asking me to come and see her. Hearing the muffled cry and incoherent words, I instantly recognised the signs of delayed grief, a testament to an unbearable loss 5 years previously, that she had not, or could not, have dealt with at the time, but one that had now demanded her acknowledgement.

8.2.2 Stella

Stella was a lovely 32-year-old lady, who had been diagnosed with a brain tumour, for which she had received treatment over several years. She was married, and had two young children, both under 5 years old. The last time I had seen Stella was during the remission period of her illness. She had been relatively well, and had been enjoying life with her family. My conversations with her at this time had revealed her anxiety and fears in regard to her illness. Here was a young woman who desperately wanted to live, be a wife and mother, and watch her children grow up, but suspected that this hope could be snatched away, just like that. I remember her telling me about the first time she had suspected there was something wrong, and of the headaches, and numerous visits to the doctor, who had failed to accurately assess her symptoms as a brain tumour, in a timely manner. It was evident that Stella had accepted her diagnosis, and the fact that the cancer may return despite treatment. As a mother, she had worried about leaving her family, especially her children, when they were so young. This worry came to fruition, as the cancer returned, and this time, Stella not only lost the battle, but also unfortunately lost the war. Needless to say, her death was hard for her family and friends, but especially for her husband, who not only had to cope with her loss, but would now also have to be mother and father to their two young children, who at this time would be unable to fully appreciate their mother's passing. It is understandable that following the death of someone so young, and especially when children are involved, the individual's death will be a significant tug on the heart strings. Coincidentally, Stella died on the same day, a Sunday, but in a different hospital to David, whose case study is illustrated next.

8.2.3 David

David was a 34-year-old gentleman, who had been diagnosed with liver cancer (primary disease source, uncertain). At the time of his death, he had left a son and a partner. David had been a prominent member of the Akan Football Club that had been developed by a group of friends in 1972, a club whose physical base had long since disappeared, but whose memory was kept alive by the regular remembrance social occasions that had been frequented by remaining club members and their family over the years. Following the news of David's diagnosis, the Club had organised a social occasion, a barbecue, to which all club members, plus their families and friends, were invited. The day was extremely hot, and while barbecuing in such heat had been quite surreal, it was nevertheless an enjoyable day. There was a large turnout of people, who ate, drank, joked and laughed, despite the occasion's sad undertone. David had looked well a little slimmer, perhaps, but still healthy. He had smiled a lot, and seemed to have enjoyed spending time with his friends, as they revisited past memories and experiences, and had indulged in their mirth. Sadly, I did not see David after that, but we were kept apprised of his progress, which sadly ended with the notification of his death that had occurred on a Sunday afternoon, several months after his barbecue event. As I think back on this situation, the fact that David's death occurred on the same day as Stella's albeit in different hospitals, that they were both so young and that their subsequent funerals took place in the same week was poignant and thought-provoking.

8.2.4 Dianne

Dianne was a lovely lady, who at 45 years old had been previously diagnosed with ovarian cancer. Dianne was a teacher. She had two children, a son, who was still in school, and a daughter, who was training to become a teacher like her mum. Dianne had been a school friend, but unfortunately, we did not see each other as often as we used to. The last time I saw Dianne, she had been working in a local school, from which she had accompanied the children in her class to the weekly swimming lessons at the local leisure centre. We had spoken about our respective families and how they were getting on, and she told me how proud she was of her daughter and the fact that she was training to become a teacher. She had also talked about her son, and her wish to support him throughout his remaining years at school.

I remember receiving the call from another school friend to inform me that Dianne had been diagnosed with cancer, and was being treated for this. She was unsure whether Dianne was still in hospital or had been discharged home, but in my need to speak to her, I proceeded to track her down via the local tertiary care hospital and finally found her at home. Even though I had not seen Dianne for a while, contact had not been uncomfortable. We managed to have a long conversation about her diagnosis, on which she was quite philosophical about its ensuing impact on her life. Dianne had admitted to feeling lucky to be alive, and was looking forward to making a full recovery. She spoke about her daughter, and of her wish to live long enough to see her graduate, and of her son, who she would like to see settled, once he had completed school. We had also spoken about many other things including school days, had agreed to my visit the following week, and as per her request would I make her an apple pie.

It is two days before the planned visit, and I am getting ready to leave home for my nursing shift, which was due to start at 1.30 p.m. The phone rings; it was Dianne's sister; she was calling to inform me that Dianne had died suddenly, earlier that morning. I can remember feeling as if the stuffing had been knocked out of me, being quiet for a while, as tears ran down my cheeks, and Dianne's sister saying, 'Hello, are you ok? … I'm sorry to have given you the news in this way'. I asked her how Dianne had died. She explained that while getting out of bed, she had collapsed to the floor, with her son present. Due to the suddenness of this occurrence, I knew instantly that she had suffered a pulmonary embolism—the 'silent killer'. Silly, I know, but all I could think of was that I was supposed to make her an apple pie. In receiving the news of Dianne's death, I had felt cheated out of meeting up with her. The memories of our past life—school, and later having children, and thoughts of unfulfilled dreams—abound, specifically her wish to see her daughter graduate and her son finish school, a wish that was cruelly denied. On the day of Dianne's funeral, as I observed her family, especially her daughter and son, school friends and many others, I was suddenly overcome by a heightened sense of mortality and a feeling that I was running out of time.

8.2.5 Mara

Mara had been a vibrant 43-year-old lady, who had been diagnosed with ovarian cancer. She was married to Clarence and was the mother of seven children, ages ranging from 3 years to 20 years plus, when she died. Mara was a very independent lady, who had had strong religious beliefs, ones that had influenced her decision not to have a blood transfusion, even though it was considered necessary to improving her health outcomes. As an alternative approach to managing her cancer, Mara had been convinced that an oral course of iron medication, combined with systemic chemotherapy, would be an effective treatment. It was initially, but alas, its effect was short-lived. Realising her fate, Mara had attempted to put her house in order, initially by arranging a social gathering to say her final goodbyes to her family and friends, to whom she had delegated specific duties relating to the gathering. The occasion was lovely, although quite sombre. Nevertheless, in respect for Mara's wishes, we ate, drank, laughed and even danced, which in looking back had been in accordance with her wishes. Several months down the line, Mara sadly succumbed to her illness, which at 43 years old was considered by her family and her friends to be much too soon to depart this world. Her overriding wish was that Clarence would be there for their children, a wish that over the years was well and truly granted. Her children and grandchildren had all grown up cherished, and well loved by their father, until his recent death from pancreatic cancer, aged 67 years old, in 2018.

8.2.6 Verona

Verona had been a feisty lady, who at 43 years old had been diagnosed and treated for breast cancer in 1997. She had three children, the youngest 3 years old at the time. I remember when she told us about her diagnosis—she was positive that she would beat the cancer. Verona had had a subsequent mastectomy, followed by systemic chemotherapy, prior to which she had shaved off her hair. Her explanation for doing so was that she was going to lose it anyway, so why not shave it off. This was not a problem; a shaved head looked good on Verona. For nearly 5 years, she battled this cancer and had succeeded—at least that is what we all thought. She looked terrific, her hair had grown back and she was hopeful of a long and eventful life.

However, in 2001, now 47 years old, Verona's hopes for a long and eventful life were cruelly crushed as the cancer reinstated its claim to her life. I remember the day I realised that the cancer had returned. It was December, and Christmas was fast approaching. For the first time ever, I had decided to go away for the festivities and was all set to travel to Spain. I remember telephoning Verona to see how she was, and to tell her that we would be away for Christmas and hoped she and the family would enjoy the festivities. By the tone of her voice, I could tell immediately that something was wrong. I asked her if she was ok, to which she had replied, 'Yes, I'm ok Bev', but I didn't believe her. 'No, you're not', I said, 'What's wrong?'. 'I'm ok', she repeated, 'Go on holiday, and have a nice time, we'll talk when you return'. Despite the sinking feeling in the pit of my stomach, I decided not to push her.

Feeling somewhat deflated, I went on holiday as planned. Christmas was a bittersweet occasion, since Verona was on my mind all the time. On our return from holiday, the first thing I did was to call Verona. She was now open to revealing the latest developments in her health. The cancer had indeed returned, and seemingly more aggressive. 'Oh, Verona', I said, as the tears ran down my cheeks. Listening to me cry, in true Verona style, she had tried to reassure me. 'It's ok Bev, it's disappointing, but you know me, I'll continue to fight'. And fight she did. In the short time that she was given, she had undergone further treatment with chemotherapy, but her response this time around had been less positive. During Verona's admission to hospital, I visited her frequently. I remember, on one visit, she was sitting in the middle of her bed, legs crossed and closely pulled up in front of her. Looking sad, and almost on the verge of tears, her body language had given a voice to her unspoken fears. Sitting at the other end of the bed, facing her, I asked if she was feeling ok, to which she responded by shaking her head. She took an orange from the fruit bowl in her locker, and with her head bowed attempted to peel it. I asked her if she would like me to peel it for her, and she more or less shoved it towards me. I peeled the orange and returned it to her, but her disinterest in eating it was clear, as she played with the segments. Later during the visit, she became quite agitated. I asked her if she was in pain, and she nodded yes. She had been prescribed regular analgesia, but was now experiencing breakthrough pain. I asked her if she wanted me to speak to the nurses on her behalf regarding her pain control, and again she nodded yes. In speaking to the charge nurse, I explained that Verona was experiencing breakthrough pain, and asked could she have a stat dose of analgesia. I went on to suggest that in light of the evident increase in breakthrough pain, would it be prudent to consider a morphine pump. My concern was that at this stage of her illness, Verona should not be experiencing any pain. The charge nurse agreed to this, and after confirming with Verona and the Breast Care CNS, a pump was subsequently prescribed.

As part of Verona's ongoing management, she had been referred to the local hospice, to which she had made several days' visits while she was in the community. Not only did she enjoy these visits, but also her participation in various activities, aromatherapy and massage, had been a therapeutic distraction. Being registered with the hospice had also ensured that in her last days, she would be guaranteed admission. Sadly, Verona did not return home. Her condition had deteriorated significantly during this hospital stay, and consequently the decision was made to transfer her to the hospice. Unfortunately, on the day of transfer, her condition worsened to the point that it was unlikely that she could make this final journey. With the nurses' acknowledgement of her worsening condition, Verona was instead moved from the four-bedded cubicle to a single-room cubicle to enable her family and friends to spend time with her in her final hours. She was well loved, a fact that was verified by the vast number of visitors. While the cubicle was not ideal in terms of space, we had nonetheless attempted to make Verona's last hours as comfortable and as dignified as we could. With family and friends taking turns to sit by her bedside and hold her hand, she died peacefully at 02.30, on seventh January 2002, a date which was significant for my son Owen, not only because it was his first 'close-up' experience of seeing someone who had known him all his life pass away, but it was also his birthday. Her death was heart-rending then, and is to this day.

8.2.7   Beatrice

Beatrice was in her 60s; she had always been shy of revealing her exact age. Beatrice was diagnosed with and treated for colorectal cancer. She is married, with two grown-up sons. I remember Beatrice's accounts of her symptoms leading up to her eventual near collapse at the train station. For months, she had been feeling unwell and experiencing symptoms of feeling weak, tired and a lack of energy, symptoms that she jokingly attributed to her being extremely unfit, and needing to do something about it. Although in light of the extreme tiredness and lack of energy, it had occurred to her that she might be anaemic. In hindsight, this near collapse had been most fortunate, since subsequent assessment and various diagnostic tests did confirm that she was extremely anaemic, and that this was due to excess bleeding, as a result of having colorectal cancer, for which she received surgery.

On visiting Beatrice in the hospital, she had looked well, and with appropriate analgesia in place was relatively pain-free. In speaking to her recently about her diagnosis and how she had felt about the news, I was not surprised by her answer, or of the matter-of-fact way in which it was given. Beatrice explained that at the time, she had tried to remember if she had updated her will. This was important, as she needed to ensure that her family would be ok—a remark which I believe echoed her unspoken fear of death and her need to be prepared. Fortunately, Beatrice recovered well from her surgery. She now has regular yearly check-ups, with CT scans, which I am sure give her cause for concern, as she anxiously awaits reassurance from the doctor that her scan is clear. Today, my friend remains in relatively good health, and long may this continue. As a cancer survivor, she has decided to take a positive outlook on life, and as such ensures that she enjoys quality time with her family and friends. Beatrice's situation reminded me of two of my patients, while working in the colorectal ward in 1996, and how they had felt following the receipt of their diagnosis and subsequent treatments.

8.2.8 Glenn

Glenn was a 60-year-old gentleman who had been diagnosed with intermediate-risk, locally advanced prostate cancer at 54 years old that had later progressed to the advanced metastatic stage. Glenn was a social worker; he was married and had three children, one grown up and two who were still at school. Glenn loved life, and had a great enthusiasm for travel. I remember attending his 50th birthday, and his obvious delight, as his family and friends had helped him to celebrate this important milestone. Four years later, he was diagnosed with prostate cancer. Glenn had been a dear friend, and a frequent attender to the local gym. However, while we had undertaken many training sessions together, I had not been aware of his diagnosis of prostate cancer. Glenn was over 6 feet tall, and while he was not excessively overweight, he had strived to keep his weight in check with frequent exercise. The next time that I had seen him at the gym, he had looked extremely well. Having utilised the services of a personal trainer, he had lost approximately 2 stones in weight, an achievement, which on congratulating him he had attributed to his efforts to improve his fitness level. Of course, I accepted his explanation, why wouldn't I? It was not until the news of his diagnosis had been revealed that I had put two and two together.

In the undertaking of my master's degree in 2012, I elected to explore the awareness of men of African descent of their risk of prostate cancer. Unbeknown to me, my husband had informed Glenn of my intention, and as a result he had offered to be the pilot participant for my research study. The interview had revealed that as a result of Glenn's diagnosis of prostate cancer, he was very eager to pass on his experience to others, mainly to increase awareness among men of African descent of their risk of prostate cancer and highlight the importance of being involved in screening programmes, specifically having the prostate-specific antigen (PSA) test at the appointed age (40 years old, for black men) to detect the disease in early stages, and accordingly secure earlier treatments and more favourable health outcomes. Glenn's need to pass on his knowledge and experience of prostate cancer was passionately embraced. During the interview, he had stated that he wished he had been more aware of his risks of prostate cancer, especially as a man of African-Caribbean descent. He believed that increased awareness would have enabled him to access a more expedient diagnosis and treatment that would possibly have extended his life, or more importantly cure the disease. Acknowledging that he was at the end stage of his illness, Glenn's main wish was to ensure that his daughter and his son had completed their studies, and to make provisions for them and his wife— a wish that was granted. Glenn's participation in the pilot study provided valuable insight into his experience of being diagnosed and treated for prostate cancer, but sadly he had not lived to see the completed project. He died peacefully in the hospice (the same one as Aaron, case study 1), a few weeks after his 60th birthday. His attempt to increase awareness among his friends and other men of African and African-Caribbean descent had been successful, since many had taken up the offer to be screened for prostate cancer.

While Glenn had not been a member of the Akan Football Club, he was nevertheless a staunch supporter. As I later learnt, a couple of club members had been diagnosed with prostate cancer, for which they had received treatment and had progressed reasonably well. Sadly, two members had subsequently died, one of whom was James, in October 2019.

As an African-Caribbean woman, married to an African-Caribbean man, this is a topic area in which I will continue to have a vested interest.

Pancreatic cancer is an extremely aggressive disease, which, due to the lack of early significant symptoms, is usually diagnosed in the later stages of its development. The survival of someone with stage I disease is significantly better than one with stage IV. Overall, approximately 1 in 64 patients is alive at 5 years post-diagnosis. For patients with locally advanced disease, the median survival is 8 to 12 months, whereas those with widely metastatic disease have a median survival of 3 to 6 months. Diagnosed in later stages, the treatment of choice is usually chemotherapy. However, since chemotherapy can have a huge impact on the individual's health and quality of life, appropriateness to receive treatment is very reliant on the individual's fitness status.

8.2.9   Eleanor

Eleanor was a 66-year-old lady who had been diagnosed with advanced pancreatic cancer. She had three sons, two of which are still living, and Aaron who unfortunately died in 1984, aged 12 years (see case study 1). In attempts to fight this cancer,

Eleanor had accepted offers of various treatments including chemotherapy, which initially provided some benefits, but due to the toxicity of the drug, and the daunting effects on her health, she had declined further treatment—a decision that had resulted in her death in 2018, 34 years after her son Aaron's death.

8.2.10 Clarence

Clarence was a 67-year-old gentleman who had been diagnosed and treated for advanced pancreatic cancer. With his first wife, Mara, they had seven children and a number of grandchildren, whom he loved with a passion. Clarence was an extremely sociable individual, with a remarkable zest for life, and was well loved by his family and friends. In his attempt to fight the disease, Clarence consented to various treatments that included chemotherapy and radiotherapy. These treatments had afforded him a decent extension to his life that had enabled him to put his affairs in order. Unfortunately, Clarence lost his fight with cancer in 2018, 13 months after his diagnosis and 25 years after his first wife Mara's death (see case study 5).

8.3   Too Close: Family

8.3.1   Berenice

Berenice, my aunt, is a lovely 80-year-old lady, who was diagnosed with breast cancer in 1997 (the same year as Verona, case study 6), at an age of 57 years. She has five grown-up children and grandchildren. For the treatment of her cancer, Berenice had undergone surgery, and subsequently chemotherapy. However, as a result of having chemotherapy, she had suffered some hearing loss and had developed diabetes, among other things, such as emotional difficulties in the early stages of her recovery. As with most people, Berenice had been quite shocked to be diagnosed with cancer, and had found the subsequent treatments quite daunting on her life and quality of life. Nevertheless, she had quickly gained perspective on her situation, in that, despite the effects of treatments, she was grateful to be alive. I must say that over the years, I have admired Berenice's positivity towards her diagnosis and her determination to survive. Based on some of the conversations that had transpired between us, she had struggled emotionally during the early stages of her recovery. One indication of this struggle had been an incident that had occurred in the early hours of the night, when perspiring profusely she had been forcibly awakened by vivid thoughts of visions of death. Even though it has been 23 years since Berenice was diagnosed and treated for breast cancer, as a cancer survivor, I know that a fear of recurrence is never far from her mind, and that this fear is only assuaged by the yearly check-ups and ensuing reassurance from the doctor that the cancer had not returned. Berenice, now 80 years old, continues to have a positive outlook on life. She believes that what will be, will be, and as such lives life to its fullest. Long may she continue.

8.3.2   Myrna

Myrna, my mum, was 80 years old when she was diagnosed with pancreatic cancer in May 2016. She has seven grown-up children, grandchildren and great grandchildren. She was an insulin-dependent diabetic, but unfortunately a lack of appetite and accordingly a poor nutritional status had meant that diabetes was poorly controlled in the later stages of her illness.

Years before her diagnosis, I can remember Myrna repeatedly saying that her body did not feel right. With this feeling, combined with numerous visits to the local hospital and the subsequent diagnostic tests that revealed no conclusive proof of what the problem might be, she had come to the conclusion that the doctors were neither listening to nor taking her concerns seriously. However, in 2015, a CT scan did reveal a 2 cm mass in her pancreas that had resulted in her being referred to the local tertiary care centre for a biopsy. A magnetic resonance cholangiopancreatography (MRCP), a special type of MRI scan, was also performed to further support a diagnosis. Myrna had had several admissions to hospital in the intervening weeks prior to her diagnosis, with subsequent discharges, after which the intervals between readmission to hospital became shorter each time. I remember clearly the penultimate admission, which was around 11 pm, to the local hospital's A&E department. Myrna had a high temperature, increased pain and, due to her not eating, worryingly high blood sugar levels. A rapid intravenous infusion of saline and paracetamol had provided some immediate relief, but clearly there was something amiss.

Eventually, Myrna was discharged home, but unsurprisingly was readmitted for what was to be the last time. While at home, Myrna had reported experiencing excruciating pain that while concentrated in her lower back had also radiated around to her right and left flanks. The ambulance was called and she was accompanied to the hospital by her sister, who accordingly informed the family of this latest development. On visiting Myrna in the ward, she had been relatively pain-free following the receipt of a morphine injection, but she still seemed frightened which on further prompting had revealed that because the pain was so severe, she was terrified of its return. By now, I believe that Myrna had her suspicions of the seriousness of her situation, but had not voiced her fears openly. At this point, I too became convinced of the gravity of the situation. The nurses and doctors had taken good care of Myrna. They had been successful in stabilising her pain, and had attempted to manage her diabetes, which in view of her poor nutritional status was not an easy task. Myrna had remained in hospital, and when we next visited, she had been transferred to another ward that was more appropriate for treating her condition. She seemed more comfortable, and was in no apparent pain. During the intervening weeks, the doctors attempted to discharge Myrna home again, but each time, discharge was cancelled since she was clearly not well enough. At this point, we were still awaiting the biopsy result from the tertiary care centre, which was received a few days before the diagnosis. The results had confirmed the previous CT scan indication of a 2 cm pancreatic mass. Sadly, the mass was now at an advanced stage that had spread to her liver, and hence the choice of treatments available to her was limited. While chemotherapy was the feasible choice, in view of Myrna's poor nutritional status and poorly controlled diabetes, it was felt that she would not be able to tolerate the drug's incurred toxicity. The only feasible option, therefore, was a palliative approach to controlling her pain and other relevant symptoms.

Myrna was given the diagnosis on tenth June 2016, and 16 days later she was gone. The speed of her demise was startling. It was as if she had just let go. Myrna had strong religious beliefs, and it was clear that these had played a big part in her acceptance of the news of her diagnosis and its implications for her life. It was clear to me that having her suspicions confirmed had taken away any hope of recovery, and with the evident fear of her previous experience of that awful pain returning, lingering was not a comforting thought. Myrna had embarked on her journey home to her Lord, and while this was an outcome that had evoked much sadness for everyone, for me, it was a mixed blessing. Though she was no longer with me, she was in no more pain, and she was now at peace.

In hindsight, I found myself wondering if, in the early stages, Myrna had been correct in thinking that there was something wrong with her. I remember, on tenth June 2016, my visit with her in the evening following the receipt of the diagnosis—a diagnosis which, while not surprising to her, was still alarming in view of the late stage of the cancer. Sitting by her bed, I quietly apologised for not being there when she was told the news, and asked her how she was feeling. It took her a while to answer me; in fact I had to repeat the question twice. Finally, in answer to my question, she had reiterated her previous remark, 'I've been telling these doctors for years, that my body does not feel right, but they did not listen'. I tried to explain that they had listened, but the tests that were conducted needed to be more specific, in terms of which organs or sites to scan to identify the cancer. Maybe, in this case, there is an element of guilt, as I wonder if more specific tests would have secured a more positive outcome.

Honesty   As a nurse, and knowing what I did about pancreatic cancer, I accepted the reality of Myrna's situation and accompanying fallout. As experienced in practice, there comes a time when total honesty is imperative to enable the individual to put their affairs in order (Anderson 2019, Part 1). In this instance, there had been some reluctance on the doctor's part to be totally honest with Myrna about her diagnosis and the resulting prognosis. As a daughter and a cancer nurse, my need to intervene had been heightened, and as a result I had managed to convince the team to be honest with Myrna … my mum.

Understandable Fears   Before my mum was diagnosed with pancreatic cancer, a close friend's relative, who was only in her early 60s, and also a long-standing insulin-dependent diabetic, had died of pancreatic cancer after a short illness. Hearing the news of her death was very surprising, since the last time I saw her, she had seemed so well. The fact that she was an insulin-dependent diabetic did make me wonder if there was a link between the two (insulin and pancreatic cancer), and whether this warranted further exploration. For me, my suspicions of a link between diabetes and pancreatic cancer had made me question whether this was to be my fate, even though I was not yet on insulin. Some might argue that I am being irrational, but this is a question that had continued to worry me, so much so that I was prompted to discuss my concerns with my GP. In his attempt to reassure me, he had explained that while my concerns are understandable, the likelihood of me developing pancreatic cancer as a result of my diabetes is highly unlikely. Despite the GP's assurances, I am not fully convinced.

Sod's and Murphy's Law Sod's and Murphy's laws are axioms that 'if something can go wrong, it will', with the further addendum … that it will happen at 'the worst possible time'. This may simply be construed as 'hope for the best, expect the worst'. While Sod's law is somewhat similar to Murphy's law, there is a twist— Sod's law carries a sense of being mocked by fate. Sod's law is related to the idea of the unlucky sod, an average person who has bad luck. Of these two laws, Murphy's law is by far the more commonly used. The notion that 'if anything can go wrong, it will' is the simplest version of a notion that has been expressed in numerous ways. Explanation is accessed from (Grammarist 2014).

The reader may be wondering why I have chosen to refer to these laws, and how they are relevant in this context. Basically, in dealing with difficult situations (those encountered at work and within the wider circle), thoughts of both Sod's and Murphy's laws often come to mind, although my interpretation of their meaning is slightly more cynical. In this instance, I imagine that I am happy, and everything is going well, then along comes 'Sod and Murphy', to put the 'kibosh' on things. They appear to be playing a game, from which they derive much fun and laughter, but it is not a game, and there is certainly no laughter. Nevertheless, envisioning such a scenario does seem to capture the overt cynicism, and to a certain extent helps to deflect the seriousness of the situation, for a while at least.

In this instance, my cynical interpretation of Sod's and Murphy's law relates to my son Owen who at 35 years old was at the stage in his life where he was ready to share his life with his long-term partner. To set in motion steps to make this dream come true, he had moved back home in April 2018 to enable him to save for a property with her. However, as will be illustrated in the following case study, his dream had encountered a devastating blow.

8.3.3 Painfully Close: Owen's Story

Background The year is 2000; Owen is 17 years old, and currently studying at college. It is a very hot August day, so hot in fact that Owen was topless, only wearing trousers. As he walked into the dining room, where we were all sitting around the dining table, my eyes locked onto the lump on his right arm. I asked him how long the lump had been evident, and had jokingly suggested that his arm had looked like 'Poppye's'. Oblivious to the implication of the lump, Owen had stated that he noticed it a few days ago, but because he had no symptoms, he was not unduly concerned. As a nurse, and having some awareness of what such lumps could indicate, I made the suggestion that he goes to the GP to get it checked out. Following this check-up, the GP had been concerned about the lump, and had therefore referred Owen to the local hospital orthopaedic team for assessment and an opinion on how best to proceed. On the day of the appointment, I was working, so Owen was accompanied to the appointment by his dad. From what I was told by my husband, the consultant had taken one look at the lump, and before conducting a full assessment, including past medical history, or any scans, had informed Owen and his dad that he had a bone sarcoma—news that was understandably harrowing for Owen's dad, but seemingly not for Owen. I remember being in the ward, in the treatment room, when my colleague came in and told me that my husband wanted to see me. He had looked very sad, and was clearly very worried and anxious, as I asked him what was wrong. He looked at me, eyes tearful, voice shaky, as he told me that the doctor thinks the lump on Owen's arm is a cancer. As I hugged him, I remember thinking, NO! This is not real. If Owen had cancer, I would know, wouldn't I? Nonetheless, the seed had been planted, and while there was an element of doubt, the fear that ensued was real.

My colleague allowed me to go downstairs to see the consultant with Owen and my husband, at which point he had re-explained the news and his reasons for reaching this decision. I remember listening to the consultant, but still the news did not seem real. I remember we were then asked to take Owen for a plain-film X-ray, and that while we were waiting to have the procedure done, my husband and I, each in our own thoughts, and trying to digest the news, must have had looked quite sad, an observation that had prompted Owen's pointed question … 'What's wrong', he asked? Knowing our son the way we did, we decided to be honest, and so we explained the consultant's thoughts on what the lump might be. Owen looked us keenly in the eyes and asked, 'What does that mean, … I'm not going to die, am I?' He had then started to cry, and we hugged him tightly. We told him that we did not know, but whatever happens, we were there for him one-hundred per cent.

After the X-ray (which only highlighted the lump), we went back to see the consultant who advised us that he would be referring Owen to the specialist consultant at the orthopaedic centre, and that we should receive an urgent appointment in a few days. As we returned home, I was not unduly fearful, since the news still did not feel real. Owen was sad, but when I said to him later that day that I did not think he had cancer, he agreed, as he also did not think he had cancer. After that, there was a shift in moods, as we decided to think positive thoughts until we see the orthopaedic specialist, for which an appointment was received a few days later.

On the day of the appointment, both my husband and I accompanied Owen to the specialist hospital. Fortunately, we did not have to wait too long. I remember the consultant introducing himself and taking the diagnostic films from Owen and placing them on the viewer, which clearly outlined the lump. Seeming perplexed, the consultant asked Owen if he had recently been hit on his arm, to which he replied that he had. Owen went on to explain that he and his friends were 'mucking around' at college in the playground, and that one of them had hit him hard on his arm. He remembered that the arm was slightly painful, at the time, but had thought nothing of it. The consultant then asked Owen who told him he had cancer, to which his response was the orthopaedic consultant at the local hospital. The consultant had then said that he should not have been told that he had cancer without a full assessment and examination of the events. He went on to say that he did not think this lump was a cancer, and was in fact as a result of him being struck on the arm, and as such the swelling would subside over the next few months. We all looked at each other, the relief clearly evident on our faces. I had taken a deep breath, and quietly thanked the Lord! At this point, the importance of giving accurate information was highlighted (Anderson 2019).

Second Scare around! Owen was now 35 years old. It was April 2018, 1 week since his return home. Owen casually stated that he was experiencing some discomfort in his right upper arm, a sharp, painful prick, which he jokingly referred to as some kind of weird magic. However, he was not overly worried at this point. Over the following weeks, a definitive lump had manifested, although, in light of his previous history of an innocuous lump when he was 17 years old, and the subsequent outcomes, I was not unduly worried. However, due to the onset of increased pain and discomfort that significantly worsened overnight and was also not that responsive to analgesia, we were both quietly concerned.

It was May bank holiday weekend, and my neighbour had previously invited us to a BBQ. Owen's girlfriend was down for the weekend, and while he was still experiencing some pain, they had agreed to go to the BBQ. We were having a good time; however, around 7.30 pm, Owen and his girlfriend said that they were leaving. His arm was now much more painful, so he was going to the local A&E to get this checked out. I offered to drive them both to the local hospital, but they did not wish me to stay in A&E. Owen was checked out by the on-call clinician, who supplied him with some stronger pain medication and advised him to go to his GP. On their arrival home from the hospital, they had both looked worried and fairly anxious, because the A&E doctor was not sure what had caused the lump, or what it possibly meant. The follow-on from this was an appointment with the GP, and a referral to the same specialist orthopaedic centre, where Owen was previously seen for the innocuous lump when he was 17 years old.

2018 When Owen had told me about the lump, I thought history had repeated itself; however, following his acutely accurate investigations, we had quickly concluded that this was not the case. The symptoms were different this time around. Owen had extensively researched the probable diagnosis of osteosarcoma, identified the classical symptoms (bone pain, increasing in severity at night, localised swelling, pins and needles, loss of power/grip) and made the initial unconfirmed diagnosis of an osteosarcoma. We did not know at this point whether the cancer was in the early or more advanced stage, but he had hoped that if it was indeed cancer, it would be early, low grade/low risk and it could be effectively treated. Following the subsequent tests, it was revealed that Owen did, in fact, have a diagnosis of osteosarcoma, but reassuringly this was a parosteal (juxtacortical low grade) cancer, one that with treatment was perceived to have very positive outcomes. Nevertheless, because the cancer was in his right (dominant) arm, the implications of restricted mobility and ensuing effect on his quality of life were acutely highlighted.

The run of events following this referral is as follows:

Outpatient appointment was done with specialist consultant orthopaedic surgeon. Assessment and relevant diagnostic tests were performed. Diagnosis was received and plan of care discussed. Consultant explained that because cancer is low grade, surgery would be a sufficient treatment; hence, chemotherapy or radiotherapy would not be necessitated. While the surgical approach was explained, a titanium plate was to be installed in his upper arm, and there had been no indication that the radial nerve might be sacrificed. With all the relevant tests completed, surgery was scheduled for 18th July 2018.

Unfortunately, during surgery, the radial nerve had to be sacrificed as the tumour had grown around it; however, it was felt that it could be repaired at a later date. The outcome of sacrificing the radial nerve was that he now had a dropped wrist, i.e. which significantly reduced hand movement. Seemingly, recovery from surgery was good and pain was well controlled. Owen was happy; he had had his first pain-free night's sleep since April. After the necessary follow-up preparations were made, Owen was discharged home after 2 days. His recovery and subsequent follow-up had gone well, and the consultant had been happy with his progress. He had maintained his exercises and his pain continued to be well controlled. Then came the news that knocked him sideways. Following the multidisciplinary team review of the pathology and diagnostics, it was felt that, even though the tumour was relatively low grade, there was a high risk of local recurrence, and hence, in an attempt to minimise this risk, the decision was made to offer radiotherapy. However, the manner in which this decision was communicated to Owen was not ideal. The news should have been delivered by the CNS involved in his care, but unfortunately this did not occur. Consequently, 2 weeks later, Owen received a telephone call from the radiotherapy CNS. Thinking that he was aware of the decision to give him radiotherapy, she had called to suggest dates for this to occur. Understandably, Owen was devastated. Having not been told that radiotherapy would be necessary, he was now thinking that the cancer was much more serious than first stated, and as a result, his fears and anxiety were significantly heightened. The radiotherapy CNS was also upset. Realising that Owen did not know about the additional treatment, she apologised and attempted to reassure him by explaining the reason for this decision. Unfortunately, the damage was already done.

Radiotherapy Planned radiotherapy sessions occurred between October and November 2018. Sessions went relatively well. Towards the final 2 weeks of radiotherapy, my husband and I went on a week's holiday. On our return, Owen seemed very low in mood. When I asked him what was wrong, he said that the radiotherapy had caused significant burns to his upper arm, and that he had been experiencing a cough, which he had self-diagnosed, and concluded that the cancer had spread to his lungs. He had then started to cry, and I could see how scared he was. Both his father and I attempted to reassure him. Realising that the thought of the cancer spreading to his lungs was a real fear to him, I contacted the radiotherapy CNS, who was very helpful. I explained the situation, and we both agreed that Owen would not be reassured until he had received proof that the cancer had not spread to his lungs. The CNS had then spoken to Owen and told him that she would organise a chest X-ray as soon as possible. Seeing my son so upset, and so scared, was very hard to take.

8.4   February 2019–November 2019

My son's fear of dying had manifested in blaming me. He suggested that I was not there for him as much as I could have been. How did this make me feel? Like I had failed him in some way. In my defence, while I am his mother, I am also a human, and as such I had my own way of coping with his diagnosis. Perhaps, by trying not to delve too deeply into this highly emotional situation, and interact with him along medical lines, I had seemed distant to him. What he wanted was a mother, not a nurse who gave him medical advice. I decided at this point that I may have been too close to the situation, and in reviewing my coping mechanism, I realised that I also needed to seek an impartial perspective for Owen. As a result, I advised Owen to make contact with the Macmillan Cancer Support, who organised an appointment with a counsellor, who provided him with a degree of reassurance.

Another Disclosure   It was first April 2019, nearly a year since Owen had noticed the lump on his right arm, and nearly 9 months since his subsequent surgery. I was in the kitchen cooking, when Owen approached me. With a wistful look on his face, and shaking his arms, 'Mum', he said, 'this is just mad, … look at my right arm, and compare it to my left arm'. I looked intently at him, and could actually see the difference in movement in both arms. The right arm swung loosely, as if unhinged, while the movement on the left arm was more normal—he could move the left arm upwards and bend to his shoulder. In contrast, he could only bend the right arm half-way, since the titanium plate was restricting his range of movement, a situation which as we had later learnt was the result of the titanium plate becoming loose. While Owen had shown some amusement at this new development, I had wondered if it was just another reminder that he is a cancer survivor, as he regularly referred to himself. I asked him how he felt about this new development. 'Oh, I'm not complaining', he said, 'I am just intrigued by the movement in my right arm, it's mad. I am aware of my situation, and I am just grateful to be alive'. For me, this insight was significant, as it gave me a clearer picture of the cancer survivor's mindset, from a professional and now a personal perspective. As a cancer survivor, Owen had provided me with an up-close and personal understanding of his experience of being diagnosed with cancer, his subsequent surgery, his fear of recurrence and the perceived threat to his life. His fear is almost palpable, and if I am honest, I am just as fearful.

After further review regarding the radial nerve, it was felt that following the additional treatment intervention with radiotherapy, the nerve could not be repaired. The decision was thus made to offer an alternate procedure to repair the impact of dropped wrist and to afford him an increase in range, rotation and grip. Although Owen was advised that power/strength may never return to the original level, he was nonetheless hopeful that he would at least regain 50% of strength. Prior to this surgery, the physiotherapist had given Owen regular daily exercises to strengthen the muscle in his right wrist, with a view to improving surgical outcomes. A date for surgery was set for 07th June 2019, but unfortunately, due to the consultant's commitments, was moved to 28th June 2019. Since Owen was impatient to get on with his life, he was understandably disappointed.

One week prior to scheduled surgery, Owen reported that while at work, he felt a click at the right elbow joint. There was some pain, but it was not exactly like the pain he had experienced before surgery. Unsure of what had happened, he contacted the surgeon at the specialist hospital, who advised him to go to A&E department. A&E performed an X-ray, but this had shown nothing significant. Doctor had concluded that pain was probably attributed to his body and arm positioning while using his computer. Owen's reaction to this outcome was one that he relates to the ongoing emotional saga of his situation—yet another hoop to jump through. Though he was disappointed, he tried to remain positive.

I asked Owen how he was feeling. He said he was ok, but in my mind, I questioned whether he actually was. In voicing my uncertainty, I was surprised by his response, as it was quite aggressive. He wanted to know why I did not believe he was ok. 'Don't try to psycho-analyse me', he said '… I'm fine'. I felt quite upset, and as hard as it was had decided to pull back. This projection of fear is similar to that expressed on 27.02.2020.

Owen apologised for speaking to me the way he did, and went on to explain his reasons. Apparently, his perception of me was that I have been speaking to him as a CNS to a patient, and comparing his situation with them. He wanted me to interact with him in the moment—as mother to a son. He felt that I am not listening to him nor was I hearing what he was saying. While these words were hard to hear, I tried to understand. Even though I had tried not to take his criticisms of me personally, they still hurt. Maybe, to some extent, I am guilty of comparing his situation to that between a patient and a CNS, and if this is the case, it is a revelation that I resolved to change going forward. I believe that, unconsciously, this was my way of coping with my son being diagnosed with cancer, and undergoing a life-altering operation. I did try to explain this to Owen, but once again, I was surprised by his response: 'Mum, you need to get over it, … I am the one with the cancer, it's affecting me'. Feeling a little desperate, I countered with 'No, it affects us ALL', a response with which he seemingly did not agree. Today, I am acutely reminded that the truth hurts; in fact, it is very painful. Nevertheless, I endeavour to remain strong. I have no choice but to!

Owen's tendon swap surgery has been moved for the second time—from 07.06.19 to 28.06.19 and now 05.07.19. This situation has given me pause for thought, as I now ponder how patients must have felt when their appointments for scheduled procedures were cancelled. While I can appreciate the reasons for why such delays/cancellations may be necessary, e.g. emergencies taking priority over routine procedures, I can also appreciate why such delays will often result in an increase in fear, distress and anxiety (as a result of cancellation) for the patient. Other concerns pertain to the individual's work, which include scheduled time off work and having to reschedule same, even though it may not be convenient for the patient or the employer. Owen's increasing pain levels are worrying, especially as he was told that if the surgery had gone ahead on seventh June 2019, he may not be having this problem now. It is hard, but all I can do is reassure him. Hopefully, it will be third time lucky!

Owen's pain persists and is accompanied by evident stiffness—feels as if implement has moved. X-ray was taken, but nothing conclusive was shown. X-ray was sent to specialist consultant for review and assessment to determine if surgery on the tendon will go ahead as planned, or whether repair on upper arm will be done first. I desperately hoped that there is no further cancellation, and that surgery will proceed as planned on 05.07.19.

Three weeks after the planned time, Owen has the tendon operation on his right arm, which, by all accounts, was successful. I vividly remember, several weeks later, with hand still in plaster, the delight on his face when he asked me to observe his fingers that were peeking out above the plaster cast and bandage. 'Look Mum', he said, 'I can wiggle my fingers'. This was clear proof that there was connection to the nerves—surgery was successful. Both his dad and I were delighted.

Owen has had his routine follow-up from his previous surgery. A current X-ray had confirmed that the titanium plate had definitely moved and would necessitate another operation to reset it. I guess this explains the previous demonstration of the 'wiggly' arm movement and the feeling that something had shifted. It was disappointing, but hopefully the situation can be rectified. Owen was told that a new titanium plate would need to be constructed under CT guidance, specifically for his needs, and that surgery would occur in 4 weeks. However, as will be shown in the following recounting of the events, this would be a long process.

Emotions are running high. Owen is still 'snapping' at me. How do I feel, not great, if truth be told, but trying not to take it too personally?

July 2019—Erythromelalgia Erythromelalgia is a rare condition that causes episodes of burning pain and redness in the feet, and sometimes the hands, arms, legs, ears and face (NHS) (NHS 2020). Impact on emotions is yet another hurdle to overcome. Once again it raises the question why are all these things happening. Is straightforward step-by-step progress too much to ask for? To find that Owen had been afflicted with this condition, and moreover in the unaffected left arm, was upsetting. The condition has caused him emotional as well as physical discomfort, as well as pain, especially in his fingers. It is sad, since both hands were now affected. Since his diagnosis and subsequent treatments, Owen seems to be open to many allergic reactions. Seemingly, erythromelalgia is associated with previous removal of the radial nerve—this is the gift that keeps giving. Luckily, with treatment, the situation had improved. However, also due to the erythromelalgia, Owen has developed a tiny red cyst on his left index finger, and while it is not deemed serious, protocol recommends its removal via surgery, which was scheduled for March 2020.

On 20th November, I came home from SPA break, feeling quite relaxed, but not for long. Owen reported that surgery may be cancelled from 04.12.19, as he has an infection, for which he is being treated with antibiotics. As per protocol, he would need to be clear of infection and be off antibiotics a minimum of 4 weeks prior to performing surgery. I explained the rationale for delay to Owen, but while he understood, a further delay was upsetting, and in his frustration, he had voiced the question, 'Why are all these things happening to me?' 'Honestly', I said, 'I don't know'. He had made an appointment with the GP on 21.11.19. I offered to go with him, but he declined. Remembering his previous words—'Be my Mum, not a CNS'—I gave him a hug, and said that I was sorry that surgery may be postponed again. I do feel for him—it is a frustrating situation, one that has highlighted an image of those two imposters again—'Sod and Murphy'. Difficult as the situation was, I continually encouraged Owen to remain positive and to focus on his future life plans.

Date for surgery was postponed from 04.12.2019 to 20.01.2020, and again to 29.01.2020. Hopefully, this will be the final extension. As a learning curve, this situation has been sobering. I have been enabled to see first-hand the many dilemmas of survivorship in terms of incurred implications, such as delays in treatments and the ensuing fears of recurrence on the individual's emotions. Another revelation at this time was that the original diphyseal prosthesis would only have a life expectancy of 10 years. Imagine our surprise. Why was not Owen made aware upfront that there would be intervening surgeries to replace the prosthesis every 10 years? Unbelievable!!!

8.5   January 2020–April 2020

Yet another revelation post-dentist appointment—an X-ray has shown a bony lump in Owen's teeth, a concern that had led him to conduct the usual research on what this could be, although this time he did not think it is anything serious. In view of his situation, the dentist had advised him to seek further review and assessment, and had referred him to the maxillofacial team at the local Hospital Foundation Trust on 10.01.2020. I offered to accompany him to the appointment—an offer he initially refused. However, after some prompting from his girlfriend, he relented. I hope that it would be good news. We do not need any more negativity before scheduled surgery on 29th January to refix prosthesis in his arm. Oh Lord, when will the worries stop, more to the point will they ever stop? I prayed that 2020 will be better than 2018 and 2019.

Maxillofacial Appointment Following assessment and an X-ray, a diagnosis of a buccal exostosis was reached. A non-threatening condition that was possibly linked to a previous root canal surgery in 2015. The doctor, a senior house officer (SHO), had fully explained the diagnosis and reassured us that it was a benign condition that required no immediate action to be taken. Phew! Feeling more relaxed and reassured, Owen and I breathed. But still he looked sad, and I know that he is still a little unconvinced by the doctor's reassurances. Looking at him, a tall 6′3″ man, I still see clearly my little boy reaching out to me, arms outstretched, vying for me to pick him up for a cuddle. I wish a cuddle could now make all his worries go away. He had not eaten today ... apparently, not hungry … nervous tummy. The reminders continue. He is now journeying to his second appointment of the day, his 3-monthly check-up post-initial surgery on his arm. Another chest X-ray, knowing him as I do, he will not breathe easily, until the X-ray is confirmed clear.

My earlier thoughts that Owen was unconvinced by the SHO's explanation of his diagnosis were later confirmed that night. That evening, he came to me very serious, and asked if I was happy with the explanation from the SHO for the lump in his maxilla. I said that I was fairly convinced by the explanation received and asked wasn't he? 'I'm not sure', he said. 'Since I had the root canal surgery in 2015, I find it difficult to relate current situation to this'. 'So, what do you think, I asked him?' 'I don't know Mum', he said … 'The fact is, that since I first noticed the lump in November, it has increased in size, and that worries me'. I logged on to Google, and after some exploration got a fairly good definition and explanation of what a buccal exostosis is. This is a 'broad-based, non-malignant surface growth occurring on the outer, or facial surface, of the maxilla (upper jaw) and/or mandible (lower jaw), found usually in the premolar and molar region. Aetiology is still not established, but it has been suggested that the bony overgrowth can be because of abnormally increased masticatory forces to the teeth' (Medsinge et al. 2018). I continue to experience an upfront appreciation of Owen's fear of recurrence and the ensuing impact on his state of mind.

Day of Surgery Owen left home at 04.00 with his dad to attend for a 06.30 appointment at the specialist orthopaedic hospital. Initially, this appointment had been bumped to 12 noon, but following his pre-op appointment with the anaesthetist, and going through his assessment, the tooth infection was revealed, and after further discussions with the consultant, surgery was once again cancelled. Despite the tooth infection being treated with antibiotics, Owen was informed that it would be unsafe to proceed with surgery as planned. There would need to be a period after he had stopped taking the antibiotics, before the performance of his surgery; however, his surgery would be treated as a priority. The disappointment for myself, and my family, was significant. As I have alluded to before, 'this is the gift that keeps giving'. Is the universe trying to tell us something? I felt deeply for my son. All he wants is to move on with his life. This cancellation will result in delaying surgery for another

6–8 weeks. In this instance, I am tempted to blame Sod and Murphy, but perhaps, it is simply a case of 'very bad luck'. Either way, a further delay will affect his life in terms of work. How long will his employer keep his job open?

Owen went on to have canal re-rooting of his tooth, and the specimen was sent for histology—nothing unduly worrying. Pending surgery was now scheduled for April 2020; however, due to current situation with the coronavirus (Covid-19) outbreak, all surgeries were cancelled until further notice. Not a surprising decision, but oh, how I had hoped it would go ahead this time. Also, planned surgery to remove tiny red cyst on Owen's finger did not occur.

On 13th of April, Owen reported increased pain and discomfort in right arm, with concentration at elbow. Prosthesis now feels as if loose and dangling; if unsupported, he has to wear the sling at all times. Owen understands the reason for delay, but situation is now becoming more urgent.

Acknowledging Pain In this instance, reflection on my experience and interpretation of pain in regard to Owen highlights my inability to fully embrace the truth regarding his diagnosis of cancer. Do not get me wrong, 'I am not living in a bubble', nor am I 'burying my head in the sand', but I am his mother; hence, when he hurts, I hurt. In this situation, a cancer diagnosis is a potential threat to Owen's life. It is a reality that is much too close for comfort, and I fear that if I delve too deeply into that emotional pit, I may not be able to come back up! Therefore, in the interest of self-preservation, I do not delve too deeply. I guess I could be accused of running away from the pain (Farnam Street Learning Community 2020), but in my defence, I am choosing to visualise an alternative outcome—for a while at least.

As a cancer nurse specialist, being strong and supportive for your patients is a difficult task—but because it is an important requirement of the job, you do your level best. However, when it comes to your son, the difficulty of the task is amplified. I have found myself asking, 'Why my son?', a question which in the cold light of reasoning is countered by another, 'Why anyone's son?'. I feared that if I were to start crying, I may never stop, so I tried not to cry. However, when my son had reiterated the question, he had asked when he was 17 years old, 'Am I going to die?', I was touched to the very core. With his pain and vulnerability laid bare, I finally gave in to the tears. I embraced the pain, but still I endeavoured to be strong, not only for my son, but also for the rest of the family.

8.6   June 2020–April 2021

During this period Owen attended a number of appointments (telephone and face-to-face) pertaining to surgery to replace the prosthesis in his arm, but due to the Covid-19 situation, many of these were cancelled and accordingly rescheduled. Quite disappointing, but Owen is surprisingly calm. It is what it is!

There it is, surgery is delayed. There is a need to perform an up-to-date CT scan to ascertain whether the previously constructed prosthesis from a year ago was still appropriate for use. Rather this, than to find on the day that it did not fit. Owen calmy reassures me that he is ok with the delay.

He arrived for CT scan on 19.10.2020 only to be told that this is cancelled—the scanner broke down 45 minutes prior to appointment. In speaking to Owen, he was surprisingly calm … said that he just laughed out loud … was partly expecting something to go wrong.

For me and his dad, it was not a laughing matter, more a case of, 'You couldn't make it up', frustration.

CT was performed on 21.10.2020. Follow-up telephone appointment with consultant was planned for early November. Fingers crossed, the call will be positive. We just want his surgery performed, so that Owen can start to mobilise his arm and return to some degree of normalcy.

It was now April 2021, and like many others, due to the impact of Covid-19, Owen is still awaiting his surgery. Unfortunately, the delay has resulted in the loss of his employment.

8.7 Conclusions and Lessons Learnt

This chapter has highlighted the many implications of what a diagnosis of cancer involves from a personal perspective. I illustrated how the personal and professional interrelate in principle. In regard to Owen, as his mother, and a nurse, I have been given an up-close and personal appreciation of the costs of survival. For cancer patients, the fear of recurrence is very real and is easily heightened by delays in scheduled appointments, if the individual believes that delay will result in the cancer spreading. In Owen's case, the cancellation of several scheduled appointments has impacted his emotions significantly. While he understands the reasons for the delays, he is nevertheless disappointed, since his life has been left in limbo at a time when he desperately wants to move on with it.

A Fear of Dying In my experience, the fear of dying is greatly exemplified by a number of issues, but especially the severity of the diagnosis and the patient's age. Owen's fear of dying resonates with that of my patient Leanne (Chap. 6, pages 140–2). Owen's response of 'Am I going to die? I don't want to die' was similar to what Leanne had asked, 'Am I going to die? I can't die, what about my children?' My own fears are also heightened as I remembered the look of pain and shock on Leanne's mother's face, and imagining her fears for her daughter at that time. I have seen that same fear in Leanne's eyes as reflected in Owen's eyes, and that same feeling of impotency, which in Owen's case is clearly magnified. The demise of your close friends—people who are in your age group, who you have grown up with, who you have socialised with and who have had children at or around the same time frame—is a bitter pill to swallow, and nothing highlights your own mortality more acutely. You quickly gain perspective on what is important; none of us are invincible. Life is short, and is very precious, so live it well and to its fullest. Based on personal observations of the prevalence in cancer diagnosis over the years, it would seem that while the disease is indiscriminate of age, I have observed a definite shift towards a prevalence of diagnosis in younger age groups. From a personal perspective, I have always wondered how I would feel if someone close to me were to be diagnosed with cancer. Now, I no longer have to wonder. Having had three family members affected, I can confirm that the ensuing feelings following the diagnosis, while similar to those of my patients, are infinitely worse.

From a professional perspective, I can appreciate that my training, knowledge and experience gave me the confidence to deal with my patients' receipt of bad news and accordingly enable me to provide them with the appropriate emotional support to counter the effect of the bad news.

Chap. 8 provides a penultimate reflection on issues that incorporate uncomfortable truths, in-team relationships and new changes like Brexit and the coronavirus pandemic, and an update on previously discussed issues of concern.

References

Anderson B (2019) Reflecting on the communication process in health care. Part 1: clinical practice-breaking bad news. Br J Nurs 28(13):858. [Internet] http://www.ncbi.nlm.nih.gov/pubmed/31303035

Farnam Street Learning Community (2020) Pain plus reflection equals progress [Internet]. fs.blog. [cited 2020 Oct 13]. https://fs.blog/2018/06/pain-reflection/

Grammarist (2014) Murphy's law, Sod's law and Finagle's law [Internet]. grammarist.com. [cited 2020 Sep 29]. https://grammarist.com/phrase/murphys-law-sods-law-and-finagles-law/

Guirgis SA (2005) The last days of Judas Iscariot [internet]. Goodreads. [cited 2020 Aug 11]. https://www.goodreads.com/quotes/930474-no-parent-should-have-to-bury-a-child-no

Hull G (2017) Cancer types [Internet]. patient.info. [cited 2020 Sep 29]. https://patient.info/cancer/cancer/types-of-cancer#nav-0

Macmillan Cancer Support (2019) Macmillan Cancer Support, Osteosarcoma, Information and support [Internet]. [cited 2020 Sep 29]. https://www.macmillan.org.uk/cancer-information-and-support/bone-cancer/osteosarcoma

Medsinge S, Kohad R, Budhiraja H, Singh A, Gurha G, Sharma A (2018) Bony bump on gums: mandibular tori or cancer? Mandibulartori

NHS (2020) Erythromelalgia [Internet]. NHS.uk. [cited 2020 Aug 1]. https://www.nhs.uk/conditions/erythromelalgia/

WebMD (2020) Understanding cancer—the basics [Internet]. webmd.com. [cited 2020 Sep 29]. https://www.webmd.com/cancer/guide/understanding-cancer-basics

Penultimate Reflections

9

9.1 Uncomfortable Truths

Racism is defined as racial colour, language, prejudice, racial discrimination or antagonism directed against a person or people on the basis of their membership of a particular racial or ethnic group, typically one that is a minority or marginalised. It is a prejudice that is focused on belittling those based on the pigment of their skin, eye colour and acting on feelings to put people down (Collins 2020). My own definition of racism is of an open wound that never quite manages to heal, an innate trait that exists in all walks of life, and one that sparks elements of antisocial behaviour, that often incites pain and discomfort for those to whom the antisocial behaviour is directed. In terms of the NHS, it is an uncomfortable truth that racism is embedded in the institution, and a truth that mostly affects individuals of Black, Asian and Minority Ethnic (BAME) backgrounds, with emphasis on those of a Black background.

The following reflective accounts on my nursing journey over the past 46 years highlight some salient issues in regard to the uncomfortable truth, that is, racism in the NHS.

9.2 Highlighting Racism within the NHS

Patient Abuse towards Black Nurses In the NHS, there is the school of thought that if a patient is not of sound mind and body, that is, they suffer with a debilitating condition such as dementia, they cannot be held responsible for any expressions of antisocial behaviour. Perhaps there is some truth to this; however, I truly believe that 'what is within, will out'. What I am trying to say is that we are all capable of hiding our true feelings when necessary, but in moments of stress, letting our guard down and not consciously thinking about what we are saying, our true thoughts and feelings, with regard to racism, can surface.

© Springer Nature Switzerland AG 2022
B. Anderson, *A Uro-Oncology Nurse Specialist's Reflection on her Practice Journey*, https://doi.org/10.1007/978-3-030-94199-4_9

My earliest experience of racism when working in the NHS relates back to 1973, 4 months on from the commencement of my enrolled nurse (EN) training. While giving a bed bath to a lady in her 80s, who suffered with a degree of dementia, she first attempted to hit me, and then said, 'get your black hands off me!'. Needless to say, this experience of racial abuse, so early in my career, came as a shock, but apparently, such behaviour was not that unusual. Over the following years, there were many such experiences, where abuse such as 'black bitch', 'black bastard', and 'get your dirty black hands off me' became par for the course, as was being spat at, scratched and having to deal with patients who refused to be treated by a black nurse. Admittedly, at such an early stage in my career, this initial display of blatant racism had been uncomfortable and hurtful. Coming from a background where I was taught to confront racist comments and attitudes directed at me, and give as good as I got, I understandably wanted to retaliate verbally, but I realised that this would have been an unacceptable behaviour on my part.

Such instances of racial abuse from patients continued throughout my career in the wards, and beyond, and sad to say continue in practice to this day. While not a daily occurrence, it can occur at any time. On one such occasion, a female patient refused my help with her healthcare needs, simply because I was Black. On this occasion, excuses such as dementia were not a factor, and being of sound mind she made her feelings quite clear. She wanted to have a White nurse tend to her needs. I remember thinking that is fine with me, and went on to explain the situation to the ward manager, who became enraged by her behaviour. The patient was surprised, when the ward manager told her, in no uncertain terms, that such behaviour would not be tolerated, and that if she did not accept my help, there was no one else to help her. The ward manager's response to addressing this incident was supportive and reassuring, but if I am honest, in that particular instance, I was not worried whether the patient wanted my help or not.

'A Touching Tale' Sometimes the boot is on the other foot. I remember a Black male colleague's painful retelling of his experience as a patient, in terms of the nurses' behaviour towards him. In recounting his experience, he intimated that he felt that the White nurses were reluctant to help him wash as they did not wish to make contact with his Black skin. Knowing that as a nurse I always endeavour to provide my patients, regardless of their ethnic background, with the very best care, not only are such behaviours unacceptable, but they are also hurtful and have no place in a caring profession.

'A Similar Tale' In my earlier years, as a Black nurse in the ward, I was very aware of the situations where I had been allocated to the care of a Black patient, and had wondered if the allocation was due to the fact that I was also Black and because my White colleagues were uncomfortable about performing this task. Some may argue that I was being overly sensitive, but I am convinced that this was a conscious decision by my colleagues. This experience had raised questions in terms of the nature of the nurse as a caring professional, in that here I was willing and unflinching in regard to providing care to my White patients, whom I see as people in need of my help. After all, as nurses, tending to a patient's needs is what we do, and at the end of the day, patients are patients, regardless of their ethnic backgrounds.

Assumption of Incompetence An assumption of incompetence is another form of racial abuse, which is not unusual or uncommon. I remember interacting with relatives who had doubted my competency, simply because I was Black. At this time, I was the senior staff nurse on a 13-bed urology ward. I was working at the nurses' station, when a relative entered the ward. He looked at me, and asked if he could speak to the person in charge. I said that I was in charge, and asked how I could be of help. The smug look and the wry smile on his face indicated his evident surprise at my being in charge. While I was irked by his smugness, I did not react, nor was I rude. In that moment, I decided to respond to his negative perception of me with positivity. I looked directly at the individual and provided him, in detail, with the information he had sought. You could say that my knowledge and eloquence had been an apt vindication of my professionalism. There have been other instances of this negative behaviour. There have been patients who would openly look me up and down with a concerned look, as they contemplate being looked after by a Black nurse. While they did not vocally express these thoughts, I could feel them. However, refusing to respond to negativity with negativity, I responded with action. I performed my duties with confidence and competence, and hopefully left them to ponder their misguided perceptions. As much as I believe that such behaviour is not acceptable in today's nursing, I am also sceptical, since I further believe that these uncomfortable truths will continue being part of the lived experience of BAME practitioners, in the NHS and the wider context.

Unconscious Racism I am very aware of how many different ways in which racism can be incited, and that ignorance is usually at its core. In terms of unconscious racism, it often passes for fun, but believe me, it is not (Ford 2019). I remember that there had been a riot in which individuals from the Black Minority Ethnic (BME) background had been scrutinised in terms of their behaviour—apparently, behaviour that was perceived to be typical of this ethnic background. This subject had come up in conversation at work, and had resulted in one of my white colleagues saying to me, 'Oh, you're different', and my subsequent riposte, 'Why am I different, am I not Black?' I remember the evident embarrassment and discomfort, clarified by the vocal stumble, as she attempted to justify an innate thought. Strangely enough, I understood what my colleague was attempting to say. In her eyes, I was somehow different to other Black people, because I behaved in the 'appropriate' manner, one that was perceived to meet the imagined ideology of the expected norm. I also understood that the remark was not a conscious thought—more an unconscious display of racism. Things have improved somewhat, but in many ways are still a long way from what they ought to be, and sadly may never be.

Recruitment of Black Applicants In terms of job applications, I have often wondered if Black nurses tend not to apply for promotion and/or other various positions because they do not think they have a chance of getting the job due to their ethnicity.

In this instance, the issue of academia is highlighted. Experience has shown that Black nurses are not always recognised for their academic achievements. If I am truly honest, I had always felt that to be afforded a fighting chance, I had to be that much better, in terms of experience and academia, than my White counterparts. A conscious thought that has been backed up by actual experience. However, it is evident that despite having the equivalent or better qualifications, this did not guarantee that you would get the job. The uncomfortable truth is that if your contender is White, and even possibly less qualified, it comes as no surprise to the BME applicant if they are overlooked for the job, which is a clear case of racism based on the colour of your skin. Added to this dilemma are questions at the start of the job application process, pertaining to the ticking of the 'ethnic background box' on the job application. People from BME backgrounds are deeply suspicious of this box on forms. Studies have shown that where two application forms are filled in for the same job with the exact same details and qualifications, the applicant with the anglicised name or background progresses through the application process, while the applicant with the ethnic sounding name or background does not progress. For those of ethnic backgrounds, it is understandable why there may be a lack of faith in such a process, since many believe that being honest about your ethnic background directly impacts selection and choice. The reality is that while the intention might be to be fair and impartial, you cannot rule out bias, conscious or unconscious, and as such discrimination will prevail.

Progression up the Professional Ladder I have observed that Black staff nurses working in the ward do not progress as quickly up the professional ladder as their White counterparts, or even those of other ethnic backgrounds. Why is this I wonder? Experience has shown that there are a number of reasons. It is feasible that they may not apply for a higher position due to a lack of confidence in their abilities, a case in point which is further compounded by the fact that many will have experienced negative feedback from their peers and superiors in regard to this. In certain cases, a lack of motivation and confidence may play a role, although with encouragement and support from peers to take that initial step, if that is the individual's wish, could prove beneficial. Based on experience, in order for Black nurses to progress up the professional ladder, they have to be more assertive in their approach to seeking promotion to a higher level of practice. Notably, such an approach may not necessarily bear fruit, since it has been shown that BME nurses remain at the bottom of the ladder (Jones-Berry 2019).

If I am honest, it hurts to know that after all these years, BME nurses as a culture are still on the receiving end of such discrimination. I have personally observed traits in my Black colleagues such as a lack of self-belief and confidence, and a fear of rejection and of being made to feel that they are not good enough, that has deterred them from applying for higher positions. As an example, there was a friend and ex-colleague, an excellent nurse (and no, I am not biased), who, while not overly confident with interviews, had the knowledge, experience and skills and as a Band 5 nurse had consistently performed at Band 6 or 7 level, way above her pay grade. This had been a clear case of exploitation, in that her expertise was frequently called upon to support the less experienced Band 6 or 7 nurse to perform at that level, while she remained as a Band 5. I find this frustrating, and hugely unfair, because all it would have taken is one person, i.e. the ward manager, to believe in her and her capabilities, and in recognition of these support her to progress up the professional ladder. In my experience, providing the correct support is integral to effective leadership. Support is also crucial to elevating an individual's self-esteem, morale and self-worth, and is imperative to confidence building. Sadly, this form of discrimination continues in practice today (Jones-Berry 2019).

Harassment, Discrimination, Diversity Reports of harassment, discrimination and diversity issues among nurses from Black, Asian and Minority Ethnic (BAME) backgrounds are another worrying issue. Recent evidence has shown that the percentage of BAME staff experiencing harassment, bullying or abuse from colleagues rose from 26% in 2017 to 28% in 2018 (Ford 2019). The NHS was built on, and continues to depend on, a diverse workforce, yet as reported by the 2018 Workforce Race Equality Standard (WRES) report from the NHS England (Ford 2019), the proportion of staff from BME backgrounds in England who reported incidents of discrimination from a manager or colleague at work has risen from 13.8% to 15% between 2017 and 2018, which is in contrast to just 6.6% of White staff making a complaint (Ford 2019). According to Jones-Berry (Jones-Berry 2019), one in seven BME staff in the NHS in England experiences discrimination in the workplace. Even today, there is clear diversity regarding the fact that nurses from Black and Minority Ethnic backgrounds (e.g. Directors of Nursing, Chief Nurse) continue to struggle to reach the higher echelons of the profession, as evidence from the NHS WRES report shows (Stephenson 2019). In addition, Black and other minority ethnic staff are disproportionately less likely to be executive directors or board members or promoted, and they are more likely to be disciplined than White staff over similar issues (McCartney 2016). The WRES was introduced in 2015 to expose and help close the gaps in workplace inequalities between BAME and White staff in the NHS (Ford 2019). These issues are long-standing, and at times had raised questions in regard to whether a promotion at this higher level was genuine—that is, was it based on the individual's professional status, or was it a case of tokenism (the practice of making only a superficial or symbolic effort to be inclusive to members of minority groups). In this context, the intent of promotion of a person of BAME background would be seen as a way to deflect accusations of discriminations and create the impression that diversity within the NHS was working well (Ford 2019; Jones-Berry 2019; Stephenson 2019). However, current evidence has shown that there is still prejudice and discrimination in the NHS, less overt perhaps, but that could be because it is now more subtle.

I have found it interesting, but not surprising, that experiences of racism among BME doctors are also congruent with those of BME nurses. An article by Rao and Stephenson (Stevenson and Rao 2014) reported on their study that evaluated levels of well-being in BAME populations in England on the experiences of racism, exclusion and discrimination and how these contribute to low levels of well-being among BAME groups, including staff in the NHS. Among the concerns highlighted in this study are that there is a lack of ethnic diversity on NHS boards and in leadership roles; a lack of BAME representation of doctors at senior levels; as well as inequality in recruitment, career progression, rewards and recognition. Although BAME people make up 45% of London's population and 41% of the capital's NHS staff, just 8% of NHS Trust board members and 2.5% of chief executives and chairs are from these groups, a picture that is broadly reflected nationally. White doctors were more likely to be shortlisted for jobs and to be appointed to roles once they had been shortlisted, while Black or Black British applicants were the ethnic group least likely to secure hospital doctor jobs (2.7% success rate), followed by doctors of mixed ethnicity (3.5%) and Asian and Asian British doctors (5.7%). It was further found that while BAME staff members were, at one level, pleased to get secure jobs, at another level they see themselves in dead-end jobs which other people do not want to do, an observation that invariably impacts their assessment of the NHS as an employer and their ability to offer them job satisfaction. The study also found that BAME staff faced "disproportionate" rates of complaints and disciplinary actions, as well as problems of racist verbal and physical attacks, bullying and harassment.

A later report (McCartney 2016) revealed that a quarter of doctors working in the NHS are not British, and that a fifth of NHS staff are Black or from other minority ethnic groups. As such, measures to improve efficiency in this area must focus on ways that will make it easier, not harder, for these individuals to work in the NHS, as their leaving could severely impact efforts to deliver a service that is of the highest quality and standard.

Rao and Stephenson's (Stevenson and Rao 2014) study had concluded that a decade on since the NHS Race Equality Plan, there is little evidence of progress in achieving its goals. With its highly ethnically diverse workforce and a specific focus on people's health, the NHS ought to be an exemplar for staff well-being, but this is far from the case.

9.3   Windrush: A Key Acknowledgement

Today, the word Windrush defines the shame of a nation …, a nation that once courted, welcomed and put to work Caribbean migrants to fill shortages in Britain's labour market after World War II (Horton 2018). The import of migrant labour during 1948–1960 has been well documented by sociologists as the reason for the increase in the Black population in Britain in the 1990s and into the next millennium. On the morning of 22nd June 1948, just 2 weeks before the NHS was launched, the cruise liner Empire Windrush delivered the new arrivals from the Caribbean islands, hailing the beginning of a generation of immigrant workers who were central and essential to the functioning of the NHS (Eftekhari 2018). In the years since, many more people from around the world have come to work in the NHS. The NHS is the largest single employing organisation of the Windrush era

(Rose 1998). Today, people of Black and Minority Ethnic (BME) backgrounds make up a fifth of its workforce (Community Practitioner 2018). In June 1998, Prince Charles hosted the 50th anniversary celebration of the arrival of the 'Empire Windrush' which transported more than 6000 people from the West Indies. What is interesting is that this event had coincided with the celebration of 50 years of the National Health Service (NHS) in the UK (Rose 1998).

In terms of uncomfortable truths, I believe that it is very fitting to acknowledge the Windrush era and its link to the NHS, in terms of the amazing contributions of BAME nurses to nursing. The subject of the Windrush era came to the fore in 2018, when as well as celebrating the 70th birthday of the NHS, 2018, had also marked the 70th anniversary of the first arrivals of the Windrush generation to the UK, and accordingly their contribution to rebuilding the British economy and the country. As previously outlined in Chap. 3, Florence Nightingale, the founder of modern-day nursing, has left us a remarkable legacy, for which her contribution, specifically in the Crimean War and accordingly to nursing research, has been rightly acknowledged over the years. However, it has also been acknowledged that other nurses, who played an integral and equally important role during this period, did not receive the deserved recognition of their contribution. One such person had been Mary Jane Grant Seacole. Born on 23 November 1805 in Kingston, Jamaica, to a Jamaican mother who was a nurse and a Scottish father who was a career soldier, Mary Seacole had been a major contributor to nursing.

Not formally trained as a nurse, she learned her nursing skills from her mother. As a nurse, Mary travelled to Cuba and Panama and worked during cholera and yellow fever epidemics. In 1854, after learning about the war in Crimea, Seacole asked the British war office to send her to the Crimea as an army nurse, but she was refused even an interview because of her race and ethnicity. Mary Seacole, determined to help the war effort, funded her own trip to the Crimea, bringing supplies with her. She soon established a hospital and respite home for wounded and fatigued soldiers in Balaclava. She worked as a volunteer and did not receive any recognition or rank in the British Army. Mary Seacole was famous for battling disease and pioneering community rehabilitation (Ford 2019), and as with Florence Nightingale, who was known as the 'lady with the lamp', Mary was known as 'mother Seacole' on the battlefield, because she nursed the wounded. However, as history has shown, giving recognition to people of BME backgrounds, in or outside nursing, is not something that comes easily. Unlike Florence Nightingale, Mary Seacole received little fame or notoriety for her work or her role in the Crimean war (Ford 2020). It had taken continued efforts on campaigners' part, before her contribution was finally acknowledged with the erection of her statue in June 2016, just outside St Thomas Hospital. Many have argued that Mary Seacole is an influential figure for Black nurses; hence, it is equally important that she is remembered in the same way as Florence Nightingale. The erection of her statue in 2016 was followed in 2017 with the opening of the Mary Seacole Trust in Brixton, London, where people from BME ethnic backgrounds can continue to acknowledge her accomplishments (Ford 2019).

Covid-19 Following the onslaught of the Covid-19 pandemic, all the additional critical care hospitals that have opened in England to date have all taken the name of Florence Nightingale, i.e. Nightingale Hospitals. However, it was felt that a similar such recognition should be given to Mary Seacole, and as a result, a new temporary unit based at one community hospital was opened in her name. This only occurred after a campaign, backed by the NHS England diversity lead nurse, Yvonne Coghill, called for one of the temporary Covid-19 hospitals to be named after Ms. Seacole as a way of recognising the contribution of Black and Minority Ethnic (BME) health staff. The hospital is in Surrey and is used for people who are recovering from Covid-19 as well as other conditions.

The expectation is that the new unit will be the first of a wave of new 'Seacole Services' that will be set up to focus on patient rehabilitation as the UK passes through the peak of the crisis (Klainberg 2010). This is another way to recognise the fact that colleagues from BME communities were integral to the NHS, both during the NHS response to Covid-19 and beyond. Naming the hospital after Mary Seacole symbolises the contribution made by so many nurses and other healthcare workers, from all different backgrounds and from all around the world. It is also a small, but hopefully powerful, way to recognise and honour colleagues from minority groups, including those from the Windrush generation (Klainberg 2010). However, while it is commendable that recognition has been given to Mary Seacole at this time, it should be further noted that recognition had only occurred following strong campaign efforts, which begs the question, in this day and age, should recognition not be automatic. Essentially, what Covid-19 has done is to highlight the innate racism that is still embedded within the NHS, and frankly, I am sceptical if it can be eradicated … ever.

My Own Experience Despite the previous accounts of my experiences of racism in the NHS, I am also fully aware that I have been very fortunate, and that this was in part due to the support I had received from some very special people, personally and professionally, Black and White, who challenged me to become the best that I could be. However, while I acknowledge the support I received, I noticed that as I rose through the NHS ranks, I was almost always the only Black nurse on that journey. It should not be left to 'luck' that BAME nurses happen to find a 'few good colleagues', who are prepared to support and encourage them to progress through their nursing career.

9.3.1 Summary

In today's society, it is evident that racism is alive and kicking, and in regard to the NHS, there is evidence (firm evidence and anecdotal) to prove that this uncomfortable truth is still deeply embedded in the organisation's culture. Granted, it is not always overtly displayed, and may now be more cleverly concealed, but to those who know the sly comments and innuendos, it is always evident

(Jones-Berry 2019; Stephenson 2019; Glasper 2019). I am a firm believer that humans are imperfect beings, and that if racism is ingrained in their personality, it will surface at the opportune time, whether consciously or unconsciously. The issue of racism is one that spans many generations, and attempt to address this spurious contempt is as challenging today as it has always been. These uncomfortable truths are classic examples of reflection inciting pain and discomfort, when confronting memories of feelings that had been buried, but seemingly not forgotten. It is the twenty-first century, and while things may have improved somewhat, people of colour (specifically those from BME background) are still having to contend with antisocial behaviour, and much more so than any other ethnic minority group.

As I have said at the beginning of this chapter, racism is like an open would, one that never quite manages to heal and quite frankly I doubt it ever will. In regard to the NHS, this is a sad conclusion, since racism has no place in this organisation, and especially not in the nursing or medical professions. Racism is a form of mass destruction that all of the society suffers when it is allowed to flourish unchecked. Current and future NHS administrators, and employees, need to commit to its eradication whenever, and wherever, it raises its head within the organisation.

9.4 Current Updates

Recruitment and Retention and Staff Shortages A recent report by Glasper (Glasper 2019) revealed that the problems associated with recruitment, retention and staff shortages (principally, the shortages of nursing staff) are undeniably long-standing, and apparently little has changed in this regard. It is estimated that the shortfall of 100,000 in nursing places could rise to a quarter of a million by the end of the next decade, and since staffing shortages are directly linked to patient care and safety, shortages could lead to significant burn-out for nurses due to the increasing impact of stress. The report had further revealed that based on a Care Quality Commission (CQC) report into acute care in the NHS, for many hospitals staff recruitment was one of their greatest challenges, and that this was leading to an over-reliance on temporary and agency staff.

It is surprising to learn that despite numerous attempts over the years to limit the overuse of agency nurses (mostly due to significant costs) and to utilise the less costly nursing bank staff, it is still an uphill struggle. Could a reason for this struggle be attributed to pay, I wonder? Over the years, I have observed the differences between bank nurses' and agency nurses' ways of working. Despite doing the same (and sometimes having greater responsibility), bank nurses are paid a great deal less than agency nurses. Another observation is of pay grade. Why is it that when a senior nurse of Grade 6 or 7 works in the bank, their pay grade is reduced to that of a 'D' Grade, despite the fact that they may be performing duties at a Band 6 or 7? I have never received an adequate response to this question—definitely, food for thought!

Overseas Recruits Glasper's (Glasper 2019) report had also emphasised that the interim plan to address shortages must acknowledge the need to recruit nurses from abroad, and should further address nursing vacancies, especially in the primary care and community, mental health and learning disability settings. The hope is that nurturing its staff and securing adequate recruitment and retention strategies will help the NHS to grow in the future. However, as I reflect forward, I wonder how the need to recruit nurses from abroad will fare in light of Brexit, and the new 'points-based' immigration rules.

Factors Deemed Necessary to Improving the NHS Image A recent report by Campbell (Campbell 2019) revealed that funding constraints and growing staff shortages have continued to exert more pressure on those working in the health service, and consequently less and less people are wanting to work in it. The report had further revealed that record numbers of 'burnt-out' NHS staff in England, many of whom are nurses, are quitting because of the non-existent 'work-life balance' where they spend too much time at work and not enough time at home with their family. There is also the constant issue of 'pay and reward', specifically unpaid overtime. In my experience, working unpaid overtime, or more to the point continually working extra hours and not being paid for this time, is a long-entrenched unspoken expectation of doctors and nurses, not only in the UK, but also in most healthcare establishments worldwide. It was a common theme that I had observed from delegates from around the world, during my attendance at the International Conference on Cancer Nursing (ICCN), in Panama in 2014. Working unpaid overtime relates to nurses and doctors, although in the case of doctors the report has shown that even when this overtime is acknowledged, and for which they receive payment, this extra payment often results in increased taxation, a situation that meant they were no better off financially. It is no wonder then that many were left feeling demoralised, demotivated and uninspired to continue working these additional hours.

Retention of Experienced Nurses Thinking back to my time in the urology ward in the 1990s, I remember the poster on the wall in the staff room inviting nurses who were approaching retirement to consider extending their working life to participate in training and supporting students and nursing colleagues with various learning activities within the clinical area. However, it would seem that for the health organisation, securing these nurses continues to be a difficult exercise. I am wondering, if possible, whether reasons for this difficulty could be attributed to the fact that following the completion of what might have been some arduous and stressful years in nursing, retirement was seen by those approaching this juncture as a dream realised; thus, for the majority of nurses, an invitation for its extension may not be eagerly embraced. Of course, for those experienced nurses who may be open to consider offers to extend their retirement, there are other reasons why they may do so. Over the years, I have seen nurses retire, sometimes before their 60th year, but due to inadequate financial planning for their retirement were forced to return to work in the bank. Likewise, there are those who elected to continue working past retirement age (myself included), because they wanted to. Nevertheless, I can appreciate the potential benefits to the Trust if the services of these nurses could be retained. In May 2020, as I watched the daily morning news programme on BBC 1, entitled 'Saving our NHS Nurses', it was interesting to note that in acknowledging the challenges faced by newly qualified RNs, and in an attempt to provide them with the required support, for one particular NHS Trust, the 'retention and reuse' of previously retired senior nurses had borne fruit. As I embark on my own retirement, and reflect on the level of experience that I have accrued over the years, I can appreciate the benefits of this type of retention scheme and hope that it will continue to progress going forward.

Based on the evidence, thus far, I believe that there is a great need to improve the image of the NHS, the objective being to make it a more attractive organisation, one in which prospective applicants, namely nurses and doctors, will want to work (Campbell 2019; Johnson 2015). The dedication shown by doctors and nurses during the Covid-19 pandemic has been recognised by the British public, and has resulted in a much improved image of the NHS, notwithstanding the issues that need to be addressed.

Smoking Update It is 14 years since the measure was imposed to phase out smoking altogether in the NHS apart from the mental health sector. However, as I have observed over this time, policing this ruling has proven to be an extremely difficult task. During 2019, as I moved between hospital sites, I often saw individuals (nurses, patients, visitors and other healthcare workers) stealing a smoke, not outside and away from hospital grounds, but inside—in car parks, behind trees and even by the front wall of the hospital, next to the sign that clearly states, 'No smoking anywhere on hospital grounds!' For healthcare workers, some attempts had been made to cover uniforms or other visible evidence of them being a healthcare worker, but often these are still visible. In this case, it could be argued that such blatant flouting of the rules is being disrespectful to the Trust. What is more worrying is the endless cigarette butts, overspilling from the allocated bins onto the ground and the pavement—not an aesthetically pleasing sight. In light of the overwhelming evidence regarding the implications of smoking and smoking-related illnesses (Babjuk et al. 2015; Vahr et al. 2015), I have attempted to increase peoples' awareness of the health implications, specifically in regard to bladder cancer, with the publication of various articles that included The Bladder Cancer series (Anderson and Naish 2008a, b, c, d), Anderson (Anderson 2009; Anderson 2013) and the subsequent update, Anderson (Anderson 2018a, b). However, despite these ongoing observations, 'No smoking' campaigns have achieved some successes in the reduction of the number of people who smoke.

9.5   Change and its Continued Impact

Final in-Team Furore At this stage in my career change has proven to be an unwelcomed imposition that has had a significant impact on my motivation as a practitioner, who has always enjoyed both caring for her patients and the interactions with them. My zest for learning has been overshadowed by petty nuances such as going behind peoples' backs with complaints and poor communications. Sadly, experience has shown that while they may work in a compassionate profession, nurses can be very dispassionate, specifically to their colleagues. Of course, this observation is not a generalisation of all nurses—the majority are clearly compassionate and actually make the job bearable and enjoyable. On my last few days of working, I had noted an evident streak of malice—a notation that I would not have anticipated at the end of my nursing journey. The recent issues regarding complaints and the ensuing team ructions have taken their toll. There is a definite disquiet within the CNS team, one that I hope will soon improve. Improvement will require a more concerted effort by the management to communicate more effectively with their staff and to work towards establishing a working environment that is conducive to motivating individuals to come to work each day. If I am truly honest, this final furore was very upsetting, but as I was reminded by a colleague, 'the people who care would always care'.

Reflection on my Academic Journey I am extremely proud of my academic achievements, and strongly believe that the learning gained has contributed to my professional development and accordingly the nurse I became, especially in the MUCNS era. I suppose I was always destined to go down the academic path, which I started during secondary school with the undertaking of the Certificate of Secondary Education (CSE), and later the EN training, progressing to colleges for ordinary level (GCSE 'O' Level) study, to the enrolled nurse conversion course, and finally to university for the completion of my nursing diploma, BSc and MSc projects.

Publications In terms of my journal publications, I can honestly say that this has been an extremely gratifying experience, in which my previous aversion to writing improved significantly, both grammatically and intellectually. As I became more engaged with my feelings, there was more substance to the story telling, and accordingly my journey to becoming an intuitive practitioner. The insight gained into some very difficult situations has enabled me to draw on the available literature, which garnered its evidence base from the best research—to fully appreciate the physical and emotional aspect of cancer on the individual and to provide them with the best support befitting their needs. My personal growth as a CNS and my knowledge in this field have certainly benefitted from this activity, specifically in regard to cancer, where I believe that I have captured the essence of what a diagnosis means for an individual. I am also very aware of what it means to be part of the support network for these patients and their families, in what could be arguably described as some of the most difficult moments in their lives. A further benefit, as a result of these publications, has been the receipt of numerous invitations to write for respective journals or to join the editorial board, invitations which while flattering I had to decline. However, as an existing reviewer for the British Journal of Nursing (BJN) magazine, I will endeavour to continue this role for as long as it is deemed appropriate.

9.6 Brexit

In terms of change, I could not avoid addressing the subject of Britain's exit (Brexit) from the European Union (EU), and what it could potentially mean for the NHS. The then Prime Minister, David Cameron, gave in to demands based on the commitment given in the Conservative Party manifesto to hold a referendum on Britain's 40-year membership of the EU. The referendum was held on 23rd June 2016, and resulted in the shock result of a 51–49% split in favour of leaving the EU, in 3 years on 29th March 2019. This was a decision where, for the Leave group, immigration and self-determination were key factors. For the Remainers, the fear of isolation and the impact on trade and free movement were high on their list of concerns. Following the referendum results, due to the complexity of the negotiations Brexit was not achieved as scheduled on 29th March 2019, nor on the subsequent date of 31st October 2019. However, a change in the Conservative Party leadership, followed by a general election proposed by the new leader, Boris Johnson, on 12th December 2019, resulted in an outright win, and parliamentary majority, for the Conservatives. This gave the new Prime Minister the green light to move forward with Brexit in 2020, and accordingly the UK left the EU on 31st January 2020, and entered the 'Transition Period' until 30th June 2020, where talks about what kind of 'deal' can be agreed took place.

There are those who believe that a 'no-deal' Brexit poses many challenges for the UK, some specifically to the NHS, and their efforts to deliver optimal care to patients. The most immediate challenges were perceived to impact areas such as the recruitment and retention of doctors, nurses and other health professionals, and the negotiation of new reciprocal arrangements for accessing healthcare both for the EU nationals living in or visiting the UK and for the UK nationals living in or visiting the EU.

Ongoing challenges facing the NHS include severe financial pressures, increased workloads, increased waiting times for both primary care and specialist services and shortages of health professionals in many key areas. Now added to these challenges are the potential restrictions on the freedom of movement for health professionals between the EU and the UK, as a result of Brexit. For decades, the NHS has faced shortages in its clinical workforce and has relied heavily on overseas trained doctors, nurses and other health professionals to fill these gaps. This reliance on overseas trained staff will not end in the foreseeable future (Health Tech Digital 2018) and Brexit will do little to improve this situation. The UK is a world leader in medical research and benefits from EU initiatives such as the Innovative Medicines Initiative and Horizon 2020. The belief is that after Brexit, the UK will be considered a third-party collaborator, so will be unlikely to lead these types of programmes, or be able to design programmes. Furthermore, around 75% of UK researchers work abroad. If one of the anticipated impacts of Brexit is to restrict free movement, then it is vital for the government to deliver an agreement to ensure that the UK medical research does not lose out, and to make sure that the UK remains a key player in future research. Those of us who work in the NHS, and who take the delivery of optimal care for patients seriously, are understandably worried—not just for patients, but also for family, friends and in fact the UK population as a whole—particularly those who are less well placed to seek care elsewhere, i.e. in the private sector. We can only wait and see what, if any, kind of 'deal' will be reached, and if it will deliver the promised fruits to the NHS (i.e. £350 M per week).

Brexit—A Personal Perspective My view on the decision to leave the EU is that the proposal split the UK right down the middle, hence the 'too close to call' referendum result. While there was increasing pressure to leave the EU, based around the many promises made about the 'benefits' of leaving, as illustrated in previous account, there was also much evidence produced on what impact a vote to leave would have.

As a nurse who has worked in the NHS for over 46 years, and who feels strongly about securing and maintaining good healthcare for everyone, I emphatically believe that the implications of the UK's departure from the EU will be far-reaching, and will affect all areas of the UK, specifically the National Health Service (NHS). Certainly, there is an ongoing need to improve internal management, and implement a 'joined-up' approach with the care and mental health sectors, to stop the abuse of the NHS (in terms of immigration, care of the elderly and other issues), but likewise we must remember that we are reliant on trade with our EU counterparts in terms of medications and research, and must therefore address the implications of not being able to secure a seamless service for our citizens. In a democratic society, people are within their rights to vote for what they believe in. Nevertheless, I do believe that the referendum result to leave the EU was clearly a surprise to David Cameron's government, and as such no actual strategies were in place to manage the immediate issues thrown up by a potential leave outcome.

What intrigues me the most is that for many years, the NHS has been blatantly used as a political pawn in the government's attempts to promote their various endeavours. In the 2019 budget, the Prime Minister promised that the NHS budget will increase by £20.5 billion over the next 5 years—a sum which Theresa May had said that would partly come from a Brexit dividend (O'Brien-Pallas et al. 2004). On 14th November 2019, Boris Johnson had maintained that Brexit was still the most viable option for the UK populace. The 'Vote Leave' campaign had promised a £350 million a week injection of funds for the NHS; this was one of the biggest promises made by the Vote Leave group (Health Tech Digital 2018), and I believe that it swayed many people, who were undecided to vote to leave the EU. Personally, I believe that these campaigns were in very poor taste, and were 'economical with the truth'. The government has consistently professed that peoples' health is at the forefront of the caregiving agenda, but based on years of austerity, underfunding, removing incentives for student nurses and denying nurses the smallest of wage increases, this is evidently not the case.

I fully appreciate that the Brexit agenda is extremely complex, and that no one knows for sure what the negotiations will mean for Britain, the EU and both populaces. It is an uncertainty that only in time will the true implications be revealed. Personally, I am highly in favour of 'the freedom of movement clause' (a key factor in the referendum), which allows individuals to move freely, in terms of employment, living and holidaying within the UK and EU countries. Furthermore, those of us who work in the NHS, and who take the delivery of optimal care for their patients seriously, are understandably, and I believe rightly, worried about what the future holds for the NHS.

Thoughts on my Retirement As I near the end of this journey, it is difficult not to feel somewhat apprehensive. Endings and new beginnings have long been interchangeable, with the end of one journey and the beginning of another. Mine is the end of a nursing career and a journey that spanned 46 years plus, and the beginning of a time to appreciate past exploits and focus on pastures new. There is the opportunity to have siestas/catnaps, which in those moments in the day I had longed for, but due to pressures of work could not indulge. At this vision, I can but smile, since I think that life has other plans for my new-found freedom. It is time to 'take the time to stand a stare'; to interact with and fully appreciate my family, especially my gorgeous grandchildren, and to treasure the moments, good or bad, happy or sad; and to rekindle relationships with friends to their previous frequency. I am further along the continuum, that is, life, being 65 years old, and I feel extremely fortunate and truly blessed. Blessed, because I have observed many, including friends and family, who have not been fortunate to reach this milestone. Gone too soon, before reaping the joys of their retirement. So, in the years to come, I pray that I will have the opportunity to reflect on times gone by, to treasure the memories and to appreciate life to its fullest.

9.7 Countdown

03.10.2019 It was Thursday, and my final MDT and final goodbyes to the team. Outside the room, I was saying goodbye to one consultant whose suggestion in regard to my retirement had echoed that of O'Brien-Pallas et al.'s (O'Brien-Pallas et al. 2004) study, to retain experienced nurses who were approaching retirement. Her remark, 'Oh Bev, all that knowledge and experience is now lost to us, would you not consider, coming back on a Bank Nurse basis, to support nursing students and newly qualified nurses?' The truth is that I am tired, and with the recent disquiet in practice, I am feeling a little disillusioned. I am afraid that for me, nursing is simply not the way it used to be, and while I have loved giving back to the profession in terms of my knowledge and experience, to my patients, students and my colleagues, I am no longer inspired by the same challenges it presents. In this instance, I am reminded of a family member's words several years ago; when I was feeling a little frustrated with nursing and had posed the question in regard to when it would be appropriate to stop work, she said, 'Bev, your body will tell you when it is time to go'. How right she was! Having worked 5 years over my actual retirement date, and considering where I am at in my nursing journey, I believe that I have done more than my fair share. So, while I was flattered by the consultant's remark, the answer had to be no.

I was in the nurse's office; the time was approximately 15.15, when the phone rang; it was my friend's daughter—she had rung to inform me that her uncle, James, a dear friend who retired 5 weeks previously, and only 4 weeks from his 69th birthday, had been the victim of a sudden and untimely death. A death, which in my opinion, cruelly cheated James out of time to enjoy his retirement and its promises of a fulfilling and enjoyable stage of his life, with his family and friends. In this instance, looming thoughts of 'Sod's and Murphy's laws' abound, and I quietly prayed, 'Please Lord, grant me the time to enjoy my retirement, my family and my friends'. James's subsequent funeral was even more sobering, since the occasion had highlighted just how much he had actually missed out on. Thinking of James has reminded me of colleagues who had previously retired and had not lived long enough to enjoy the fruits of their retirement. Who, having released 'the shackles of the NHS', had been denied the opportunity to enjoy this new-found freedom? The freedom to 'stand and stare', and knowing that time, for the most part, is theirs to do with as they wish.

08.10.2019—Final Actions It was my final day and looking around at the environment that had consumed a significant part of my working life and time, I guess it is inevitable that I should feel a little sad. However, there is also a sense of relief; the past 2 years had not exactly been smooth sailing. On this final day, the way I was made to feel by certain colleagues will remain with me over the intervening years.

As my good friend and an ex-nurse had intimated in a WhatsApp message on my last day of working, 'it is time to lay down the gauntlet and be free of the shackles of working for the National Health'. Thinking on this comment, it has been a long journey, so while still thinking about the consultant's entreaty, it is definitely time to go.

10.10.2019—Black History Month—Final Presentation Black History Month has long been an integral part of the Black culture; hence, when I had received the call from the library manager, asking if I would consider doing a presentation to mark the event, I had jumped at the chance. The presentation was to a group, comprising nurses and doctors, and other healthcare workers, on the undertaking of the previous research project entitled: African and Afro-Caribbean men's experiences of prostate cancer (Anderson et al. 2013) and subsequent outcomes. This included the Panama experience and the follow-up study (Anderson and Marshall-Lucette 2016). The presentation was well received and I was proud to have been asked to present something that was so important to Black men and on how they deal with being diagnosed with prostate cancer.

9.8   Post-Retirement Update

17.11.2019 First report of Covid-19 in China confirmed by a whistle-blower.

25.11.2019 It was 25th of November 2019, 7 weeks since my retirement, and as I lay in my foam-filled bath (yes, one of those inspirational moments), following my gym session and with the usual book in hand, my trail of thoughts returned to the last 3 months of my nursing journey, but specifically on the last 4 weeks, and the incident that had incited much pain and discomfort. As I reflect, I can feel the anger rising, because I had elected not to full-on confront the individuals concerned, at the time. I am feeling very annoyed with myself. In hindsight, I should have been more assertive in voicing my concerns, to ask the individual who gave her the right to speak to me in the manner that she did. However, in hindsight, if I had challenged her, I might have lost control, and that would have been counterproductive. It was certainly not the way I had imagined my last few weeks of working, and the incident did put a huge 'dampener' on what should have been a little sad but happy experience. Fortunately, it did not cancel out, or overshadow, all the other wonderful memories and experiences.

12.12.2019 In November 2019, Boris Johnson had voiced his wishes for a general election—a proposal that other parties were strongly against while a no-deal vote, and clarity in regard to what this would mean for the UK, in principle, was still on the table. However, while there was some scepticism regarding an election at this time, the date was set for 12th of December 2019, again a date which many believed would not be welcomed in view of its proximity to Christmas. However, here we are—it is 12th December 2019, and the British people have spoken loudly and extremely clear—Boris Johnson has secured his role as Prime Minister with a landslide victory—a vote to leave the EU trumps the day—the Conservatives have won. This victory had given Boris Johnson the green light to pursue leaving the EU by the end of 2020, possibly with a deal in place. What this holds for the UK is anyone's guess. Only time will tell if the country has made the correct decision. Watch this space!

29.01.2020 Two cases of coronavirus (aka Covid-19) reported in the UK.

31.01.2020 Final day, seemingly we have 'Brexited' the European Union!

28.02.2020 First death from Covid-19 in the UK, in this case the individual had not gone abroad.

9.9   Conclusion and Lessons Learnt

This chapter addressed a number of issues that have, and continue to have, a significant impact on the NHS. It has highlighted the 'uncomfortable truth', that is, racism, and more importantly that little has changed in this regard. The recent Covid-19 onslaught has brought the issue of racism within the NHS to the forefront, with the deaths of significant numbers of BAME NHS employees. This antisocial behaviour is perhaps now more cleverly masked, but is still deeply embedded in the NHS culture. A fundamental change in peoples' attitudes is desperately needed. I hope for the best outcome, but I am prepared if it is not achievable. The evidence has shown that efforts to improve the NHS and the nursing image must work towards establishing an environment in which prospective employees will be attracted to work in. A key strategy to achieving this objective is in addressing the long-standing issues of pay and reward, recruitment and retention which lead to staff shortages and an increased workload, resulting in a poor 'work-life' balance for NHS employees, which in turn completes the cycle back to recruitment and retention issues, etc. It is time to break this cycle. Despite numerous health education and promotional campaigns to raise peoples' awareness of the risks of smoking to their health, in terms of cost, this behaviour continues to be a major bugbear for the NHS. No smoking campaigns need to continue. It might be useful to direct a campaign towards NHS staff, to encourage them to give up smoking. I believe that non-smoking NHS staff can set a good example to members of the public.

Chapter 10 provides a final reflection of my practice journey that includes a rounding up of the issues discussed throughout the book with a current update on the most salient issues.

References

Anderson B (2009) Understanding the role of smoking in the aetiology of bladder cancer. Br J Community Nurs 14(17):385–392

Anderson B (2013) Detecting and treating bladder cancer. Br J Nurs 22(11):628–628. [Internet]. http://www.ncbi.nlm.nih.gov/pubmed/23899731

Anderson B (2018a) Bladder cancer: overview and disease management. Part 1: non-muscle-invasive bladder cancer. Br J Nurs 27(9):S27–37. [Internet]. https://doi.org/10.12968/bjon.2018.27.9.S27

Anderson B (2018b) Bladder cancer: overview and management. Part 2: muscle-invasive and metastatic bladder cancer. Br J Nurs 27(18):S8–20. [Internet]. https://doi.org/10.12968/bjon.2018.27.18.S8

Anderson B, Marshall-Lucette S (2016) Prostate cancer among Jamaican men: exploring the evidence for higher risk. Br J Nurs 25(19):1046–1051. [Internet]. https://doi.org/10.12968/bjon.2016.25.19.1046

Anderson B, Marshall-Lucette S, Webb P (2013) African and Afro-Caribbean men's experiences of prostate cancer. Br J Nurs 22(22):1296–1307. [Internet]. https://doi.org/10.12968/bjon.2013.22.22.1296

Anderson B, Naish W (2008a) Bladder cancer and smoking. Part 1: addressing the associated risk factors. Br J Nurs 17(18):1182–1186. [Internet]. http://www.ncbi.nlm.nih.gov/pubmed/18946399

Anderson B, Naish W (2008b) Bladder cancer and smoking. Part 4: efficacy of health promotion. Br J Nurs 17(21):1340–1344. [Internet]. http://www.ncbi.nlm.nih.gov/pubmed/19060816

Anderson B, Naish W (2008c) Bladder cancer and smoking. Part 3: influence of perceptions and beliefs. Br J Nurs 17(20):1292–1297. [Internet]. http://www.ncbi.nlm.nih.gov/pubmed/19043336

Anderson B, Naish W (2008d) Bladder cancer and smoking. Part 2: diagnosis and management [internet]. Br J Nurs 17:1240–1245. [cited 2020 Oct 1]. https://doi.org/10.12968/bjon.2008.17.19.31466

Babjuk M, Burger M, Zigeuner R, Shariat S, Van Rhijn BWG, Compérat E, et al. (2015) Guidelines on Non-muscle-invasive Bladder Cancer (Ta, T1 and CIS [Internet]. uroweb.org. p. 1–42. https://uroweb.org/guideline/non-muscle-invasive-bladder-cancer/

Campbell D (2019) NHS England losing staff in record numbers over long hours—study [internet]. The Guardian. [cited 2020 Oct 10]. https://www.theguardian.com/society/2019/feb/16/nhs-england-losing-staff-in-record-numbers-over-long-hours-study

Collins (2020) Definition of "racism" [Internet]. [cited 2020 Jan 20]. https://www.collinsdictionary.com/dictionary/english/racism

Community Practitioner (2018) Celebrating the unsung BME heroes [internet]. Community Pract 91:18. –undefined. [cited 2020 Oct 10] https://www.communitypractitioner.co.uk/opinion/2018/05/celebrating-unsung-bme-heroes

Eftekhari H (2018) Celebrating black history month. Br J Card Nurs 13(11):567–567. [Internet]. https://doi.org/10.12968/bjca.2018.13.11.567

Ford M (2019) Yvonne Coghill: "cultural transformation" is needed to tackle racial inequality. Nurs Times 115(10):8–9

Ford S (2020) NHS reveals first Covid-19 rehab hospital named after Mary Seacole [internet]. Nurs Times. [cited 2020 May 19]. https://www.nursingtimes.net/news/coronavirus/nhs-reveals-first-covid-19-rehab-hospital-named-after-mary-seacole-04-05-2020/

Glasper A (2019) Will the NHS improvement interim plan help solve the nursing staff crisis? Br J Nurs 28(14):950–951. [Internet]. https://doi.org/10.12968/bjon.2019.28.14.950

Health Tech Digital (2018) What does Brexit mean for the NHS? [internet]. Health Tech Digital. [cited 2020 Oct 1] https://www.healthtechdigital.com/what-does-brexit-mean-for-the-nhs/

Horton R (2018) Offline: a Caribbean consciousness. Lancet 391(10132):1757. [Internet]. https://linkinghub.elsevier.com/retrieve/pii/S0140673618310304

Johnson S (2015) How has nursing changed and what does the future hold? The Guardian

Jones-Berry S (2019) Racism in the NHS: are things getting better or worse for BME staff? [Internet]. Nurs Stand. [cited 2020 Mar 3]. https://rcni.com/nursing-standard/newsroom/analysis/racism-nhs-are-things-getting-better-or-worse-bme-staff-152681

Klainberg M (2010) An historical overview of nursing. In: Klainberg M, Dirschel KM (eds) Today's nursing leader : managing, succeeding, excelling. Jones and Bartlett Publishers, Sudbury, MA, pp 24–28

McCartney M (2016) Racism, immigration, and the NHS [internet]. BMJ:i4477. [cited 2016 Aug 15]. https://doi.org/10.1136/bmj.i4477

O'Brien-Pallas L, Duffield C, Alksnis C (2004) Who will be there to nurse? JONA J Nurs Adm 34(6):298–302. [Internet]. http://journals.lww.com/00005110-200406000-00009

Rose FG (1998) Black and ethnic minority elders! Who cares? Health and social care needs of black and ethnic minority elders by the statutory services. Manage Clin Nurs 2(4):111–115

Stephenson J (2019) Profiles: nurse leaders from BME backgrounds. Nurs Times 115(10):10–11. [Internet]. www.nursingtimes.net

Stevenson J, Rao M (2014) Explaining levels of wellbeing in BME populations in England [Internet]. [cited 2020 Oct 10]. https://www.leadershipacademy.nhs.uk/wp-content/uploads/2014/07/Explaining-levels-of-wellbeing-in-BME-populations-in-England-FINAL-18-July-14.pdf

Vahr S, De Blok W, Love-Retinger N, Thoft B, Turner JB, Villa G, et al. (2015) Evidence-based Guidelines for Best Practice in Urological Health Care Intravesical instillation with mitomycin C or bacillus Calmette-Guérin in non-muscle invasive bladder cancer [Internet]. [cited 2020 Oct 25]. https://nurses.uroweb.org/wp-content/uploads/EAUN15-Guideline-Intravesical-instillation.pdf

A Final Reflection of my Clinical Practice Journey

10

As I reflect on this journey, I am reminded of times gone by, and the way things used to be. That we have come a long way, and witnessed many changes. We could not have prevented them, nor could have we foreseen their subsequent impact on the nursing profession, or on healthcare delivery over the years.

When I reflect back to 1973, I am reminded of a young, inexperienced 18-year-old woman, entering the world of employment, in which she was keen to learn and gain experience, but at the same time wary of the journey's unknown path. I remember trying to get my head around the concept of having to look after individuals who, in many cases, were old enough to be my grandparents, or even great-grandparents, and worried that I did not have either the life experience or the know-how to provide them with the care they deserved. Yes, you eventually learn, and you acquire the skills, but in the beginning, it is a frightening prospect, although, with the appropriate support from your peers, it is one that becomes less so. During the 2 years of pupil nurse training, I clearly remember feeling the support from within the group, and my tutor's reassuring words of wisdom when dealing with 'difficult' colleagues in the ward (i.e. I should not take remarks too seriously, that it is not my fault), which in hindsight did help initially. At such a young age, it is understandable that you take such remarks personally, and would often think it was your fault.

My memory of my first experience of poor communication, the ensuing pain and discomfort, the way I had felt and the staff nurse's words provided an essential platform for my learning and in informing future practice. I have always believed that you should treat people the way you would wish to be treated—no more, no less— and that a crucial part of this is respect. I was recently told that I am a stickler for respect. I admit I am, but do not think this is necessarily a bad thing. I believe that showing respect to those with whom we interact throughout life is a duty, albeit a duty that is incumbent on such respect being returned. The memories of my first experiences of death and cancer are still vivid in my mind, as is the 'last office duty' procedure, of which the colour purple has remained indelible in my mind as a permanent reminder of death, and what it signified.

© Springer Nature Switzerland AG 2022
B. Anderson, *A Uro-Oncology Nurse Specialist's Reflection on her Practice Journey*, https://doi.org/10.1007/978-3-030-94199-4_10

Cancer Management Then and Now Cancer is a complex illness that demands equally complex management. My memory of cancer management in the 1970s and 1980s is of a disease that was not as fully understood as it is today. As such, it evoked much fear and anxiety in those afflicted by the disease, as well as in their loved ones. Sadly, these feelings are still as distressing today, as they were then. There have been significant changes in cancer management, of which today's holistic approach to determining care is deemed crucial to securing successful health outcomes (Doyle and Henry 2014; Duffin 2016). Pain management has progressed in terms of efficacy, typically in ensuring that those patients who are at the end stage of their illness (end-of-life care) experience a good death (Weston 2015). Advancements in technology have also meant that there have been some incredible improvements in treatment interventions. With regard to urological cancer, pioneering treatment for metastatic bladder cancer, with immunotherapy (Powles et al. 2014; Anderson 2018), and the use of robot in the performance of various surgeries (BBC Newsround 2020) are just two such advancements that have secured significant improvements in both patient and practice outcomes. The prevalence of cancer in an ageing society, and increases in longevity, combined with continued pressure from government targets, has meant that the NHS efforts to deliver high-quality, cost-effective and compassionate care to the public have been, and still are, an extremely challenging task (Doyle 2008).

Summarising the Changes to Nursing, Nurse Training and the Nurse's Role Without question, nursing, nurse training and the nurse's role have evolved significantly over the last 50 years, and technology, research and academia have played a central role in this evolution. However, with such advancements, questions have emerged asking whether nursing and the true essence of caring have been diluted (Patterson 2012). Thinking back on my enrolled nurse (EN) training, and remembering the admission of Tom, the newly qualified Project 2000 RN (*Chap. 3, pages 59–60*), and his reservations in terms of whether the level of training and hands-on experience had adequately prepared him to perform the role, I can appreciate his concerns. While this comment may be subjective, I truly believe that the EN training was very in-depth. In fact, I would go as far as to say that we were trained to 150% competency, and due to the level of hands-on experience, our practical nursing skills were second to none, a conclusion that was validated in a report by previous ENs, who had been converted to RN status (O'Dowd 2008). These nurses believed that the EN training and the amount of hands-on experience received had made them a much more rounded nurse, with better clinical skills that stood them in great stead for their role (O'Dowd 2008). They also believed that their training was in stark contrast to today's nurses, who mostly observed, and for the most part, that is all they did (O'Dowd 2008). As a previous EN, I can honestly say that I truly appreciate the training I received, and see it as the foundation on which the principles of practice were built. Admittedly, there have been moments when I pined for elements of the good old days, but I can also appreciate the many advancements made in practice over the years (Cipriano 2010).

Changes to the Nurse's Role   The literature suggests that the traditional perception of the nurse's role has now been transformed into something far more complex than that of 50-years ago (Patterson 2012; O'Dowd 2008; Cipriano 2010; Johnson 2015; UKEssays 2018). Today, the nurse's role is more dynamic, and the increased requirements for those working at an advanced practitioner (ANP) level have meant that today's nurses have to be more academically driven and infinitely more tech-savvy (Paton 2020). Today's ANPs are consultants, researchers, nurse leaders and matrons (UKEssays 2018), and are a key support for doctors, specifically those in a more junior role. More importantly, these ANPs are patient advocates, and as such are central in the delivery of care to their patients. However, despite these admissions, the rising demand for academia and higher academic status has attracted some scrutiny in terms of whether these nurses were in fact 'too posh to wash' or had lost some of their ability to care (Cipriano 2010; UKEssays 2018). The demand for higher academic status has also rightly raised questions in regard to pay, and whether the remuneration received is accurately reflective of the individual's status or their worth. Increasing workloads and diminished staffing levels, combined with current challenges, such as an ageing population and rising patient demand, have undoubtedly increased the pressure on today's nurses (UKEssays 2018).

Scrutinising the MUCNS Behaviour and Changes to the Role   As I reflect on those early years (1970s and 1980s), when I was young, naïve and I suppose still immature, I can see why some may have viewed my character as tempestuous and forthright. In fact, reference to my forthright behaviour back then was recently made by my very good friend, Lor, which in all honesty is a fair assessment of my character at that time. However, over the intervening years, I have grown, mellowed and hopefully less naïve. As a human being and a nurse, I acknowledge that I am not perfect. I have made mistakes, but would like to think that I have learned from them. In dealing with challenging situations, I have learned to choose my battles carefully, and to only act after I have garnered all the supporting evidence. I believe that I have become the nurse that I first visualised 46+ years ago—a caring and compassionate practitioner, who was able to admit when she was wrong, but was equally capable of standing her ground when she was right, a nurse who was able to recognise injustice, and abuse of power, and had the courage to challenge these behaviours.

I can honestly say that achieving the MUCNS role 14 years ago was hugely satisfying. While I found working in cancer stressful, and emotionally draining at times, the learning and the experience I gained have been immensely rewarding, both personally and professionally. My role as key worker was very important, in terms of providing the appropriate support to patients following their receipt of a cancer diagnosis. This support required providing the time to listen to them, and to recognise the non-verbally expressed fear that was often so clearly expressed by the individual's body language: an inability to make eye contact, the tears welling in their eyes (and their trying hard not to give in to them) or the forced smile, followed by them stating that they were 'ok', when they clearly were not. In this instance, being able to explain and reassure, and seeing the difference your support makes, was for me a most rewarding experience.

However, since 2017, the impact of changes made to my MUCNS role have become evident. The one-to-one patient interaction, and my ability to provide the necessary level of support to my patients, was no longer as it had been previously. My MUCNS role comprised looking after all urology cancers (i.e. bladder, kidney and prostate); as previously explained, testicular and penile cancers were usually managed at other secondary or tertiary care centres. While the decision to allocate treatment of these cancers to CNS-specific sites had been made in the belief that this would improve ways of working, and ultimately patient experiences and outcomes, the decision also meant that my involvement in the care of prostate and kidney cancer patients was significantly reduced, with my role now mainly focused on bladder cancer. Based on my observations on practice, I believe that making the tumour sites CNS specific has created a state of single-mindedness towards care, in that each CNS tended to focus on a particular set of patients. While this might not have been the intention, I found that this change in practice, to a 'stovepipe' way of working, was to some extent counterproductive, in terms of continuity of care and working as one team. It also contributed to increased tension and stress within the clinical environment. It was at this moment that I realised that the MUCNS role was sadly no longer the one that had inspired, challenged and rewarded me, from a job satisfaction perspective, over the last 14 years.

Covid-19 As I reflect on the current pandemic, I am humbled as Covid-19 rages across the world. In all of its 72 years, the NHS has not had to deal with a health emergency so virulent and damaging to so many. Literally overnight, Covid-19 has totally changed what people perceived as their normal day-to-day life. The impact on the economy has been far-reaching, with financial security impacted and predicted to suffer from the effects of Covid for some time. Arguments rage over whether Covid-19 is a phenomenon of nature, or a man-made event. Irrespective of its origins, Covid has forced us all to pause, and think about life as we know it. It has also shown that despite questions being raised about the core purpose of nursing, and what is truly at its heart (Patterson 2012), based on observations of nursing during the pandemic, it would appear that we have not lost the capacity for compassion, or indeed the ability to care (O'Dowd 2008; Cipriano 2010).

Uncomfortable Truths Even in such surreal times, the uncomfortable truth, that is, racism, has raised its ugly head. According to McCartney (McCartney 2016) despite an NHS constitution that promises equal treatment regardless of ethnicity, racism remains a lived truth for BAME NHS staff. This is a truth that has been brought to the fore by Covid-19 pandemic, whose onslaught has highlighted the true feelings of many individuals towards people of a BAME background. Evidence has shown that BAME nurses are being selected to work in the coronavirus wards in greater proportions than their White counterparts (Ford 2020). This despite it being known that, because of the prevalence of increased comorbidities, such as diabetes and heart problems within the BAME community, they are at an increased risk of contracting the virus, and consequently mortality rates are disproportionately higher among this group of people (Ford 2020). As a nurse from a BAME background, I find these revelations disturbing, but what is even more upsetting is that such blatant discrimination comes as no surprise to those of the BAME background. The sad truth is that for BAME NHS staff, racism in some form is an expectation. The surprise for many would be if it did not surface.

10.1 Summary

July–December 2020 Well, here we are—we have been through the lockdown. With the cautious loosening of lockdown, and the opening up of certain businesses, we now observe 2 m distancing in shops, etc. Wearing a mask is compulsory in supermarkets, shops, trains and buses, and public areas where 2 m distancing is not achievable. This legislation carries a £100.00 fine for those who do not comply.

Observation of both success and any violations of the rules is followed by reassessment and readjustment (i.e. potentially reinstating lockdown), as necessitated. The hot summer weather prompted a rush to congregate on a beach. This in turn prompted Prime Minister Boris Johnson to restate the lockdown rules. Inevitably, there was further tightening of lockdown rules due to Covid spikes in certain areas in England.

The worldwide search for a vaccine continues. In the UK the Oxford vaccine is in the trial phase. The benefits of treating Covid-19 sufferers with dexamethasone have been recognised, and it has improved symptoms and outcomes.

Testing – A 'world beating' test and trace was implemented in the UK, at great cost and with much fanfare. However, to date, its performance has failed to meet expected success rates.

Once again, the Covid-19 onslaught has raised questions in regard to people of BAME backgrounds and their contribution to the Covid-19 crisis. In the earlier months, it was interesting to note that Covid-19 advertisements (TV and billboards) featured hardworking Caucasian NHS staff on the Covid-19 'frontline'. This was despite the disproportionate number of deaths among frontline BAME NHS staff. At best this was classic unconscious bias, at worst racism. Whether due to belated recognition of this fact or an afterthought, finally the first advertisement featuring a Black nurse was produced to raise peoples' awareness of the importance of testing for Covid-19.

As a result of the recent spike in new cases of Covid-19, and deaths, the 'rule of 6' (no more than 6 people together at any one time in an external location) is implemented. Other rules include: maximum numbers for weddings reduced from 30 to 15 people—quite a knock-on impact on emotions for the bride, groom, their family and friends, as well as wedding organisers, in light of the significant loss of funds.

October 2020 It is October 2020, 10 months since the UK officially left the European Union. However, due to the onslaught of Covid-19, and the uncertainty it presents, the time frame for the UK/EU negotiations has been pushed back. Nevertheless, the Prime Minister is adamant that Brexit will not be delayed. The UK transition period ends on 31st December 2020; I had hoped with a deal, this now seems increasingly unlikely. We can only wait and see what happens in the coming months.

Covid-19 is still a very real threat. Lockdowns are instigated in some areas, and tightening of the rules is seen in others. News of the possible launch of a vaccine in November 2020 is briefed. The possibility of another surge in Covid cases is quite depressing, especially with the potential impact on the NHS, which bears the brunt of any Covid spikes.

The continual loss of jobs signifies a bleak Christmas ahead for significant numbers of people. This combined with lockdown rules that prevent the yearly get-together with families and friends will make the situation even more daunting. Christmas is about coming together to celebrate and appreciate the people in our circle, and sharing in the festivities. Not being able to see my children and grandchildren is an extremely bleak thought. Frankly, if this is to be the new norm, I am hugely dismayed. It is a prospect we have to reluctantly accept, and try to manage as best as possible, or allow ourselves to fall into despair and depression.

Black History Month 2020 What is going on? So much hidden/buried Black history revealed in terms of Black endeavour and fortitude, often in the face of overt racism. Black successes and contributions to science and technology, which should not have taken Covid-19 to force acknowledgement. The revelation of Kofoworola Abeni Pratt, Hon. FRCN (1915–18 June 1992), a Nigerian-born nurse, who was the first Black nurse to work in Britain's National Health Service (NHS) in 1946. Her memoirs reveal that even then, incidents of White patients not wanting to be nursed by a Black nurse were commonplace, and unfortunately have remained an ever-present problem within the NHS (Pratt 1915).

'Black Lives Matter' While the BLM movement had been around for some time, two separate events raised its visibility to national and subsequently international prominence. The Covid-19 pandemic struck the UK in early 2020. Investigations in the intervening months showed that people from a BAME background, in the UK and elsewhere, were dying from the virus in greater numbers than non-BAME people. The investigations raised a number of issues around race. One was that BAME medical staff felt that they were being put into the 'frontline' to look after Covid-19 patients in greater numbers than their White counterparts, leading to increased mortality among BAME doctors and nursing staff. In addition, the social conditions that BAME people live under were identified as a potential contributary factor to the higher mortality rate. These same factors exist in the USA, with similar outcomes for BAME communities. However, it was the horrific killing of George Floyd that brought BLM to worldwide prominence. George Floyd's killing sparked an outpouring of anger leading to worldwide demonstrations against racism, in all its forms, and an overspilling fury that shone a light on the systematic racism experienced by people of colour, on a daily basis, around the world, and accordingly brought increased pressure for change.

13.12.2020 The Brexit talks were extended by 17 days, in the hope of securing a deal with the EU. Seemingly, no one wants to be seen as the party who 'walked away' from the negotiating table—the first to give in and admit defeat. Many Brexiteers would admit that the implications of a no-deal Brexit are too far-reaching to accept, especially the impact of enforced changes on business and free movement.

The UK left the EU on 31st December 2020. The Brexit talks resulted in a positive outcome, but with reservations for many. It is, nevertheless, a result which at the end of 4 years of talks and negotiations has provided a breathing space for continued negotiations down the line.

The Vaccine The search for a vaccine resulted in not one, but two main vaccines Pfizer-BionTech and the AstraZeneca-Oxford vaccines. The roll-out of the immunisation programme (targeting the most vulnerable as a priority) which commenced on eighth October 2020 with the Pfizer vaccine provided a ray of hope of successfully securing improvements to bring a deadly virus under some degree of control.

March–July 2021—Brexit and Covid-19 Update Following the UK's exit from the EU on 31st December 2020, with a deal in place, the UK experienced early teething problems. These problems have continued, and are not only having an impact on trade with the EU, but have also impacted food and goods distribution across the UK. The problems appear to be caused by a gross miscalculation of the problems that would be encountered, combined with a lack of pre-planning to address post-Brexit issues, and consequently the UK is unprepared to manage the fallout.

The immunisation programme continues to make great strides. However, the proliferation of new Covid-19 variants is proving challenging, and has raised questions in terms of the vaccine's efficacy. Nevertheless, the trend in both new infections and deaths is down, sufficiently enough to warrant a cautious exit from lockdown.

The latest addition of new vaccines is reassuring in terms of maximising the vaccination programme and hope for success. From a personal perspective, Brexit plus Covid-19 is the perfect storm that heralds uncertain times ahead, not just for the UK's economy, health and life as we previously knew it, but also internationally, for the rest of the world.

Revisiting my Initial Thoughts on Retirement It is one year since my retirement, and I reflect back on my initial plans for this period of my life, which were to interact more with and to fully appreciate my family, especially my gorgeous grandchildren; to take the time to plan new adventures, appreciate past exploits and rekindle relationships with friends; or to take the time to 'stand and stare' at life and have siestas and catnaps when I felt like it. I had hoped to see whether life would have other plans for my new-found freedom, and seemingly it does. While at this moment I am tempted to think that 'Murphy's law' (whatever can go wrong, will go wrong!) is having a final meddle with my life, I am also smiling at the irony of life and the uncertainty of its promise for a tomorrow that may never come. As I have acknowledged over the years, and was reminded in October 2019 by James's untimely death, life is short and time is precious. As Chaucer said, *'Time and tide wait for no man'*. In other words, 'Time stops for no one' (Lemon 2005). As such, I believe that you should enjoy life to its fullest, each and every day. My retirement so far has been eventful, but I am hopeful that now that I have completed my project, it will slow to a more relaxing tempo. Although with Covid-19 still dictating the rules of play, life as we knew it is unlikely to return anytime soon, and I believe that it will be a case of adjusting to a new normal, whatever that may be! To the very end, change has been, and will always be, unrelenting; all we can do is to embrace its insistence.

10.2   Conclusion and Lessons Learnt

As I near the final pages of this project, I am amazed that in 2018, the NHS celebrated its 70th birthday and that I have been working for this organisation for over 46 of those 70 years! An achievement for which, I believe, the writing of this book is a fitting acknowledgement. In this context, reflection is an activity from which I have benefitted both personally, in terms of my family and my friends, and professionally, in terms of my patients and the resulting health and practice outcomes. The process of reflection has highlighted memories of hard work, team spirit, patient interactions, challenges, achievements and pride, and forging of long-term relationships, and also memories of both personal and professional losses, fear and pain and a heightened awareness of one's mortality that forces one to quickly gain perspective on what is important in life, a journey, which, in the early years, had incited much **FUN**, a stark difference to today's nursing, which could arguably be described as one that incites tension, stress and decidedly less fun (O'Dowd 2008). I would hope that today's trainee nurses have as much fun, if not more, at the start of their careers than I had, before the real work starts.

It has been a journey, throughout which technology and research have achieved groundbreaking improvements in healthcare. Over the course of this journey, I believe that I have acquired a rich tapestry of learning that has enabled me to adapt to the challenge of working in an ever-changing National Health Service.

One of the reasons for writing this book was to devise a beneficial point of reference, from which individuals, both within the healthcare profession and the wider circle, could access information on the art of reflection, and its usefulness, in terms of exploring their feelings and understanding their meaning, in terms of their personal and professional growth. Hopefully, I have achieved this objective.

References

Anderson B (2018) Bladder cancer: overview and management. Part 2: muscle-invasive and metastatic bladder cancer. Br J Nurs 27(18):S8–20. [Internet]. https://doi.org/10.12968/bjon.2018.27.18.S8

BBC Newsround (2020) Florence Nightingale: where did modern nursing first begin? [internet]. BBCnewsround. [cited 2020 Sep 20] https://www.bbc.co.uk/newsround/52397246

Cipriano PF (2010) The world of nursing—then and now—American Nurse [Internet]. americannurse.com. [cited 2020 Oct 24]. https://www.myamericannurse.com/the-world-of-nursing-then-and-now/

Doyle N (2008) Cancer survivorship: evolutionary concept analysis. J Adv Nurs 62(4):499–509. [Internet]. https://doi.org/10.1111/j.1365-2648.2008.04617.x

Doyle N, Henry R (2014) Holistic needs assessment: rationale and practical implementation. Cancer Nurs Pract 13(5):16–21

Duffin C (2016) Assessing the benefits of social prescribing. Cancer Nurs Pract 15(2):18–20. [Internet]. https://doi.org/10.7748/cnp.15.2.18.s19

Ford M (2020) Exclusive: BME nurses "feel targeted" to work on Covid-19 wards [internet]. Nurs Times. [cited 2020 Oct 10]. https://www.nursingtimes.net/news/coronavirus/exclusive-bme-nurses-feel-targeted-to-work-on-covid-19-wards-17-04-2020/

Johnson S (2015) How has nursing changed and what does the future hold? [internet]. The Guardian. [cited 2020 Oct 12] https://www.theguardian.com/healthcare-network/2015/mar/17/how-has-nursing-changed-and-what-does-the-future-hold

Lemon J (2005) Opening convocation remarks. Susquehanna, University, Office of the President. [Internet]. [cited 2019 Feb 10]. http://www.susqu.edu/president/convocation05.htm

McCartney M (2016) Margaret McCartney: racism, immigration, and the NHS. BMJ (Clin Res Ed.) 354:i4477

O'Dowd A (2008) Nursing in the 1970's: 'You are here to do the work, so get on with it'" [Internet]. nursingtimes.net. [cited 2020 Jun 9]. https://www.nursingtimes.net/archive/nursing-in-the-1970s-you-are-here-to-do-the-work-so-get-on-with-it-03-03-2008/

Paton F (2020) 4 positive uses of social media in nursing [Internet]. nurselabs.com. [cited 2020 Feb 11]. https://nurseslabs.com/4-positive-uses-social-media-nursing/

Patterson C (2012) Reforms in the 1990s were supposed to make nursing care better. Instead, there's a widely shared sense that this was how today's compassion deficit began. How did we come to this? [internet]. The Independent. [cited 2020 Oct 24] https://www.independent.co.uk/voices/commentators/christina-patterson/reforms-1990s-were-supposed-make-nursing-care-better-instead-there-s-widely-shared-sense-was-how-today-s-compassion-deficit-began-how-did-we-come-7631273.html

Powles T, Eder JP, Fine GD, Braiteh FS, Loriot Y, Cruz C et al (2014) MPDL3280A (anti-PD-L1) treatment leads to clinical activity in metastatic bladder cancer. Nature 515(7528):558–562. [Internet]. http://www.nature.com/articles/nature13904

Kofoworola Abeni Pratt (1915-1992) First black nurse in NHS. [cited 2021 March 06]. https://www.tes.com/teaching-resource/kofoworola-abeni-pratt-1915-1992-first-black-nurse-in-nhs-12362918

UKEssays (2018) Changes in roles and responsibilities of nurses in the modernisation of the NHS [Internet]. ukessays.com. [cited 2019 Oct 19]. https://www.ukessays.com/essays/nursing/changes-in-roles-and-responsibilities-of-nurses-in-the-modernisation-of-nhs-nursing-essay.php?vref=1

Weston C (2015) An answer to the question of what is a good death? [Internet]. mariecurie.org.uk/blog. [cited 2020 Oct 13]. https://www.mariecurie.org.uk/blog/what-is-a-good-death/48655

Appendix A: List of Publications

01	Anderson B (2005) Nutrition and wound healing: the necessity of assessment. BJN (Tissue Viability Supplement) 14(19): S30–S38
02	Anderson B, Khadra A (2006) Acute urinary retention: developing an A&E management pathway. BJN 15(8):434–438
03	Anderson B, Naish W (2008) Bladder cancer and smoking. Part 1: Addressing the associated risk factors. BJN 17(18):1182–1186
04	Anderson B, Naish W (2008) Bladder cancer and smoking. Part 2: Diagnosis and management. BJN 17(19):1240–1245
05	Anderson B, Naish W (2008) Bladder cancer and smoking. Part 3: Influence of perceptions and beliefs. BJN 17(20):1292–1297
06	Anderson B, Naish W (2008) Bladder cancer and smoking. Part 4: Efficacy of health promotion. BJN 17(21):1340–1344
07	Anderson B (2009) Understanding the role of smoking in the aetiology of bladder cancer. BJCN 14(17):385–392
08	Anderson B (2010) The benefits to nurse-led telephone follow-up for prostate Cancer. BJN 19(17):1085–1090
09	Anderson, B. (2010) A perspective on changing dynamics in nursing over the past 20 years. BJN 19(18):1190–1191
10	Anderson B (2013) Detecting and treating bladder cancer. BJN 22(11):628
11	Anderson B, Marshall-Lucette, Webb P (2013) African and Afro-Caribbean men's experiences of prostate cancer. BJN 22(22):1296–1307
12	Anderson B (2014) Challenges for the clinical nurse specialist in uro-oncology care. BJN (Oncology Supplement) 23(10):S18–S22
13	Anderson B (2015) Cancer treatment: at what cost. NRC 17(3):173–174
14	Anderson B (2016) Cancer management: the difficulties of a target-driven healthcare system. BJN (Urology Supplement) 25(9): S36–S40
15	Anderson B, Marshall-Lucette S (2016) Prostate cancer among Jamaican men: exploring the evidence for higher risk. BJN 25(19):2–7

© Springer Nature Switzerland AG 2022
B. Anderson, *A Uro-Oncology Nurse Specialist's Reflection on her Practice Journey*, https://doi.org/10.1007/978-3-030-94199-4

16	Anderson B (2017) An insight into the patient's response to a urological cancer diagnosis. BJN (Urology Supplement) 26(18):S4–S12
17	Anderson B (2018) Bladder cancer: overview and disease management. Part 1: non-muscle-invasive bladder cancer. BJN (Urology Supplement) 27(9):1–11
18	Anderson B (2018) Bladder cancer: overview and management. Part 2: muscle-invasive and metastatic bladder cancer. BJN (Urology Supplement) 27(18):S8–S20
19	Anderson B (2019) Reflecting on the communication process in healthcare. Part 1: Clinical Practice 'Breaking Bad News'. BJN 28(13):858–863
20	Anderson B (2019) Reflecting on the communication process in healthcare. Part 2: the management of complaints. BJN 28(14):927–929

Appendix B: List of In-House-Supportive Educational and Promotional Information

Continued observations and evaluations of practice have resulted in the development and implementation of the following leaflets and document into practice:

IIA—The Trial Without Catheter (TWOC) leaflet was the first leaflet to be developed while I was a senior staff nurse in the ward. It was designed to provide information on what a TWOC entailed and to inform patients prior to their catheter being removed in the ward. I have since handed this leaflet over to my nursing colleague, the urology CNS, who has updated format and implemented into practice.

IIB—The Catheter Valve (Just a Useful Device?) document was devised by me to support students' and staffs' learning in the urology ward. Content included the use of urinary drainage systems, choice of catheters and highlighting the importance of the catheter valve (CV) in the management of patients with catheters. Over the years, the use of the CV had grown in popularity and was seen as an acceptable and therapeutic alternative to leg bags for catheterised patients within the UK. In 2019, CVs have continued to prove useful in the management of catheterised patients.

IIC—The Acute Urinary Retention (AUR) Patient Information leaflet was devised and implemented into practice in 2004. It was developed in conjunction with the AUR Pathway, to provide information to those patients who presented to the A&E department with AUR.

IID—The Prostate-Specific Antigen (PSA) leaflet was devised following the development and implementation of the PSA telephone follow-up nurse-led clinic in 2006. This leaflet is now null and void since patients have been discharged back to follow up with their GPs in the primary care sector.

IIE—The Bacillus Calmette-Guérin (BCG) and Mitomycin leaflets are given to patients prior to them commencing treatment with either BCG (immunotherapy) or mitomycin (chemotherapy).

© Springer Nature Switzerland AG 2022
B. Anderson, *A Uro-Oncology Nurse Specialist's Reflection on her Practice Journey*, https://doi.org/10.1007/978-3-030-94199-4

IIF—The Bladder Cancer and Smoking leaflet: Can You Minimize the Risks? was developed as a result of the bladder cancer and smoking survey indicating that health promotion was needed in this area. This leaflet is given to patients at the time of diagnosis or when they present for their treatment in the day surgery unit, now the urology centre.

IIG—The Post-operative Mitomycin leaflet was given to patients in the ward prior to them receiving the post-operative dose of mitomycin following transurethral resection of bladder tumour (TURBT). All these leaflets were last reviewed and updated in 2017 and will be updated again in 2020.